Veterinary Herbology

NIPA® GENX ELECTRONIC RESOURCES & SOLUTIONS P. LTD.
New Delhi-110 034

About the Editor

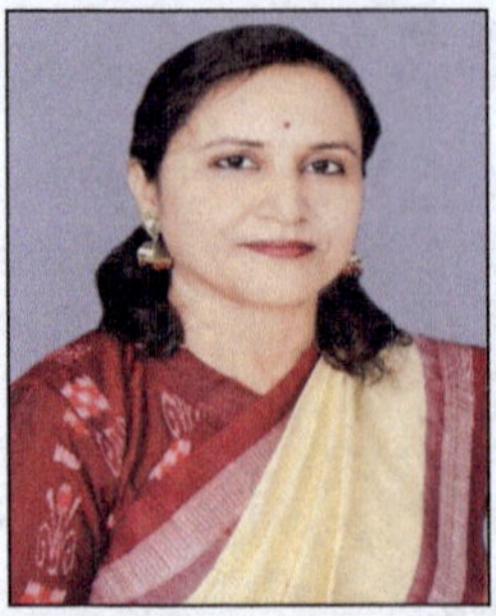

Dr. Santwana Palai has a specialization in Vascular Pharmacology, Toxicology, and Ethnopharmacology. She is a knowledgeable scientific orator. She is trained for analysis of bioactive compounds for development of high-value products and oriented on Laboratory animal Sciences. She has published 22 research papers, 25 review articles in journals, 31 popular articles in magazines, and 27 book chapters of international repute like Springer, Wiley, etc. She has been a resource person in 23 technical meetings and presented 19 oral and 17 poster presentations at national conferences. She has written 53 conference papers and orated 9 TV shows and radio talks in vernacular language for the benefit of practicing veterinarians and farmers too. She is acting as Principal Investigator for funding under the scheme "Collaborative Research Grant in Biotechnology" on "Wound healing efficacy of green nanoparticles in diabetic mice model" in collaboration with the Institute of Life Sciences, BBSR. She visualizes Veterinary Pharmacology & Toxicology as a sound platform for understanding drug action, its mechanism, and therapeutic effects in target animal species and mitigating the toxic effects of all chemical drugs/ toxicants and herbal products with a thorough understanding of aspects of toxicology. She aims to popularize alternate medication especially herbal medicaments through scientific validation, to decrease antimicrobial resistance, reduce residues of allopathic drugs in animal tissues and products along with providing cheap and safe treatments to livestock. She works keenly on natural product chemistry for novel therapeutic approaches.

Veterinary Herbology
Therapeutic Uses of Medicinal Plants for Animal Health

Santwana Palai
Department of Veterinary Pharmacology & Toxicology
College of Veterinary Science & Animal Husbandry
Odisha University of Agriculture & Technology
Bhubaneswar-751003, (Odisha)

NIPA® GENX ELECTRONIC RESOURCES & SOLUTIONS P. LTD.
New Delhi-110 034

NIPA® GENX ELECTRONIC
RESOURCES & SOLUTIONS P. LTD.
101,103, Vikas Surya Plaza, CU Block
L.S.C.Market, Pitam Pura, New Delhi-110 034
Ph : +91 11 4386 0225, 9717133558, 9540816132
E-mail: newindiapublishingagency@gmail.com
Website: www.niparesources.com

Print ISBN: 978-93-58875-37-9

ebook ISBN: 978-93-58873-57-3

Composed and Designed by NIPA®.

College of Veterinary Science & Animal Husbandry
Odisha University of Agriculture & Technology
Bhubaneswar-751003

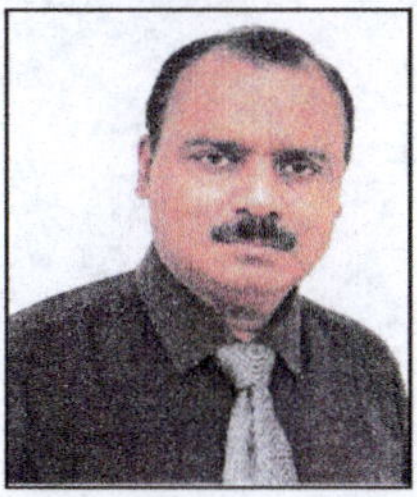

Prof. S. K. Panda
Dean

Message

It gives me immense pleasure that the book "Veterinary Herbology: Unlocking the Power of Medicinal Plants" is going to be published which covers a wide range of medicinal plant-based modalities for veterinary use. Traditional remedies derived from medicinal plants have been used to care for various diseases in animals, ranging from farmyard animals to pets. Medicinal plants hold great promise at a time when concerns about antibiotic resistance and the adverse effects synthetic drugs cause to the environment are growing. Most of these plants produce bioactive compounds with documented antimicrobial, anti-inflammatory, and analgesic activities and have established efficacy in the treatment of a wide range of conditions in animals. This suggests that the integration of evidence-based plant-based treatments designed using traditional scientific methods, in combination with scientific research, lays the way for safer and more effective treatments.

This book is of fundamental value for the veterinarian, researcher, student, or any individual involved in alternative treatment for animal health.

I congratulate the editor for compiling the book, which will kindle budding scholars and mid-carrier scientists to search for newer drugs. I express my hearty greetings to the authors from various parts of India for their commendable efforts in shaping this book.

(S.K. Panda)
C.V.Sc. & A.H.

Department of Veterinary Pharmacology & Toxicology
College of Veterinary Science & Animal Husbandry
Odisha University of Agriculture & Technology
Bhubaneswar-751003

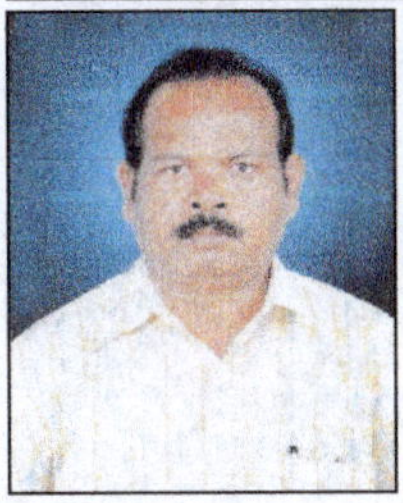

K.K. Sardar
HOD, VPT, C.V.Sc. & A.H.

Message

Traditional folk veterinary medicine is the mode of identifying, using and integrating local knowledge, related skills, and custom procedures created by people to preserve animals' health and welfare. Those traditional drug practices are becoming scarce as medicinal plants have been replaced by modem medicine. However, in the last decades, the study and use of medicinal plants in veterinary medicine have gained importance due to the emergence of antimicrobial resistance. The veterinarian practices, related to the use of medicinal plants, are still alive which is to be validated through scientific methods.

This book encompasses medicinal plants of veterinary importance which is anunderexplored field although it should be considered an alternative to improve animal health. These chapters contribution integrates established wisdom and modem science about major medicinal plants to provide an overview of the principles of therapeutic action, and safe and

effective use. The book will simplify the process of identifying medicinal plants, their pharmacologic effects, and their practical applications. The absolute clarity of the chapters will allow the readers a highly concise way to understand its application in usual practice for animal care-keeping science and conduct further research on these medicinal plants. It not only describes the therapeutic effects of medicines of plant origin, but also highlights the importance of sustainability in veterinary practice. It re-evaluates the use of plants for the improvement of health in animals in a way that offers the much-needed perspectives for those who want to improve the animal welfare in the ever-changing world.

It is a matter of pleasure to note the sincere efforts of authors of the Department of Veterinary Pharmacology & Toxicology from all parts of India & Veterinary Medicine and ARGO departments of our college. I wish them success and congratulate all of them for their efforts in shaping this book.

(K. K. Sardar)
HOD, VPT, C.V.Sc. & A.H.

Preface

The flora of India is diverse and abundant. Synthetic medications are known to be expensive, and even dangerous. Herbal remedies, on the other hand, are less harmful, less expensive, and environmentally beneficial. They have also been used by the populace for many generations. They have also been applied to routine issues in animal healthcare. Plants are the source of 25% of the medications administered globally. The biological action of medicinal plants is due to the presence of phytochemicals or plant secondary metabolites, which are byproducts of secondary metabolism that continue with their vital primary metabolism.

This book deals with a comprehensive review of conditions of veterinary importance where medicinal plant species are involved. The botanical names, distribution, plant part used, bioactive principles, and pharmacological actions are mentioned. Also, selected veterinary herbal formulations are provided. This book will contribute to the knowledge of medicinal plants from several aspects like their natural properties and pharmacological effects.

This compilation has 20 chapters covering medicinal plants effective in various diseases and conditions of veterinary importance. This book will be helpful to researchers, drug developers, drug discoverers and anybody else attempting to use botanicals to alleviate animal discomfort.

The editor expresses gratitude to each author for their prompt contributions to the published book. The editor appreciates the Medicinal Plant Knowledge Centre in Kalinga Vihar, Bhubaneswar, Smritivan Botanical Garden in Kalinga Nagar, Bhubaneswar, and Ekamravana, Bhubaneswar, for enabling us to take the scientific photos of medicinal plants that were included in this book.

This book would not have been launched without the unwavering efforts of 3rd year, BVSc & AH students (Pratyush Panda, Satyajit Mahanta, Rohit Kumar Pradhan, Ajit Kumar Nandi, Suman Pradhan, Subhashree Priyadarshini Sahoo).

Santwana Palai

Contents

Part I
Introduction and General Concepts

1

Herbal Remedies for Animal Diseases

Santwana Palai[1*], Arpita Priyadarshini[2]

[1]Department of Veterinary Pharmacology & Toxicology, College of Veterinary Science & Animal Husbandry, Orissa University of Agriculture & Technology Bhubaneswar- 751003, Odisha, India
[2]College of Veterinary Science & Animal Husbandry, Orissa University of Agriculture & Technology, Bhubaneswar- 751003, Odisha, India

Introduction

Plants have been used for ages as animal and human health cures. Ethnoveterinary medicines, a phrase that primarily refers to folk skills, beliefs, knowledge, practices, and procedures related to animal health and the treatment of various disorders in rural regions, have acknowledged the ability of plants to combat a variety of diseases. The World Health Organisation (WHO) defines traditional medicine, also referred to as herbal medicine, as "When it comes to maintaining health and preventing, diagnosing, improving, or treating physical and mental illnesses, the entirety of the knowledge, abilities, and practices derived from indigenous theories, beliefs, and experiences whether or not they can be explained as illness". Approximately 25% of contemporary medications are derived from plants that were once used in traditional medicine. The use of traditional medicine and its confirmation could result in the creation and discovery of more novel medications.

Treatment of Diseases

Diseases are the basic problems for both humans and animals. Living beings have always been fighting various diseases since prehistoric periods. According to reports, over 30–35% of losses in the animal breeding industry are caused by improper animal husbandry techniques, particularly in developing nations where rural populations rely largely on livestock. Disease concepts and their treatments vary widely. Synthetic medications are known to be expensive, toxic, and even dangerous. Also, due to financial constraints, these smallholders are unable to invest in the health of their animals with high-end costly allopathic medications. The long-term use of these synthetic medications by animal farmers is also a source of concern since it may result in the presence of residual hazardous compounds in milk, meat and egg, such as antibiotic and drug metabolites and byproducts that make people resistant to antibiotics. These kinds of problems have led to the quest for safer and less expensive alternatives to contemporary animal health care systems, such as herbal medicines.

Plants and Phytochemicals in Animal Care and Treatment

Plants are the source of 25% of the medications administered globally. Herbal medicine has been used for thousands of years to treat both humans and animals. Veterinary herbal medicines are plant-based drugs used in animal health care for therapeutic, prophylactic, or diagnostic purposes. These traditional medicines or herbal cures are less hazardous, less costly, and more environmental friendly than manufactured medications and pharmaceuticals. They are also easier to use and more sustainable.

Common issues with animal care and treatment in rural India frequently entail the abilities, know-how, practices, customs, and beliefs of local healers. Numerous animal problems, including pneumonia, bone fractures, poisoning, burning, foot and mouth disease, dermatitis, coughing, constipation, cataracts, snake bites, abdominal aches, skin diseases, and more, are reported to be cured by medicinal herbs. The use of a single remedy or plant extract can also treat more than one disease. Garlic can be used to treat skin infections, arthritis, FMD, rickets, snake bites, gastric troubles, internal parasites, etc. Similarly, turmeric can be used to treat wounds, urinary infections, gastrointestinal disorders, mastitis, and swellings.

A wide variety of pharmacologically active substances can be found in medicinal herbs, and each herb has a special combination and set of characteristics. Plants create bioactive substances called phytochemicals to defend themselves. They can be found in vegetables, nuts, whole grains, fruits, and herbs, among other meals. More than a thousand phytochemicals have been discovered thus far. Among the significant phytochemicals include carotenoids, polyphenols, saponins, dietary fibers, isoprenoids, phytosterols, and certain polysaccharides. In addition to their strong antioxidant qualities, these phytochemicals also have antiviral, anthelmintic, antibacterial, antiallergic, antidiarrheal, and antispasmodic-like qualities. Additionally, they strengthen gap junction communication, boost immunity, control gene transcription, and offer defense against prostate and lung malignancies.

Herbal Drugs can be the Source of New Drug Discovery

Medicinal and aromatic plants having ethnopharmacological usages have been used as a natural source of medicines for care and treatment for thousands of years. Several herbal preparations like powders, tinctures, macerations, inhalations, infusions, teas, tinctures, poultices, decoctions, and percolation products were the initial crude forms of these well-known medications. These traditions have passed down the precise dosage of the plant and the technique of administration for specific illnesses from generation to generation, and traditional pharmacopeias have steadily documented knowledge of therapeutic plants.

Numerous academic disciplines and research approaches have been involved in the discovery of medicinal plant medications. Plant ecologists, botanists, ethnopharmacologists, and ethnobotanists, often collect and identify the plants of interest. Since the early 19th century, when morphine was extracted from *Papaver somniferum*, the separation of active ingredients has been necessary for the use of plants as medicines. An outstanding accomplishment in the realm of medicine was the discovery of early medicines derived from medicinal plants, including digitoxin, cocaine, pilocarpine, codeine, and quinine. These substances are still recognized for their therapeutic use today after being isolated and examined for their medicinal properties.

Moreover, in addition to these preliminary discoveries, several other compounds derived from plants have been discovered in more recent years. After undergoing a great deal of research and development, these substances were eventually brought to market as pharmaceutical drugs. Extracted from the foxglove plant, digitoxin is used to treat heart conditions, including congestive heart failure. Originally discovered for its anesthetic properties, cocaine has long been utilized for blood vessel constriction and local anesthesia. The jaborandi plant yields pilocarpine, which has been utilized in medicine because it increases sweating and salivation. The opium poppy is the source of codeine and the opioid alkaloid was popularised for its ability to reduce pain as well as stop coughing.

Numerous early drugs, such as quinine and digitoxin, are being utilized in current medicine, indicating the continued significance of these plant-based substances. The continuous efforts to separate and describe pharmacologically active molecules from medicinal plants have also led to the discovery of other compounds with therapeutic promise. Part of this procedure involves comprehending these substances' modes of action, chemical structures, and possible medical uses. The implication of nature as a source of bioactive compounds can aid in the creation of innovative medications and treatments in modern medicine through ongoing research.

Using drug development approaches, herbal medicines have been standardized thus far to identify analytical marker biomolecules. Plant-based pharmaceutical research is a successful, safe, and affordable alternative to conventional techniques that use animal cell cultures or microbial fermentation. These medications derived from organic compounds in plants are simpler and quicker to reach their patients.

Herbal Products for Animal Use

Globally, the use of herbal products has significantly increased. About 70% of the animals like cattle, horses, sheep, goats, and pigs followed by poultry, dogs, and rabbits are treated with herbal treatments. This is because there are lot of research supporting the effectiveness of herbal therapies in addition to the broader trend toward using natural items to treat ailments. The importance of using natural goods is growing. When used properly, herbal solutions can offer a better solution to the negative effects of prescription medications. These can reduce the needless usage of chemical medications, such as antibiotics, to address residual issues and the increasing resistance of microorganisms. Herbal products are readily available, well-tolerated, and more effective for chronic disease conditions. They are affordable, readily available, and simple to administer and prepare. They don't leave residues in animal products, making them safe for human consumption.

Sometimes, the side effects of herbal medicines' can show negative side effects and even death due to adulteration or contamination, overdosing, or improper prescription. So, herbal medicine and dietary supplement products should undergo safety, and presumed efficacy tests.

Conclusion

Medicinal plants are making a resurgence. Compared to synthetic drugs, herbal products are safer and more secure nowadays. This knowledge of ethnoveterinary medications or medicinal plants in practice should be available to researchers and drug developers who can aid in the development of higher-quality herbal medicines, functional foods, and nutraceuticals for animals. This traditional ethno-veterinary expertise can also provide valuable insights for extracting natural extracts to create novel products for animal health and welfare. This offers fresh possibilities for conducting additional research, beginning with old customs, to find noble natural products for the health and welfare of domestic animals.

References

Chaachouay N, Zidane L. Plant-derived natural products: a source for drug discovery and development. Drugs and Drug Candidates. 2024 Feb 19;3(1):184-207.

Kuralkar P, Kuralkar SV. Role of herbal products in animal production–An updated review. Journal of Ethnopharmacology. 2021 Oct 5;278:114246.

Part II
Medicinal Plants for Specific Diseases

2

Medicinal Plants Effective in Diabetes in Animals

***Arpita Shrivastava*[1]*, Neeraj Shrivastava*[2]*, P.K. Singh*[3]**
***A.K. Niranjan*[4] *and Namrata Upadhyay*[5]**

[1&5]*Department of Pharmacology & Toxicology, College of Veterinary Science & Animal Husbandry, Rewa, Madhya Pradesh*
[2,4]*Department of Microbiology, College of Veterinary Science & Animal Husbandry Rewa, Madhya Pradesh*
[3]*Associate Professor Department of Livestock Products Technology College of Veterinary Science & Animal Husbandry , Jabalpur, Madhya Pradesh*

Introduction

Diabetes mellitus is a disease the related to metabolism of the body and malfunctioning of pancreas. Pancreas having alpha and beta cells where alpha cells produce enzymes needed for the digestion and beta cells mainly produce insulin. One important component that regulates blood glucose (sugar) levels and how it is delivered to the body's cells is Insulin. The body's cells run out of their primary energy source when insulin levels are low. Insulin voices the body's cells to engross glucose from the bloodstream. Without an satisfactory amount of insulin glucose cannot invade the cells and so it accrues in the blood, triggering hyperglycemia (high blood sugar). In retort to this ostensible starvation, the body starts flouting down supplies of protein & fat for energy, producing weight loss contempt a ravening appetite. The body efforts to remove the extra glucose by micturating. To avoid thirst, the dog drinks more and more water. Type I increased diabetes mellitus outcomes from complete obliteration of the insulin-creating beta cells. In dogs, this is the most prevalent kind of diabetes. As the name implies, insulin injections are necessary to balance blood sugar in dogs with this kind of diabetes.

Type II diabetes mellitus is characterized by either inadequate insulin production, delayed insulin secretion, or relatively insulin-resistant tissues in the dog. Type-2 diabetes (T2D), which was formerly said as adult-onset or non-insulin-dependent diabetes, accounting for 90–95% of all instances of diabetes; dogs rarely develop Type II diabetes. This complex metabolic disease is characterized by changes in insulin resistance, lipid metabolism, and pancreatic β-cell dysfunction. Pregnancy or tumors that release hormones can develop insulin resistance, which leads to type III diabetes. Although blood sugar regulation is compromised in all forms, the fundamental mechanisms underlying the illness vary. Instead of being dispersed throughout the body, glucose builds up in the bloodstream, causing hyperglycemia, or elevated blood sugar levels. Before the kidneys finally remove it, the glucose spills into the urine after reaching a specific saturation point, pulling significant amounts of water. For diabetic pets, these processes can result in severe health issues such as dehydration, elevated blood pressure, blindness, limb and foot swelling, amputations, kidney failure, and death. Since both *in-vivo* and *in-vitro* methods are used in primary and secondary screening, choosing and creating suitable methods could enhance this procedure. In-vivo methods are too costly and unreliable to evaluate hits.

Therefore, in order to carry out the necessary tasks and achieve the corresponding goals, it is now essential to develop and apply appropriate *in-vitro* screening techniques. But choosing the right *in-vitro* test for a particular assessment of cellular activity is not an easy undertaking. It necessitates a careful examination of all relevant factors. Glucose, radioisotope, genetic, calcium, cAMP, insulin secretion, and phosphoprotein tyrosine 1B (PTP1B) assays are among the assays utilised in *in-vitro* research. In the study of diabetes, animal models are essential. Preclinical animal models that faithfully replicate the pathophysiology of the human disease are crucial due to the disease's complexity. Toxic chemicals are employed in the majority of animal models used to induce diabetes which target the pancreatic β-cells.

Streptozotocin, which may cause both type 1 and type 2 diabetes, is the most often utilized chemical to cause diabetes. In addition to seriously impairing insulin secretion, high dosages can cause ketone bodies to develop and leak into the urine, which is a sign of uncontrolled type 1 diabetes. Insulin secretion is mildly impaired by low dosages. Insulin resistance developed in animals that were excessively fed a high-fat diet. In patients with type 1 diabetes, the immune system of the body targets and kills the beta cells in the pancreas that produce insulin. The hormone insulin, which is necessary for regulating blood sugar levels and the uptake of glucose by cells, is consequently insufficient.

Diagnosis of Diabetes

Up to 50% of cats and some dogs with diabetes mellitus have a drop in appetite. Hepatomegaly, or a fatty liver brought on by an increase in fat mobilisation from adipose tissue, is another clinical indication. Animals with diabetes frequently get chronic or recurring infections and have weakened resistance to bacterial and fungal diseases. Dehydration, hypovolemia, increased metabolic acidosis, anion gap, electrolyte imbalances, raised liver enzymes, hyperlactatemia, azotemia, and clinical manifestations of anorexia & vomiting are all associated with diabetic ketoacidosis. Diabetes mellitus is diagnosed based on glucosuria and chronic hyperglycemia. Insulin, Oral hypoglycemic agents and Dietary management show a vital role in the treatment of diabetes. The administration of oral hypoglycemic agents such as glipizide in combination with dietary management, sulfonylureas eg, glimepiride, glyburide, oral SGLT2 inhibitors, Acarbose, Sodium-glucose transport protein 2 (SGLT2) inhibitors, Because bexagliflozin and velagliflozin prevent glucose resorption in the proximal renal tubule, they raise urine glucose excretion, Correcting dehydration by administering IV fluids, such as lactated Ringer's solution or 0.9% NaCl (saline) solution or decreasing ketosis & hyperglycemia by administering crystalline zinc (regular) insulin maintaining serum electrolyte concentrations, especially potassium and phosphorus, by administering appropriate supplemental electrolyte solutions.

Medicinal plants are once again being explored for their potential in diabetes treatment. Numerous conventional medications have been developed from pharmacologically active compounds found in these plants. A notable example is Metformin, an effective oral agent for lowering blood glucose levels, which was developed from *Galega officinalis* for diabetes management. This plant is abundant in guanidine, a compound known for its hypoglycemic properties. However, due to the toxicity of guanidine for clinical applications, the synthetic alkyl biguanides, synthalin B & synthalin A, were presented as oral anti-diabetic medications, though their use was eventually phased out following the broader availability of insulin. Currently, more than 500 traditional plant-based treatments for diabetes are documented, but only some of them have undergone scientific and medical scrutiny to evaluate their effectiveness.

The Expert Committee on Diabetes of the World Health Organization has advised that further research be conducted on traditional medicinal herbs. The lack of clinical and scientific proof of herbal medicine's safety and efficacy is a major obstacle to its incorporation into modern medical procedures. It is essential to undertake clinical studies on herbal medications, create straightforward bioassays for biological standardization, and perform toxicological and pharmacological assessments. Additionally, various animal models are to be developed to evaluate its safety & toxicity. Identifying active components present in these herbal extracts is also of paramount importance.

Medicinal Plants used in Diabetes

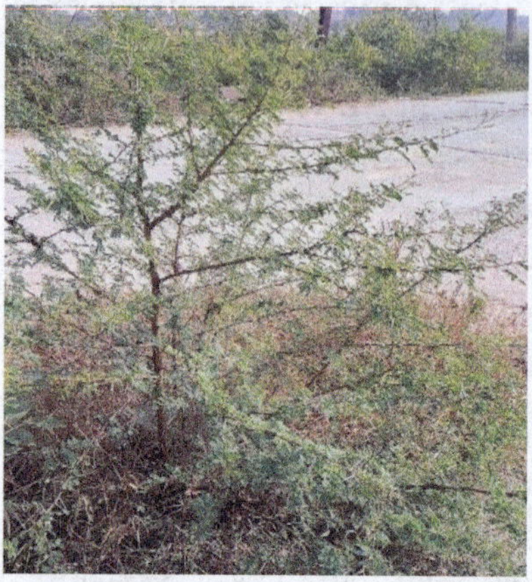

Scientific Name: *Acacia arabica*

Common Name: Babul

Distribution: Rajasthan, Gujarat, Madhya Pradesh, and Tamil Nadu

Part Used: Bark, leaves, and gum

Bioactive Principle: Tannins, catechin, gallic acid, and flavonoids

Remarks: The plant extract functions as a secretagogue to release insulin, which lowers blood sugar levels. Control rats experience hypoglycemia, whereas alloxanized animals do not. When given to healthy rabbits, powdered *Acacia arabica* seeds caused a hypoglycemic action by triggering the insulin release from the pancreatic beta cells.

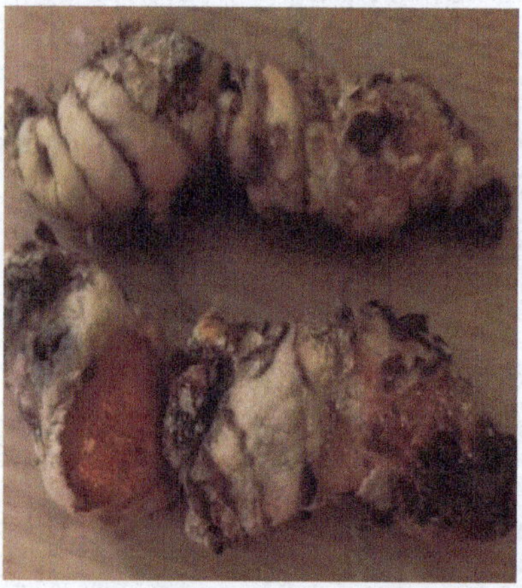

Scientific Name: *Curcuma longa*

Common Name: Haldi

Distribution: Tamil Nadu, Maharashtra, Andhra Pradesh, Telangana, Odisha, and West Bengal.

Part Used: Rhizome

Bioactive Principle: Curcumin

Remarks: Curcumin may be 400 times more effective than the popular diabetic medication Metformin at enhancing insulin sensitivity and aiding in reversal of type 2 diabetes, according to research.

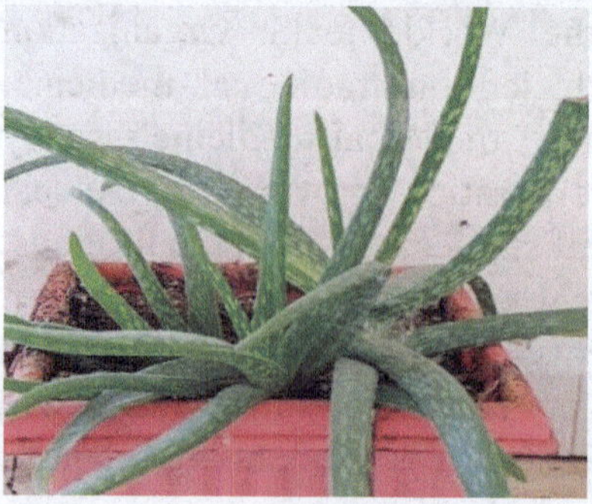

Scientific Name: *Aloe barbadensis miller*

Common Name: Aloe Vera

Distribution: Rajasthan, Gujarat, Maharashtra, Tamil Nadu, and Andhra Pradesh.

Part Used: Leaves (gel and latex)

Bioactive Principle: Aloin, aloe-emodin, acemannan, and polysaccharides

Remarks: Aloe gum extracts successfully improve glucose tolerance in healthy as well as diabetic rats. In rats with alloxanized diabetes, exudates from *Aloe barbadensis* leaves had a hypoglycemic outcome. The bitter part of the same plant caused hypoglycemia in diabetic rats whether given in single or repeated doses.

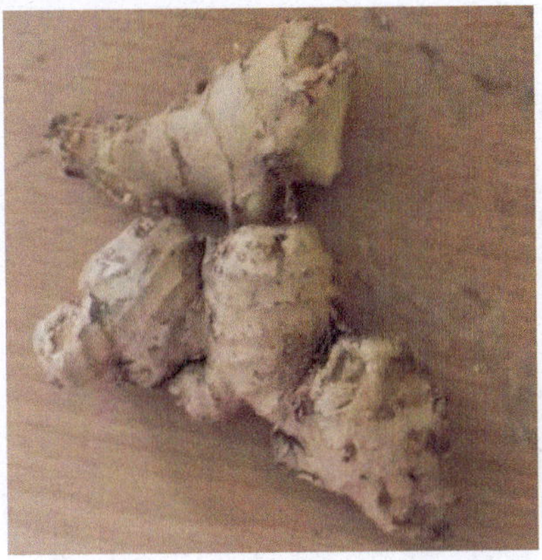

Scientific Name: *Zingiber officinale*

Common Name: Ginger

Distribution: Kerala, Karnataka, Assam, Meghalaya, and Arunachal Pradesh.

Part Used: Rhizome

Bioactive Principle: Gingerol, shogaol, zingerone

Remarks: Ginger is most frequently used as a food flavoring, but it can also be taken orally in larger doses for a variety of digestive benefits and to lower blood sugar and cholesterol levels.

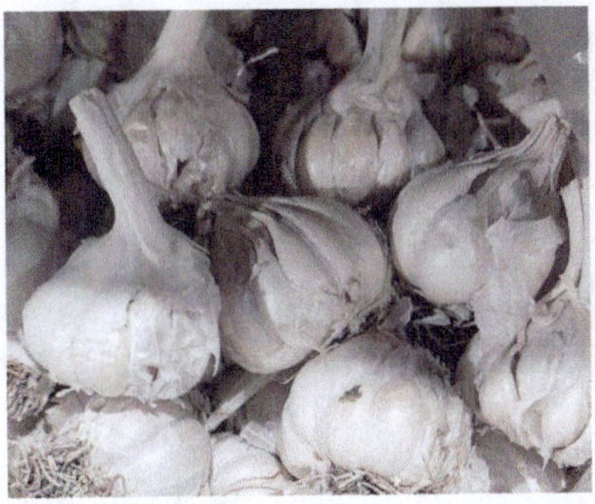

Scientific Name: *Allium sativum*

Common Name: Garlic

Distribution: Madhya Pradesh, Gujarat, Uttar Pradesh, and Rajasthan.

Part Used: Bulb

Bioactive Principle: Allicin, alliin, sulfur compounds

Remarks: Its strong smell is caused by the sulfur-containing chemical allicin, which has also been demonstrated to have strong hypoglycemic effects. higher hepatic metabolism, higher insulin release from pancreatic beta cells, and/or the insulin sparing effect are the three possible causes of this impact. When compared to sucrose controls, rabbits fed sucrose showed a substantial increase in hepatic glycogen and free amino acid content, a drop in fasting blood glucose, and a decrease in serum triglyceride levels when given an aqueous homogenate of garlic (10 ml/kg/day).

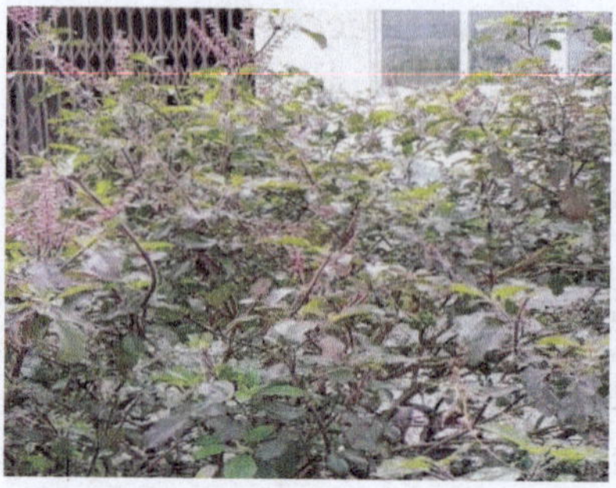

Scientific Name: *Ocimum sanctum*

Common Name: Basil Leaves

Distribution: Uttar Pradesh, Tamil Nadu, and Madhya Pradesh.

Part Used: Leaves and seeds

Bioactive Principle: Eugenol, ursolic acid, and rosmarinic acid

Remarks: Tulsi is the popular name for it. In both normal as well as alloxan-induced diabetic rats, the aqueous extract of *Ocimum sanctum* leaves demonstrated a substantial decrease in blood sugar levels.

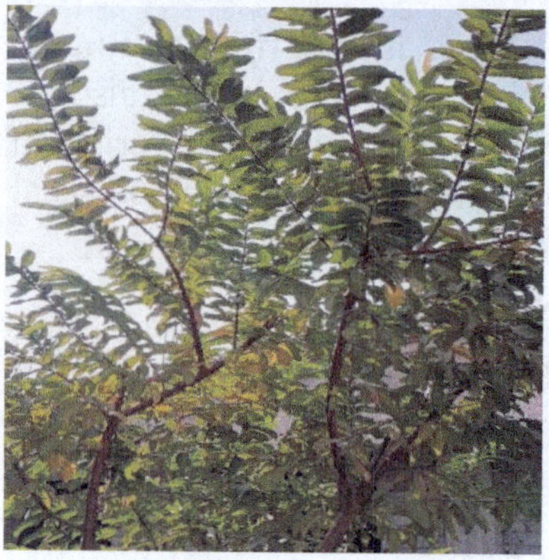

Scientific Name: *Psidium guajava*

Common Name: Guava

Distribution: Uttar Pradesh, Bihar, Maharashtra, Karnataka, and Tamil Nadu.

Part Used: Leaves and fruits

Bioactive Principle: Quercetin, lycopene, and flavonoids

Remarks: *Hypoglycaemic* activity of guava leaves have been well documented but not for guava fruit.

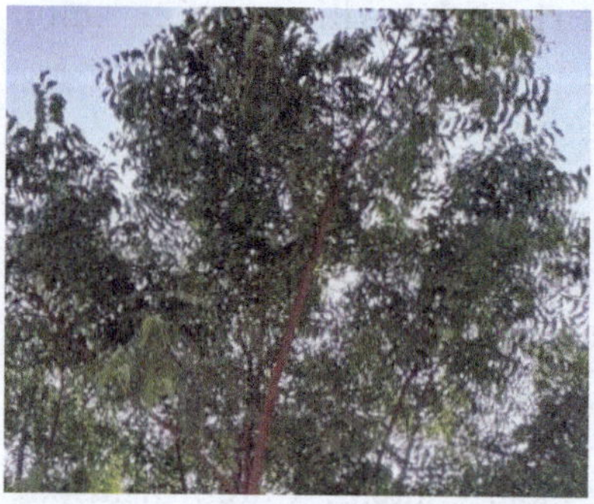

Scientific Name: *Azadirachta indica*

Common Name: Neem

Distribution: In semi-arid regions like Rajasthan, Andhra Pradesh, and Karnataka.

Part Used: Leaves, bark, seeds, and flowers

Bioactive Principle: Azadirachtin, nimbin, and nimbidin

Remarks: Aqueous-alcoholic extracts of this plant showed anti-hyperglycemic action in rats given streptozotocin. Increased glucose absorption and glycogen deposition in the isolated rat hemidiaphragm were the causes of this effect.

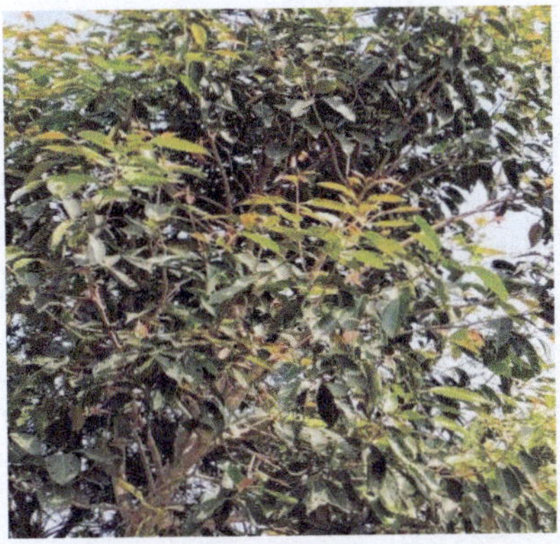

Scientific Name: *Eugenia jambolana*

Common Name: Jamun

Distribution: Bihar, Uttar Pradesh, Tamil Nadu, Maharashtra, & West Bengal.

Part Used: Leaves, seed, bark

Bioactive Principle: Anthocyanins, ellagic acid, and myricetin

Remarks: *Eugenia jambolana* kernel decoction is used as a home cure for diabetes. Blood glucose levels are lowered by the antihyperglycemic effects of lyophilized powder, alcoholic extract, and aqueous extract.

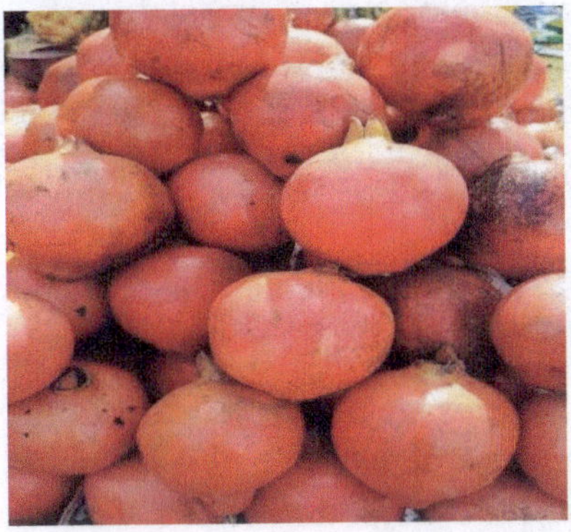

Scientific Name: *Punica granatum*

Common Name: Pomegranate

Distribution: Maharashtra, Karnataka, Gujarat, Andhra Pradesh, and Tamil Nadu.

Part Used: Fruit rind, seeds, and bark

Bioactive Principle: Punicalagins, ellagic acid, and flavonoids

Remarks: Numerous healthy compounds, including polyphenols, which have antiviral, anti-tumor, and antioxidant qualities, are present in this tasty fruit.

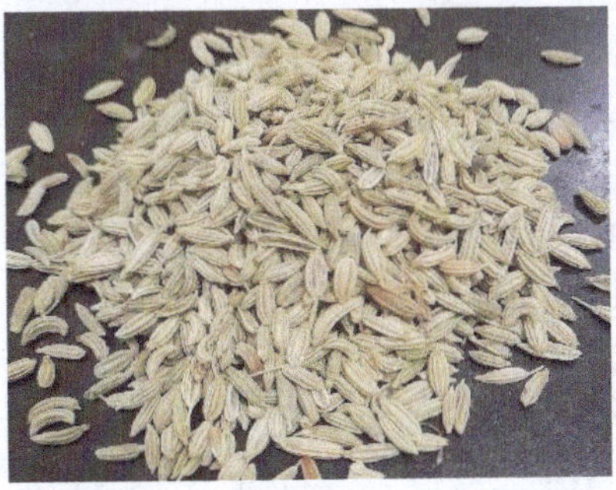

Scientific Name: *Foeniculum vulgare*

Common Name: Fennel Seed

Distribution: Rajasthan, Gujarat, and Uttar Pradesh.

Part Used: Seeds

Bioactive Principle: Anethole, fenchone, and estragole

Remarks: Fennel seed has shown hypoglycaemic activity in diabetic rats and improved pathological changes in their kidneys and pancreas.

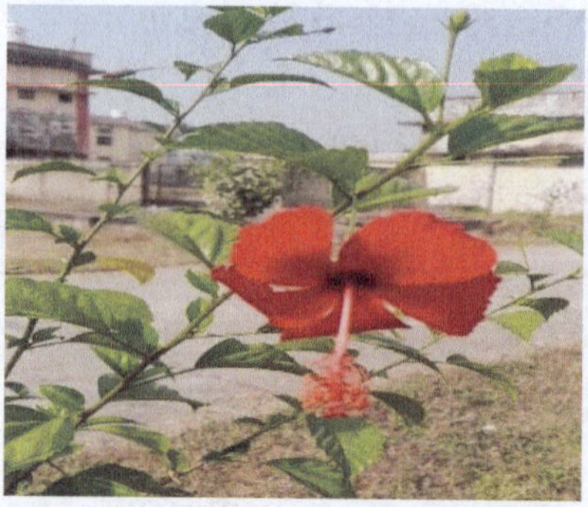

Scientific Name: *Hibiscus rosa-sinesis*

Common Name: Gudhal

Distribution: In tropical and subtropical regions.

Part Used: Flowers and leaves

Bioactive Principle: Anthocyanins, hibiscetin, and ascorbic acid

Remarks: Initiates insulin release from pancreatic beta cells.

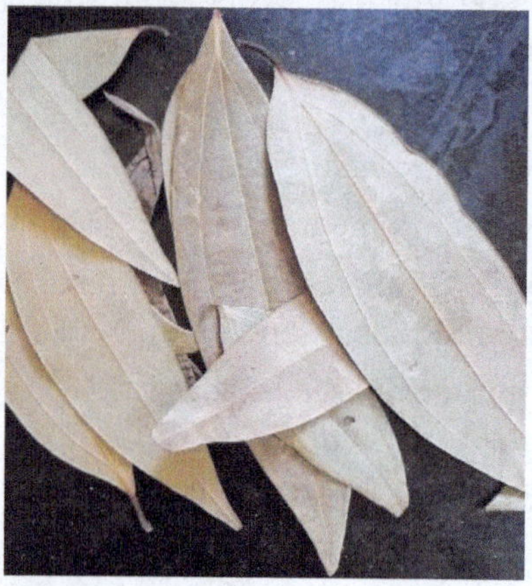

Scientific Name: *Laurus nobilis*

Common Name: Bay leaves

Distribution: North-eastern states like Assam, Meghalaya, and Manipur, and in hilly regions of Uttarakhand and Himachal Pradesh.

Part Used: Leaves

Bioactive Principle: Cineole, eugenol, and flavonoids

Remarks: At dosages as little as 500 mg, or less than half a teaspoon, bay leaf has been shown to improve the body's use of insulin. Cumin, turmeric, coriander, cloves, cinnamon, and other spices are also effective at regulating blood sugar levels.

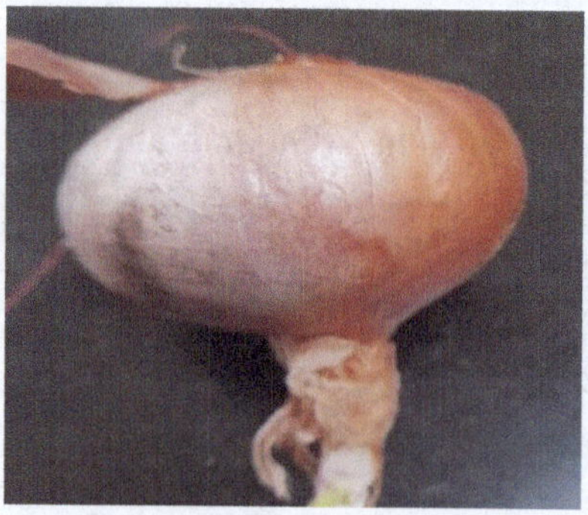

Scientific Name: *Allium cepa*

Common Name: Onion

Distribution: Maharashtra, Karnataka, Madhya Pradesh, and Gujarat

Part Used: Bulb

Bioactive Principle: Quercetin, sulfur compounds, and flavonoids

Remarks: When given to diabetic rabbits, different ether-insoluble and soluble fractions of powdered dried onion powder exhibited anti-hyperglycemic actions. When 50 g of onion juice was administered orally as a single dosage to diabetic patients, postprandial glucose levels were dramatically reduced.

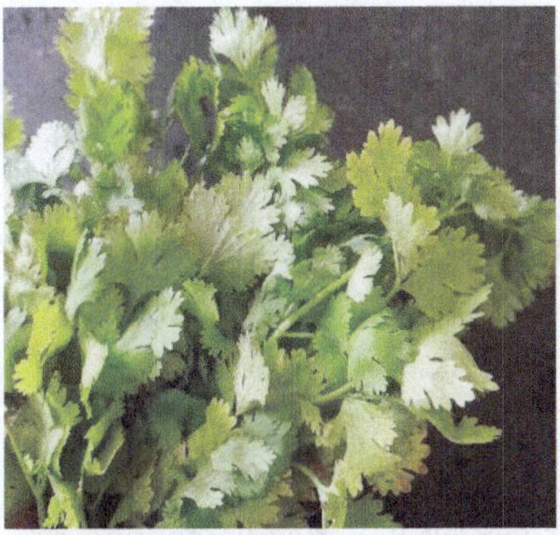

Scientific Name: *Coriandrum sativum*

Common Name: Coriander

Distribution: Rajasthan, Madhya Pradesh, Uttar Pradesh, and Gujarat.

Part Used: Seeds, leaves, and roots

Bioactive Principle: Linalool, cineole, and coumarins

Remarks: For diabetics, coriander seeds can help reduce blood sugar. Enzymes that aid in the body's processing of blood glucose can be activated by coriander. It can also stimulate insulin secretion from pancreatic beta-cells. Coriander leaves can help regenerate pancreatic β cells.

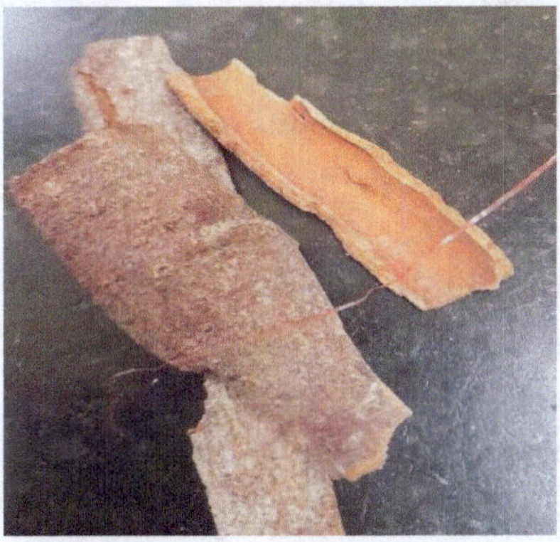

Scientific Name: *Cinnamomum verum*

Common Name: Cinnamon

Distribution: Kerala and the northeastern states, particularly in tropical forest regions.

Part Used: Bark

Bioactive Principle: Cinnamaldehyde, eugenol, and cinnamic acid

Remarks: Cinnamon bark powder is most commonly used in the diabetes condition.

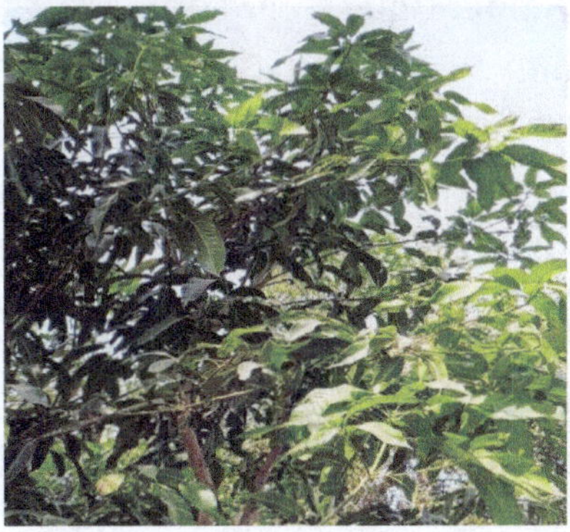

Scientific Name: *Mangifera indica*

Common Name: Mango

Distribution: Uttar Pradesh, Tamil Nadu, West Bengal, Karnataka, Andhra Pradesh, & Maharashtra.

Part Used: Leaves, bark, and seeds

Bioactive Principle: Mangiferin, quercetin, and lupeol

Remarks: This plant's leaves are utilized as an antidiabetic. when the rats were given the extract 60 minutes before the glucose, as well as when the extract and glucose were given at the same time. The findings suggest that Mangifera indica aqueous extract has hypoglycemic properties. An intestinal decrease in glucose absorption could be the cause of this.

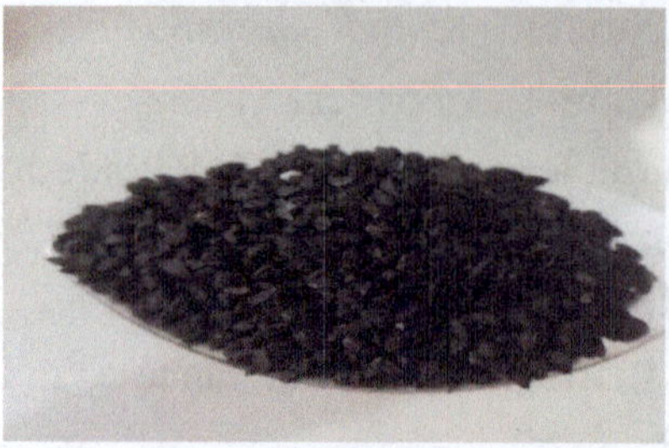

Scientific Name: *Nigella sativa*

Common Name: Kalonji

Distribution: northern India, particularly in Uttar Pradesh, Bihar, and Rajasthan.

Part Used: Seeds

Bioactive Principle: Thymoquinone, nigellone, and alkaloids

Remarks: Kalonji can help regulate blood sugar levels and may be used as an adjuvant therapy for diabetes. It can decrease insulin resistance and increase insulin release from pancreatic cells and also decrease hepatic gluconeogenesis and counteract oxidative stress.

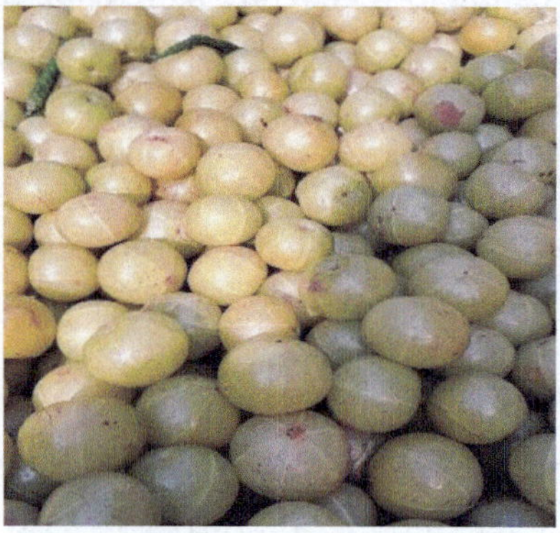

Scientific Name: *Emblica officinalis*

Common Name: Amla

Distribution: Gujarat, Uttar Pradesh, Maharashtra, Tamil Nadu, and Madhya Pradesh.

Part Used: Fruits

Bioactive Principle: Ascorbic acid, gallic acid, and tannins

Remarks: Decreases lipid peroxidation, antioxidant, hypoglycaemic.

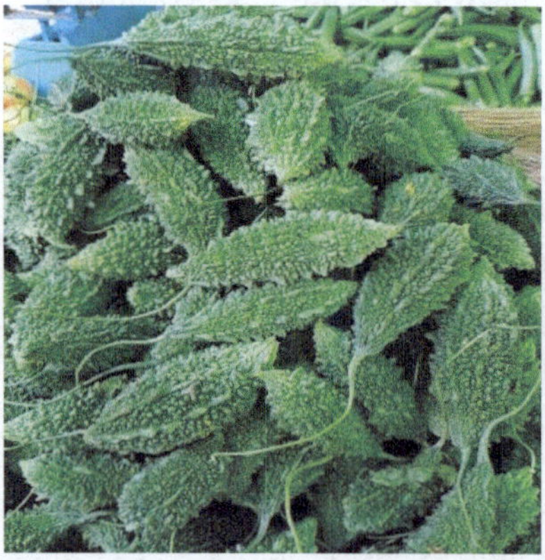

Scientific Name: *Momordica charantia*

Common Name: Bitter Gourd

Distribution: West Bengal, Bihar, Uttar Pradesh, and Tamil Nadu.

Part Used: Fruits and seed

Bioactive Principle: Charantin, momordicin, and polypeptide-p

Remarks: In several animal models, fruit pulp, seeds, leaves, as well as entire plant extracts have demonstrated hypoglycemic impact. Rats with and without diabetes both exhibited hypoglycemic and antihyperglycemic effects from ethanolic extracts. The liver's suppression of glucose-6-phosphatase in addition to fructose-1, 6-biphosphatase and activation of hepatic glucose-6-phosphate dehydrogenase activities could be the cause of this.

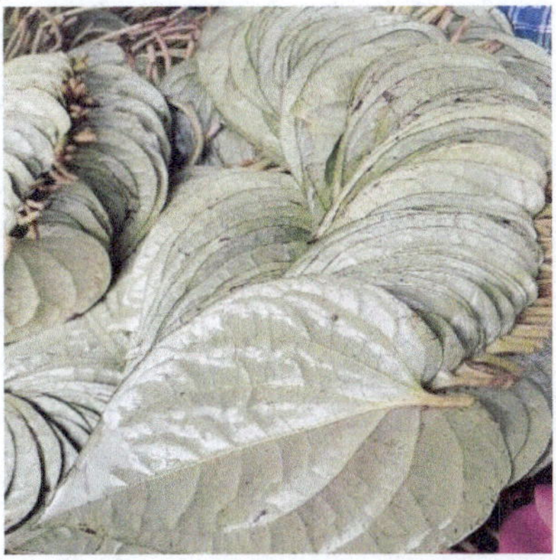

Scientific Name: *Piper betle*

Common Name: Paan leaves

Distribution: Assam, Odisha, Andhra Pradesh, Tamil Nadu, and West Bengal.

Part Used: Leaves

Bioactive Principle: Eugenol, chavibetol, and isoeugenol

Remarks: Blood sugar management is aided by the anti-diabetic qualities of paan leaf. After eating, chewing paan leaves can lower your risk of developing diabetes and prediabetes. Betel leaf improves insulin sensitivity and lowers blood sugar levels.

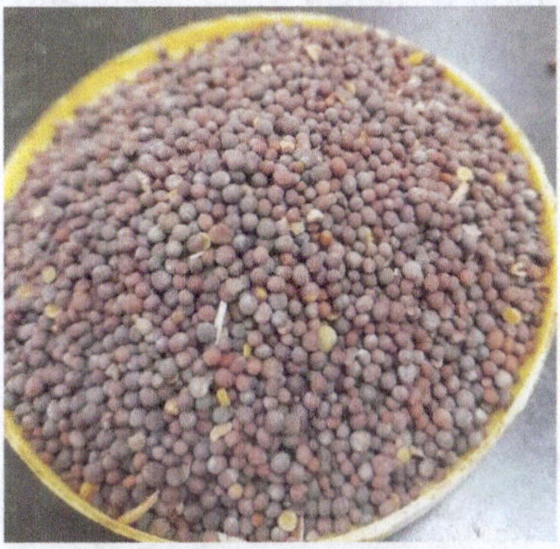

Scientific Name: *Brassica nigra*

Common Name: Mustard

Distribution: Rajasthan, Uttar Pradesh, Haryana, and Madhya Pradesh.

Part Used: Seeds

Bioactive Principle: Glucosinolates, isothiocyanates, and sinigrin

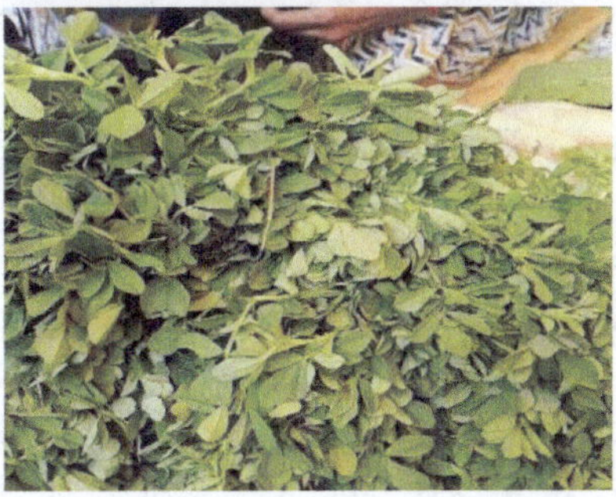

Scientific Name: *Trigonella foenum graecum*

Common Name: Methi

Distribution: Rajasthan, Gujarat, Madhya Pradesh, and Uttar Pradesh.

Part Used: Seeds and leaves

Bioactive Principle: Diosgenin, trigonelline, and galactomannan

Remarks: Blood glucose levels in normal as well as diabetic rats decreased in a dose-dependent manner when 2 and 8 g/kg of plant extract were administered orally. Additionally, giving diabetic rats fenugreek seeds enhanced their metabolism of glucose and restored normal creatinine kinase activities in their liver, skeletal muscle, and heart.

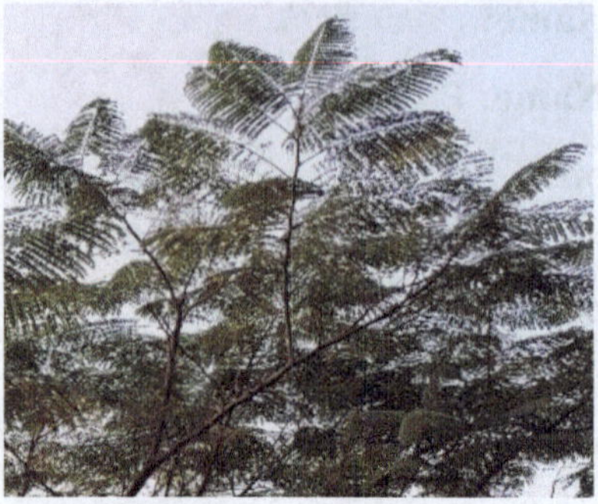

Scientific Name: *Butea monosperma*

Common Name: Palash

Distribution: Rajasthan, Uttar Pradesh, Madhya Pradesh, Bihar, and Odisha.

Part Used: Flowers, bark, and seeds

Bioactive Principle: Butrin, butein, and flavonoids

Remarks: It also show antihyperglycemic effect.

Herbal Drug Formulations

On the recommendation of their doctors, diabetic patients regularly utilize a variety of formulations that are available in the market.

1. ***Diabecon*** is said to boost muscle glucagon & hepatic levels, enhance peripheral glucose utilization, encourage beta cell regeneration & repair, & raise C peptide levels.

2. ***Epinsulin*** has epicatechin, a benzopyran, as an active ingredient and is sold under the Swastik formulations brand. Epicatechin raises the islet's cAMP concentration, which is linked to a higher release of insulin. By raising cathepsin activity, it contributes to the transformation of proinsulin into insulin.

3. ***Bitter gourd powder:*** It decreases the sugar levels in the blood and urine. It cleanses blood and strengthens the body's defenses against illnesses.

4. ***Diabetes:*** Daily which effectively and safely Improves Sugar Metabolism.

5. ***Gurmar powder:*** Blood sugar swings are avoided by an anti-diabetic medication that inhibits the intestinal absorption of saccharides. Additionally, it correlates the metabolic processes of the kidney, liver, and muscles. Gurmar has the ability to lower blood sugar and increases insulin secretion.

6. ***Diabeta***- is a blend of established anti-diabetic ingredients enhanced with strong immunomodulators, antihyperlipidemics, anti-stress, and plant-based hepatoprotectives. For almost a millennium, fenugreek has been a part of traditional formulas. Both cultured islet cells and an animal model are used to investigate the mechanism of this antidiabetic medication.

7. ***Chromium:*** It is employed in the process of glucose metabolism. may aid in lowering type 2 diabetes patients' fasting blood glucose levels.
8. ***Vitamin B1:*** Thiamine is another name for vitamin B1. Thiamine deficiencies are common in diabetics. Some consequences from diabetes may be exacerbated by this.

Conclusion

The antidiabetic properties of medicinal plants can be attributed to the presence of flavonoids, terpenoids, phenolic compounds, & coumarins. These bioactive constituents have demonstrated the ability to lower blood glucose levels. Notable examples of commercially available antidiabetic medications derived from natural sources include acarbose, Pycnogenol, voglibose, and miglitol. The active compounds sourced from these plants operate through various antidiabetic mechanisms, such as the inhibition of α-glucosidase, α-amylase, & protein tyrosine phosphatase actions. A significant benefit of herbal medications is their relatively low incidence of side effects, which has prompted numerous researchers to explore the development of new therapeutic molecules for diabetes management.

References

Kaoud Hussein. Diabetes in Animals Facts and Explanations 2017.

Kumar S, Mittal A, Babu D, Mittal A. Herbal Medicines for Diabetes Management and its Secondary Complications. Curr Diabetes Rev. 2021;17(4):437-456. doi: 10.21 74/ 157339 9816666201103143225

Modak M, Dixit P, Londhe J, Ghaskadbi S, Devasagayam TP. Indian herbs and herbal drugs used for the treatment of diabetes. J Clin Biochem Nutr. 2007;40(3):163-173. Doi : 10.3 164 /jcbn.40.163.

Zeugswetter FK, Luckschander-Zeller N, Karlovits S, Rand JS. Glargine versus regular insulin protocol in feline diabetic ketoacidosis. J Vet Emerg Crit Care (San Antonio). 2021;31(4):459-468. doi:10.1111/vec.13062

3

Medicinal Plants Effective in Tumour in Animals

Nisha, A.R., Varsha B., Archana, A. and Sudhakar, S.

Department of Veterinary Pharmacology and Toxicology
College of Veterinary and Animal Sciences, Mannuthy, Thrissur-680 651
Kerala Veterinary and Animal Sciences University

Tumour in Domestic Animals

Tumours in domestic animals, much like in humans, can occur in various tissues and organs. These can range from benign growths (non-cancerous) to malignant tumors or cancerous. Their causes, types, diagnosis, and treatments depend on the animal species, breed, age, and environmental factors. Common tumours in dogs are mammary tumours, skin tumours, lymphoma, osteosarcoma and hemangiosarcoma. In cats lymphoma, squamous cell carcinoma, mammary tumors and fibrosarcomas are reported. In cattle, squamous cell carcinoma, lymphosarcoma and papilloma are common. In horses, sarcoids, melanomas and squamous cell carcinoma are common. In small ruminants (sheep and goats) lymphoma and skin tumours are reported. In pigs, lymphoma and melanomas are commonly reported. Diagnosis of cancers are done by physical examination, cytology, biopsy, imaging: X-rays, ultrasound, CT, MRI and blood Tests.

Cancers Induced in Lab Animals

Causes and risk factors

- Genetic predisposition: Some breeds are more prone to specific tumours (e.g., Boxers and mast cell tumours in dogs).
- Hormonal influence: Unspayed females are at higher risk for mammary tumours.

- Environmental factors: UV exposure, exposure to carcinogens, or chronic irritation.
- Infectious agents: Viruses like FeLV in cats or BLV in cattle.

Induction of Tumour in Lab Animals

Cancers induced in lab animals are typically used in research to study cancer biology, assess the effectiveness of treatments, and investigate prevention strategies. Scientists can induce cancers in lab animals through various methods, depending on the type of cancer being studied.

1. Chemical carcinogens

Chemical agents are used to induce mutations or damage in cells, eventually leading to cancer. Examples include polycyclic aromatic hydrocarbons (PAHs), N-nitrosamines, Aflatoxins, and Benzo[a]pyrene etc

2. Radiation

Exposure to ionizing radiation like Gamma rays or X-rays and Ultraviolet (UV) light, can induce cancer in lab animals by causing DNA damage.

3. Genetic engineering

Genetically modified animals, especially mice, are used to study specific genetic mutations linked to cancer. Transgenic animal models in which oncogenes (e.g., *MYC*, *RAS*) overexpressed. Knockout animal models in which tumour suppressor genes (e.g., *p53*, *BRCA1*) inactivated.

4. Viral oncogenesis

Certain viruses are used to induce cancers in animals like SV40 virus, Human papillomavirus (HPV, Epstein-Barr virus (EBV)) which are associated with lymphoma studies.

5. Cell or tumour implantation

Cancerous cells or tissue fragments are implanted into animals as Xenografts. Allografts and Orthotopic models are also available.

6. Diet-Induced Models

Specific diets can promote cancer development like high-fat diets which are linked to colon or breast cancer or carcinogenic contaminants which induce gastrointestinal or liver cancers. Commonly used animals are mice and rats.

Most frequently used due to their genetic similarity to humans, short lifespan, and ease of handling. Hamsters, rabbits, and zebrafish are occasionally used depending on the research goals. Non-human primates are rarely used but can provide insights closer to human physiology. These models allow researchers to understand the mechanisms of cancer development and evaluate the safety and efficacy of drugs or therapies in a controlled environment. However, ethical considerations and animal welfare regulations are critical in these studies.Bottom of Form

Drugs Used in The Treatment of Cancers

Cancer involves a wide range of drugs that target the disease in various ways. These drugs are categorized based on their mechanism of action and the type of cancer they are used to treat. Chemotherapeutic agents work by killing rapidly dividing cells. These drugs can target cancer cells but may also affect healthy cells, leading to side effects. Examples of the drugs are Alkylating agents like Cyclophosphamide, Ifosfamide, Busulfan and Melphalan. Antimetabolites like Methotrexate, 5-Fluorouracil (5-FU), Capecitabine and Cytarabine. Platinum-Based Drugs like Cisplatin, Carboplatin, Oxaliplatin. Topoisomerase Inhibitors like Irinotecan, Topotecan and Etoposide. Mitotic inhibitors like Paclitaxel, Docetaxel, Vincristine and Vinblastine. Targeted drugs specifically interfere with molecules involved in tumour growth and progression like Tyrosine Kinase Inhibitors and Monoclonal Antibodies are also being used. Hormonal Therapy used for cancers that depend on hormones for growth, such as breast and prostate cancer. Epigenetic Modulators modify the expression of genes involved in cancer. Each type of cancer may require a specific combination of these drugs, often personalized to the patient's genetic makeup and disease progression.

Medicinal plants Used in Cancer

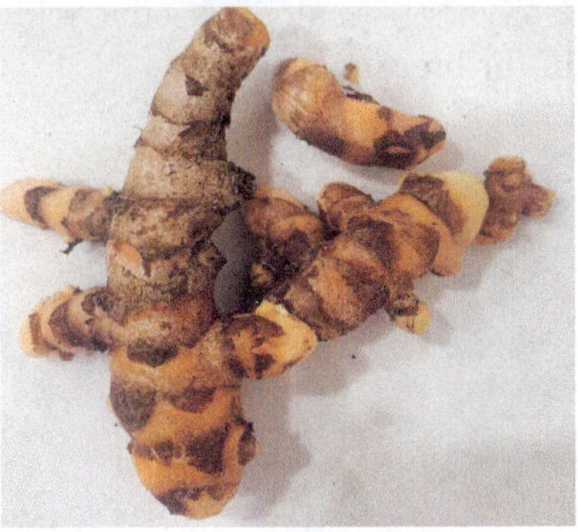

Scientific name: *Curcuma longa*

Common name: Turmeric

Distribution: South east India

Part used: Rhizome

Bioactive principles: Curcumin

Remarks: Downregulates NF-kB and AP-1 (inhibits cancer cell survival and proliferation)

Scientific name: *Azadirachta indica*

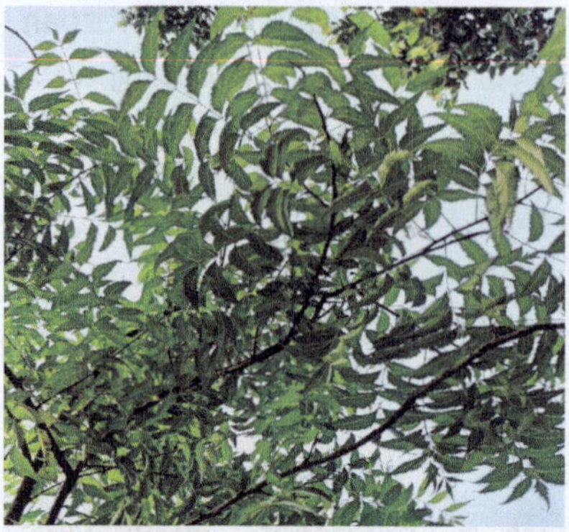

Common name: Neem

Distribution: Southeast Asia

Part used: Leaf, seed, flower

Bioactive principles: Azadirachtin, Nimbolide

Remarks: Induces apoptosis in tumour by increasing Bax and caspases in leukemia and breast cancer

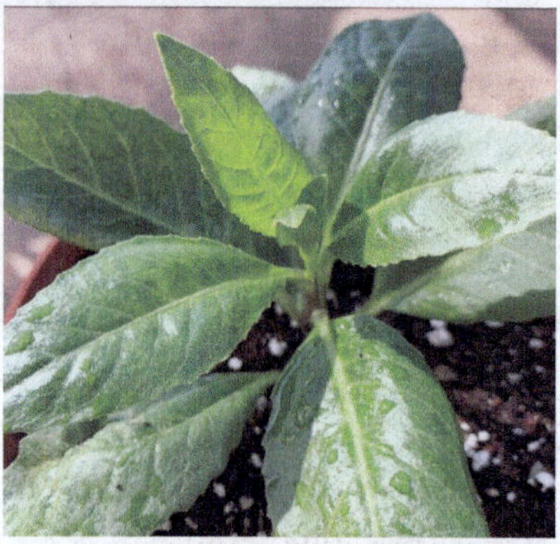

Scientific name: *Gynura procumbens*

Common name: Gynura, Longevity spinach

Distribution: South east Asia

Part used: Leaves

Bioactive principles: Flavanoids, phenolic acids, thaumatin like proteins

Remarks: Ethanolic extracts suppress matrix metalloproteinase (MMPs)

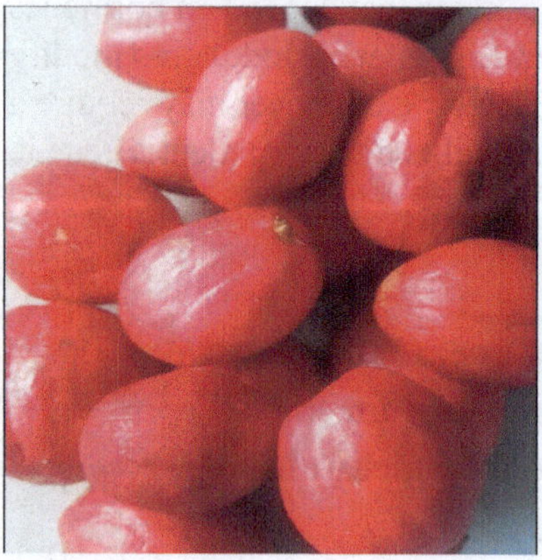

Scientific name: *Phaleria macrocarpa*

Common name: Mahkota Dewa

Distribution: Indonesia

Part used: Fruit, Leaf

Bioactive principles: Gallic acid

Remarks: Synergistically used with Doxorubicin for breast cancer

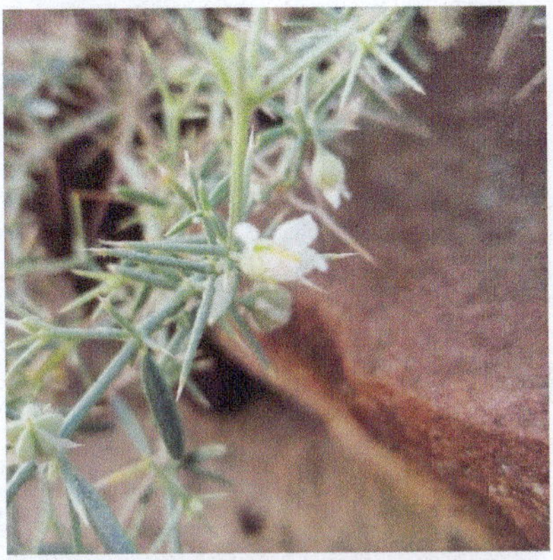

Scientific name: *Fagonia cretica*

Common name: Panchaga, dhamasa

Distribution: Europe, Africa, West Asia, India

Part used: Whole plant

Bioactive principles: Alkaloids

Remarks: Aqueous extracts induces cell cycle arrest in breast cancer cells

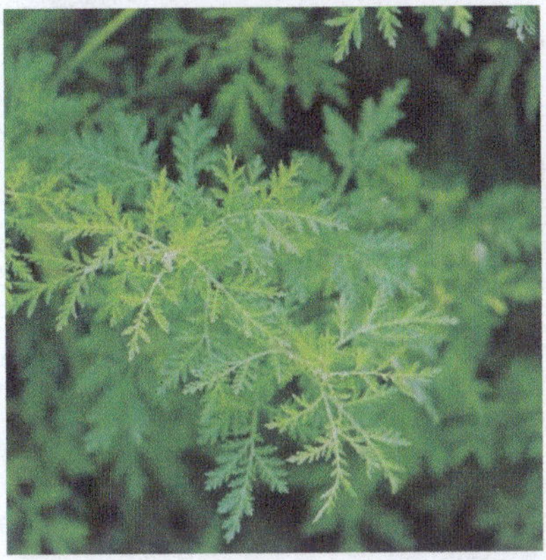

Scientific name: *Artemisia annua*

Common name: Sweet worm wood

Distribution: Asia, Europe

Part used: Leaves

Bioactive principles: Artemisinin

Remarks: Antiangiogenic effect, inhibits VEGF expression

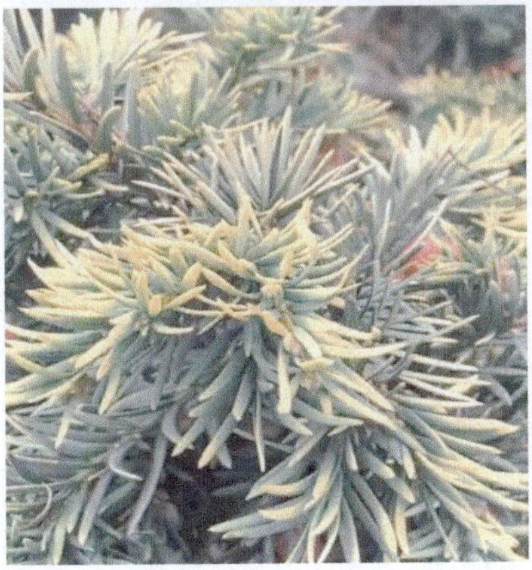

Scientific name: *Taxus baccata*

Common name: European Yew

Distribution: Southern Europe, South west Asia

Part used: bark, branch tips

Bioactive principles: Paclitaxel (Taxol)

Remarks: Inhibits microtubule function during mitosis

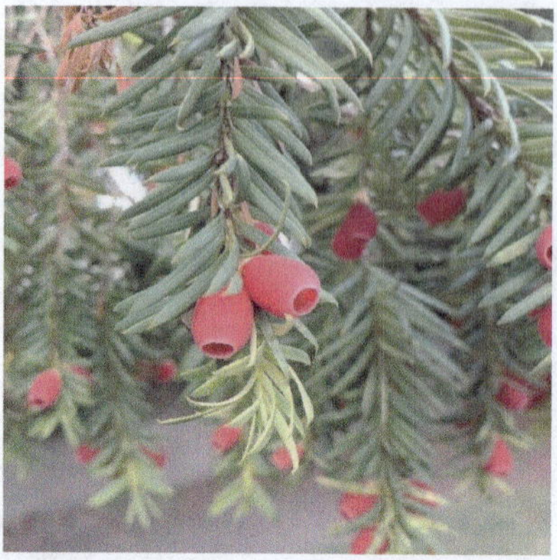

Scientific name: *Taxus brevifolia*

Common name: Pacific yew

Distribution: North America

Part used: Bark

Bioactive principles: Docetaxel

Remarks: Inhibits microtubule function during mitosis

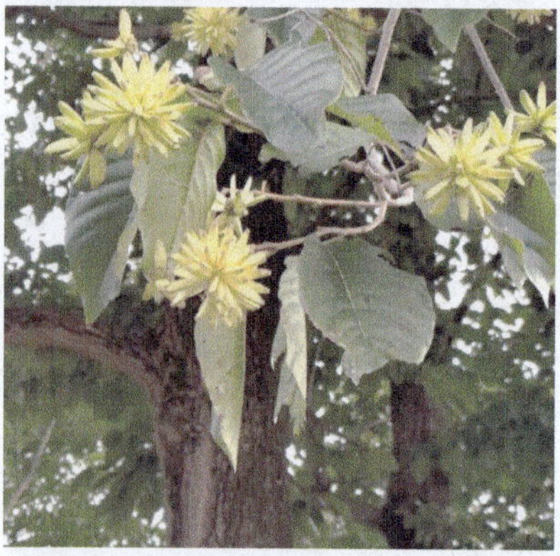

Scientific name : *Camptotheca acuminata*

Common name: Camptotheca

Distribution : China

Part used : leaves, bark, fruits, roots

Bioactive principles: Camptothecin

Remarks: Stabilizes topoisomerase I-DNA complex

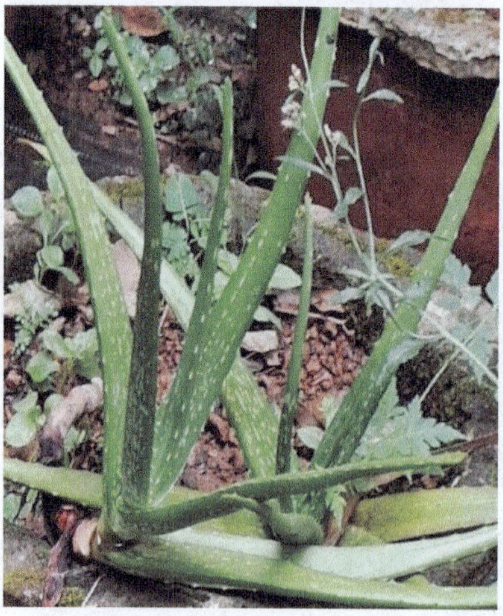

Scientific name : *Aloe barbadensis miller*

Common name: Aloe Vera

Distribution : Tropical and subtropical regions

Part used : leaves

Bioactive principles: Anthraquinones

Remarks: Induces apoptosis and inhibits tumor growth and has antioxidant property

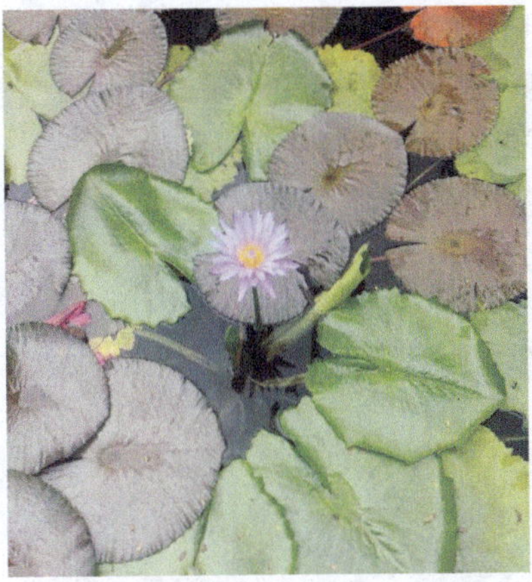

Scientific name : *Nymphaea nouchali* var. *caerulea*

Common name: Blue lotus

Distribution : Africa, Asia

Part used : flower

Bioactive principles: Alkaloids, flavonoids, glycoside

Remarks: Induces apoptosis and inhibits cell proliferation

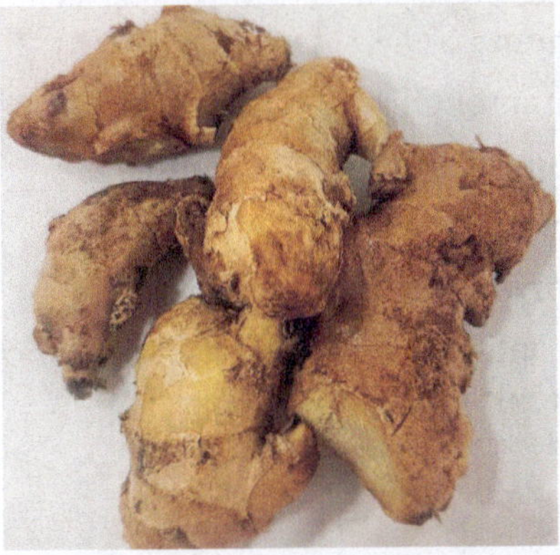

Scientific name : *Zingiber officinale*

Common name: Ginger

Distribution : Asia, widely cultivated globally

Part used : Rhizome

Bioactive principles: Gingerol

Remarks: cell cycle arrest in G0/G1 phase

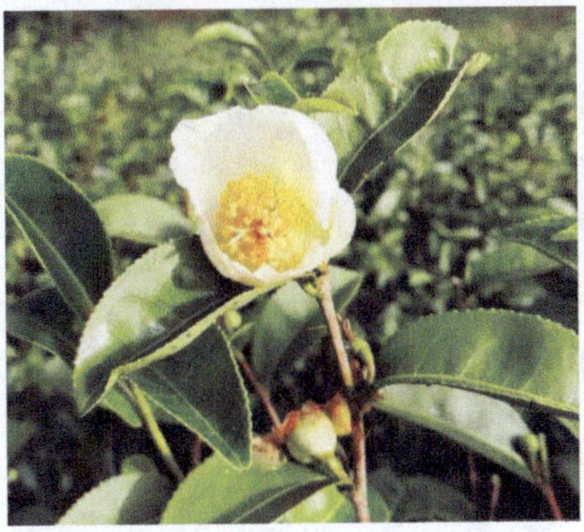

Scientific name: *Camellia sinensis*

Common name: Green tea

Distribution : East Asia

Part used : Leaves

Bioactive principles: Epigallocatechin gallate (EGCG)

Remarks: inhibits angiogenesis and has antioxidant property

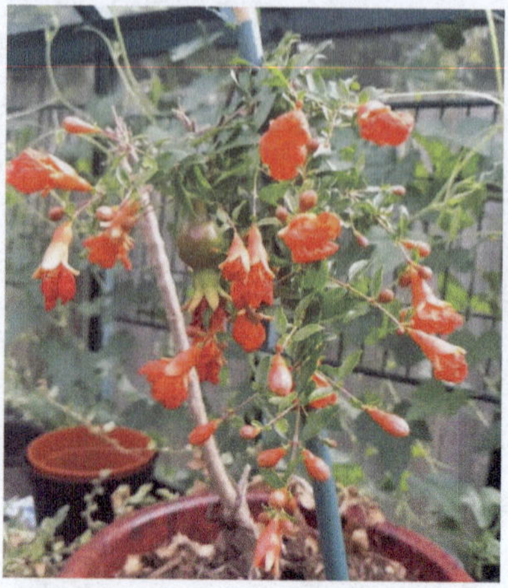

Scientific name : ***Punica granatum***
Common name: Pomegranate
Distribution : Mediterranean region
Part used : Seeds
Bioactive principles: Punicalagins
Remarks: Antioxidant effects and induces apoptosis

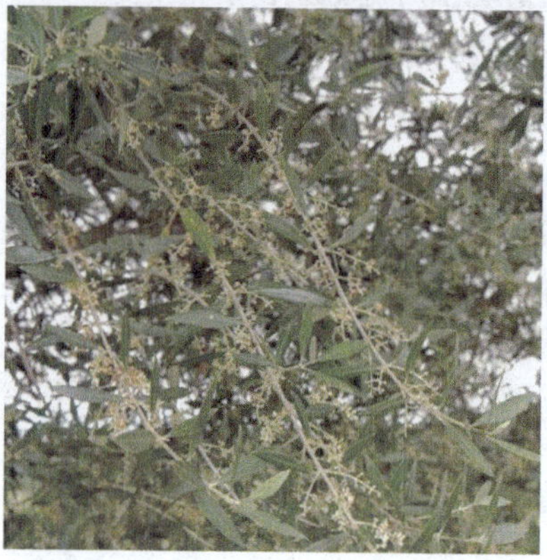

Scientific name : *Olea europaea*
Common name: Olives
Distribution : Mediterranean region
Part used : Leaves , Fruits
Bioactive principles: Oleuropein
Remarks: anti-proliferative and apoptotic effects in breast (MCF-7) cell line

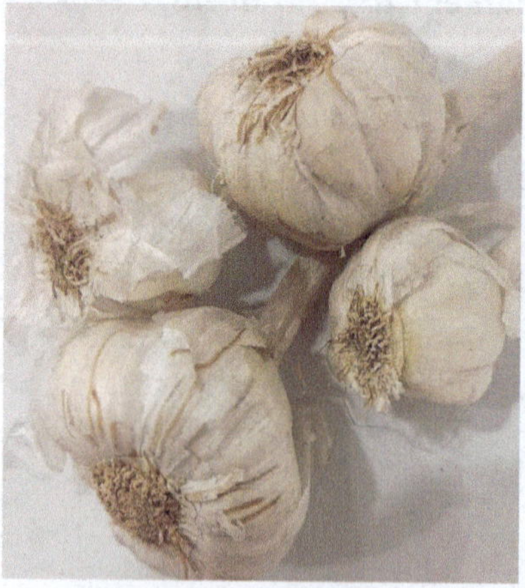

Scientific name : *Allium sativum*
Common name: Garlic
Distribution : Worldwide
Part used : bulbs
Bioactive principles: Allicin
Remarks: Cell cycle arrest at G1 phase

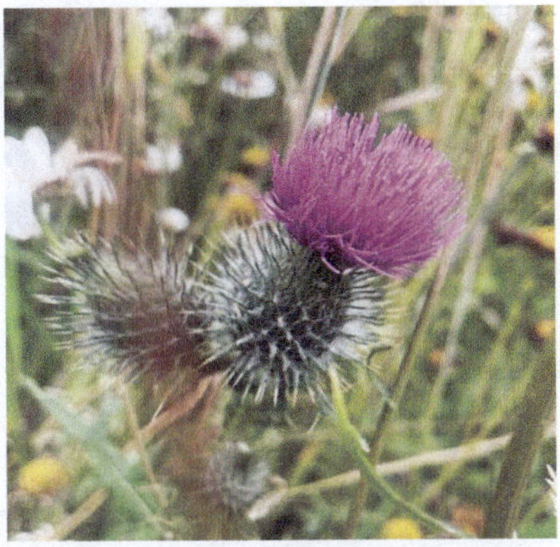

Scientific name: *Silybum marianum*

Common name: Milk Thistle

Distribution : Mediterranean region

Part used : Seeds

Bioactive principles: Silymarin

Remarks: Protects liver cells and induces apoptosis

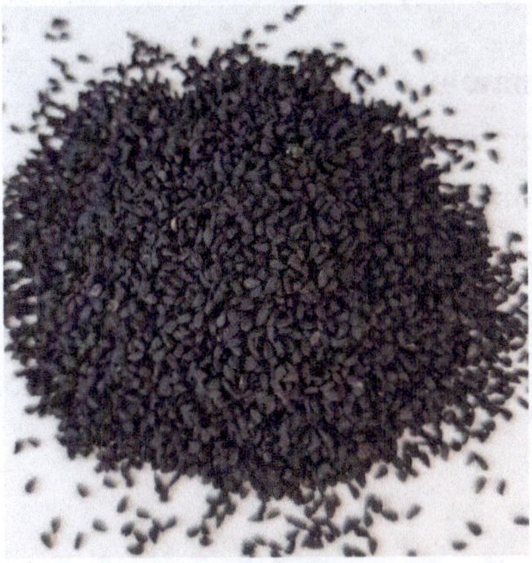

Scientific name : *Nigella sativa*

Common name: Black Seed

Distribution : Middle East, South Asia

Part used : Seeds

Bioactive principles: Thymoquinone

Remarks: Decreases Bcl2 antiapoptotic protein

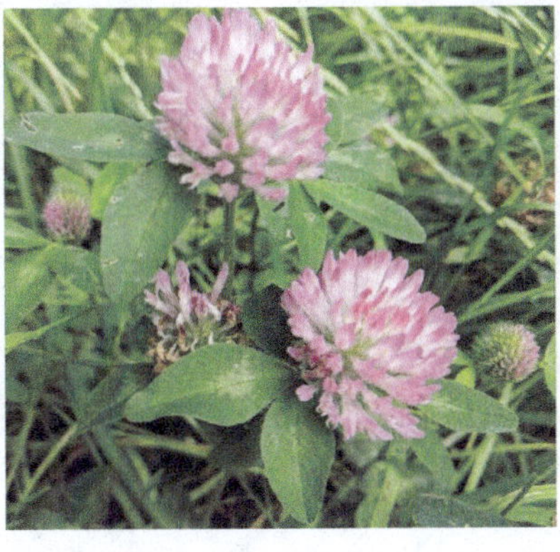

Scientific name: *Trifolium pratense*

Common name: red clover

Distribution : Europe, North America

Part used : Flower

Bioactive principles: Isoflavones

Remarks: Modulates estrogen activity and induces apoptosis

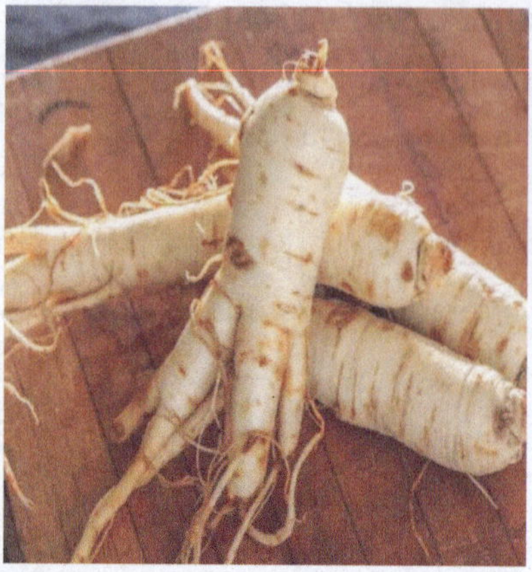

Scientific name : *Panax ginseng*

Common name: Ginseng

Distribution : East Asia

Part used : Rhizome

Bioactive principles: Ginsenosides

Remarks: Enhances immune function and induces apoptosis

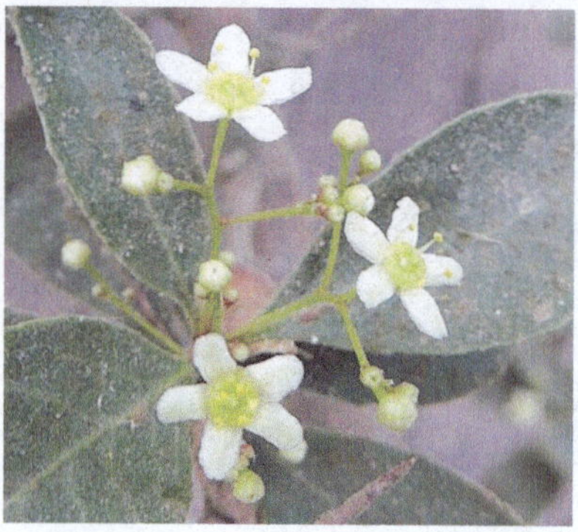

Scientific name: *Maytenus serrata*

Common name: Maytenus

Distribution: Asia, Africa

Part used: roots

Bioactive principles: Maytansine

Remarks: Inhibits microtubule assembly by binding to tubulin

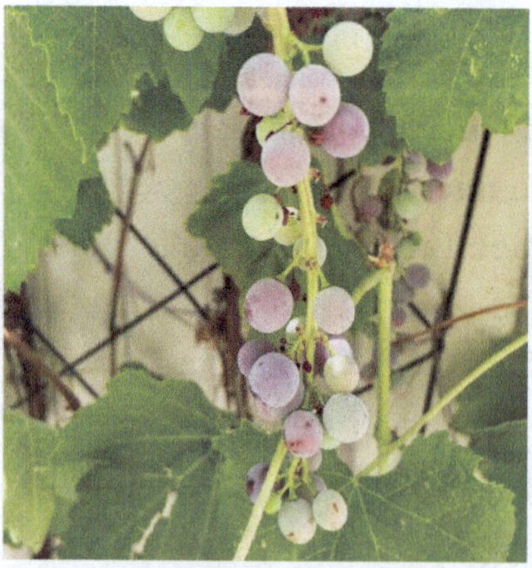

Scientific name: *Vitis vinifera*

Common name: Resveraterol

Distribution: Worldwide

Part used: Seeds of grapes

Bioactive principles: Resveratrol

Remarks: Antioxidant and inhibits *Bcl2*

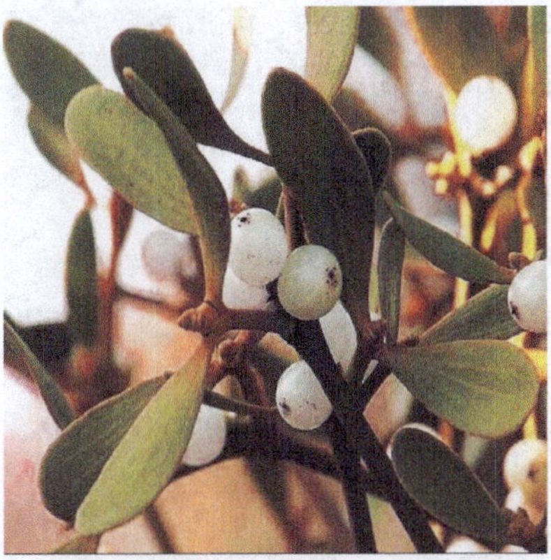

Scientific name: *Viscum album*

Common name: Mistletoe

Distribution: Europe, Asia, and parts of Africa

Part used: Aerial parts (leaves and stems)

Bioactive principles: Viscotoxin, lectins

Remarks: Immune modulation and supportive care in chemotherapy; studied in breast, lung, and gastrointestinal cancers

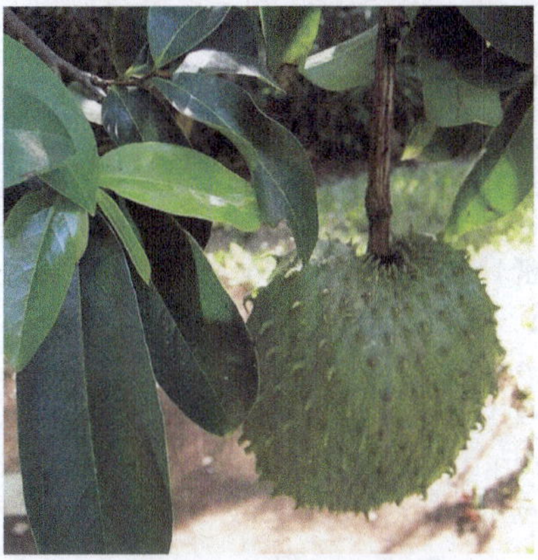

Scientific name: *Annona muricata*

Common name: Soursop

Distribution: Tropical and subtropical regions

Part used: Fruit, leaves, and seeds

Bioactive principles: Acetogenins

Remarks: Cytotoxic to cancer cells; potential to reduce tumor growth; studied in pancreatic, breast, and prostate cancers

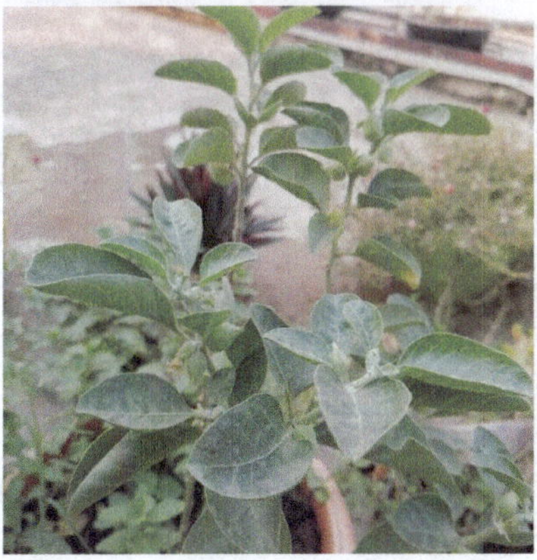

Scientific name: *Withania somnifera*

Common name: Ashwagandha

Distribution: Native to India, the Middle East, and parts of Africa

Part used: Roots and leaves

Bioactive principles: Withaferin A

Remarks: Adaptogen, stress relief, and potential anti-tumor effects; studied in breast, prostate, and lung cancers

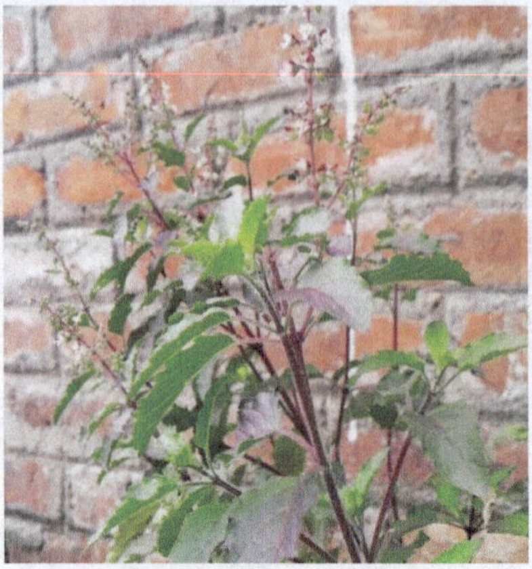

Scientific name: *Ocimum sanctum*

Common name: Holy Basil

Distribution: Native to India and Southeast Asia

Part used: Leaves and seeds

Bioactive principles: Eugenol, ursolic acid

Remarks: Antioxidant, anti-inflammatory, and anti-tumor properties; studied in skin, lung, and oral cancers

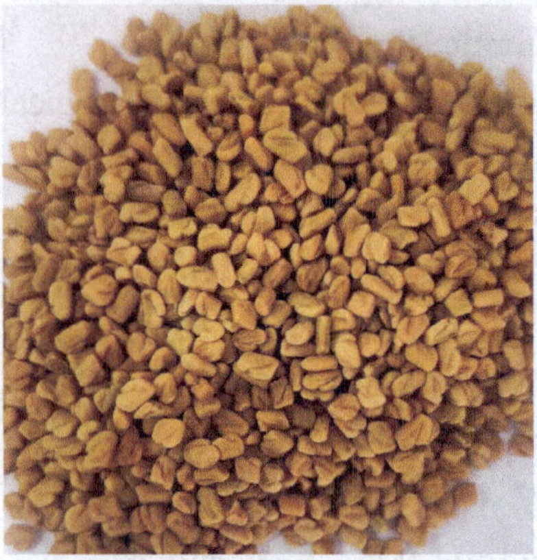

Scientific name: *Trigonella foenum-graecum*

Common name: Fenugreek

Distribution: Native to the Mediterranean region, widely cultivated worldwide

Part used: Seeds and leaves

Bioactive principles: Diosgenin

Remarks: Cytotoxic effects on cancer cells and anti-inflammatory properties; studied in breast and prostate cancers

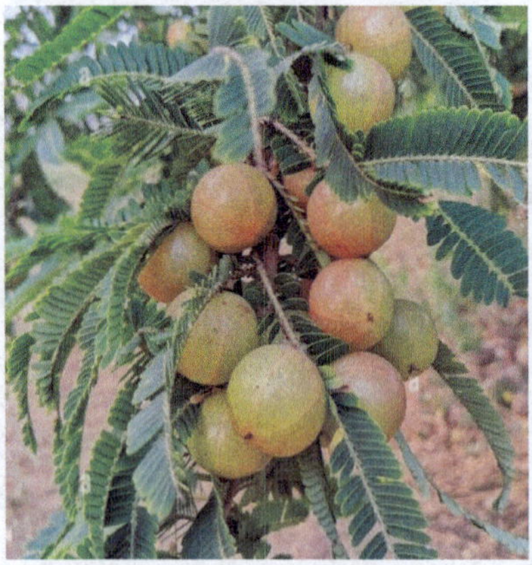

Scientific name: *Emblica officinalis*

Common name: Indian Gooseberry

Distribution: Native to India and Southeast Asia

Part used: Fruits

Bioactive principles: Phyllemblin, ellagic acid

Remarks: Antioxidant and anti-cancer properties; studied in liver, stomach, and lung cancers, as well as various cancers in palliative care and clinical research

References

Bartoszek A. Mutagenic, carcinogenic, and chemo-preventive compounds in foods. Chemical and functional properties of food components. 2002:307-36.

Desai AG, Qazi GN, Ganju RK, El-Tamer M, Singh J, Saxena AK, Bedi YS, Taneja SC, Bhat HK. Medicinal plants and cancer chemoprevention. Current drug metabolism. 2008 Sep 1;9(7):581-91.

Gezici S, Şekeroğlu N. Current perspectives in the application of medicinal plants against cancer: novel therapeutic agents. Anti-Cancer Agents in Medicinal Chemistry (Formerly Current Medicinal Chemistry-Anti-Cancer Agents). 2019 Jan 1;19(1):101-11.

Govind P, Madhuri S. Medicinal plants: better remedy for neoplasm. Indian drugs. 2006;43(11):869-74.

Greenwell M, Rahman PK. Medicinal plants: their use in anticancer treatment. International Journal of Pharmaceutical Sciences and Research. 2015 Oct 10;6(10):4103.

Gupta DK, Singh R, Gupta N, Shrman K. Neoplasms in dog and cat. InIntroduction to Diseases, Diagnosis, and Management of Dogs and Cats 2024 Jan 1 (pp. 363-376). Academic Press.

Hardisty JF. Factors influencing laboratory animal spontaneous tumor profiles. Toxicologic Pssathology. 1985 Feb;13(2):95-104.

Sharma H, Parihar L, Parihar P. Review on cancer and anticancerous properties of some medicinal plants. J Med Plants Res. 2011 May 18;5(10):1818-35.

Workman P. Animals in experimental neoplasia. Br J Cancer. 1998;77(1):1-0.

Wu HC, Chang DK, Huang CT. Targeted therapy for cancer. J Cancer Mol. 2006 Apr 15;2(2):57-66.

4

Medicinal Plants Effective in Arthritis in Animals

Vandana Singh[1] and Anuj Singh[2]

[1]*Department of Veterinary Pharmacology & Toxicology, COVAS, Kishanganj Bihar Animal Science University, Patna*

[2]*Department of Animal Nutrition, COVAS, Kishanganj, Bihar Animal Science University, Patna*

Introduction

Arthritis, a condition characterized by inflammation of the joints, is prevalent among livestock species, particularly in older animals or those subjected to intensive farming conditions. It results in pain, reduced mobility, and diminished productivity. Herbal plants with anti-inflammatory and analgesic qualities are being investigated as a result of the increased interest in natural therapies, even if treatments like non-steroidal anti-inflammatory medications (NSAIDs) and corticosteroids have been utilized to manage arthritis in livestock. This chapter addresses the use of herbal plants to treat arthritis in cattle, including a summary of the best plant-based remedies, their modes of action, and the scientific data that backs them up.

Pathophysiology of Arthritis in Livestock

Arthritis in livestock is primarily caused by joint degeneration, trauma, infection, or autoimmune disorders. The inflammation of the synovial membrane leads to the discharge of cytokines that cause inflammation, which degrade cartilage and cause pain. The condition significantly impacts the animal's ability to move, affecting their overall well-being and productivity. In farmed animals, arthritis can lead to decreased milk production, reduced growth rates, and compromised meat quality, thus representing a significant economic loss.

Models of inflammatory joint disease in animals

To assess possible treatments and comprehend the pathophysiological processes of inflammatory arthritis, animal disease models are quite beneficial. Rats and mice are the most used animal species for this purpose, either as inducible models where arthritogenic stimuli can be given to develop the disease or as strains that cause arthritis on their own.

Models of spontaneous arthritis

Although it has been reported that several rodent strains are prone to developing spontaneous arthritis, experimental research has mostly concentrated on a small number of genetically altered mouse strains, particularly TNF-transgenic (TNFtg) and K/BxN mice, which exhibit full penetration and consistent disease progression.

The K/BxN model

K/BxN mice with the I-Ag7 MHC-II allele have a T-cell receptor transgene specific for a peptide generated by the common enzyme glucose-6-phosphate isomerase (GPI).

Around three to four weeks of age, autoimmune disease first appears as joint inflammation, which develops into complete inflammatory-erosive arthritis over the course of four to eight weeks. The main source of the disease seems to be anti-GPI autoantibodies, since K/BxN serum or even anti-GPI monoclonal antibodies produced from K/BxN can induce arthritis in other mouse strains.

The model of TNF-transgenic mice

TNFtg mice, which were developed in the early 1990s, have offered crucial proof that TNF plays a role in inflammatory arthritis. They lack post-transcriptional regulatory mechanisms and express a human TNF gene. In comparison to multicopy transgenics, the 3647-strain TNFtg mice have longer lifespans (more than a year under proper husbandry), slower illness development (13–16 weeks from commencement to maximum severity), and delayed initiation of joint inflammation (3-4 weeks of age vs. 6-8 weeks). Due to their delayed growth and late beginning, single-copy TNFtg mice are especially well-suited for studying pathways linked to preclinical illness stages and growing chronicity. Therefore, TNFtg mice are a great model to study the inflammatory pathways caused by TNF in diseases.

Models of inducible arthritis

Rats and mice are used in well-established systems to experimentally develop inflammatory arthritis in a variety of species. In these models, arthritogenic signals can be caused by passively supplied autoreactive antibodies or sera, nonspecific inflammatory agents such various adjuvants, or immunization processes that use particular antigens that break down self-tolerance.

Adjuvant-induced arthritis and associated models

Adjuvants such as pristane, squalene, and complete or incomplete Freund's adjuvant (CFA, IFA) can consistently cause arthritis when given intradermally to sensitive strains of rats (such Lewis or DA rats) or intraarticularly to presensitized rats or mice.

In the majority of cases, After a few days of treatment, the illness appears and peaks in severity in a few weeks and then usually goes into remission, which in certain protocols can be reversed with additional treatments. The strain and arthritogenic signal affect the severity and progression of the disease. For instance, arthritis caused by antigen-free adjuvants such as IFA or pristane is significantly less severe and widespread than arthritis caused by CFA.

Collagen-induced arthritis

The most used experimental model for arthritis is collagen-induced arthritis (CIA).

Immunization with type II collagen, usually derived from cows, results in inflammatory arthritis in genetically vulnerable rats, rabbits, mice, and other species.

According to a standard mouse technique, polyarthritis appears a few weeks following CFA-emulsified collagen immunization Within two weeks of starting, CFA-emulsified collagen vaccination reaches its peak clinical severity and then persists in a chronic form.

Antibody-induced arthritis

Early experimental evidence of the direct pathogenic role of humoral immunity in arthritis was provided by the discovery that serum from mice and rats injected with collagen may passively cause arthritis in recipients. The same technique is commonly used to create acute, transient arthritis in mice or rats in models such as K/BxN serum-transfer arthritis and collagen-antibody-induced arthritis (CAIA).

According to these models, arthritis develops without the assistance of B and T cells and is brought on by the accumulation of immune complexes in the joints, the recruitment of neutrophils, and other innate inflammatory components. The models are ideal for studying acute mechanisms because of the quick, consistent, and severe inflammatory response in the joints

Experimental techniques for examining animal models' reactions to pain

The two main components of animal behavior models to pain are measurement of behavior that is thought to be indicative of that pain state and experimental treatment meant to create a pain-like condition. Experimental evaluation of pain and its alleviation after antinociceptive medication delivery can be done using these models.

In general, measuring pain-suppressed or pain-evoked behaviors is the basis for experimental evaluation of pain in animal behavioral models. In the absence of pain, pain-evoked actions can happen extremely infrequently, but they can become more frequent after alleged nociceptive stimulation. Footpad withdrawal, jumping, flinching, and licking are a few examples. Pain-suppressed behaviors, on the other hand, are those that happen frequently when there are no unpleasant stimuli present and that lessen in intensity or length following exposure to a negative stimulus.

Locomotor activity, nesting, eating, and balance and motor coordination are examples of natural behaviors that may be impeded under this circumstance. Pain reactions to typically unpleasant stimuli, hyperalgesia (an increased sensitivity to low-grade painful stimuli), or allodynia (a painful reaction to a normally non-noxious stimulus) can all result in measurable behavioral changes.

Treatment of Traumatic Arthritis

Physical treatment, systemic and intra-articular anti-inflammatory drugs, and rest can resolve mild osteochondral fractures and mend major articular fractures.

Acute traumatic synovitis and capsulitis are treated with rest and physical rehabilitation exercises such swimming, passive flexion, ice application, and cold water treatment. NSAIDs, such as phenylbutazone, are frequently taken orally or intravenously and may lessen synovial inflammation. Numerous medications have been administered intra-articularly. The strongest anti-inflammatory drugs, corticosteroids, work well for acute traumatic arthritis. In order to reduce inflammation and promote healing, biologic therapies such Autologous protein solutions, autologous conditioned serum, and platelet-rich plasma are also being used more and more.

Surgical treatment to prevent the development of osteoarthritis, major intra-articular fractures that disturb joint congruity, such as distal metacarpal and metatarsal condylar fractures, proximal phalanx sagittal articular fractures, and third carpal bone slab fractures, should be corrected.

Herbal treatment with medicinal plants having Anti-Arthritic Properties

Numerous herbs have been found to have medicinal promise for reducing livestock arthritic symptoms. Because of their analgesic, antioxidant, and anti-inflammatory qualities, these herbs are frequently employed in traditional veterinary care. Some of the most researched herbs are listed below:

Scientific name: *Zingiber officinale*

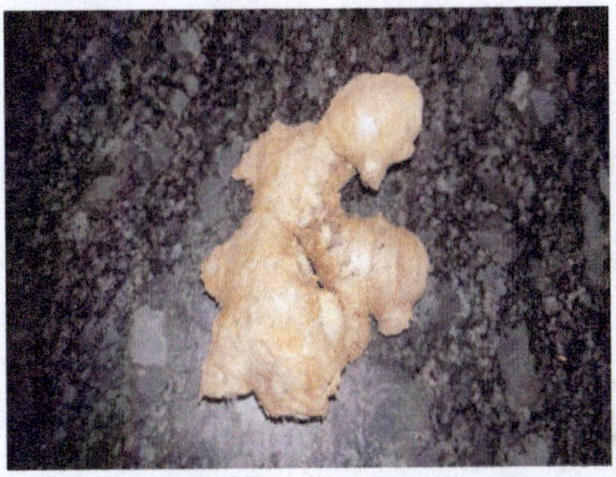

Common name: Ginger

Distribution: Madhya Pradesh, Karnataka, assam, kerela, Meghalaya , northeastern states.

Parts used: stem

Bioactive principles: Gingerol, 6-shogaol

Remarks: helps to reduce swelling, pain, and inflammation associated with arthritis and also helps in improving joint function and reduce cartilage deterioration.

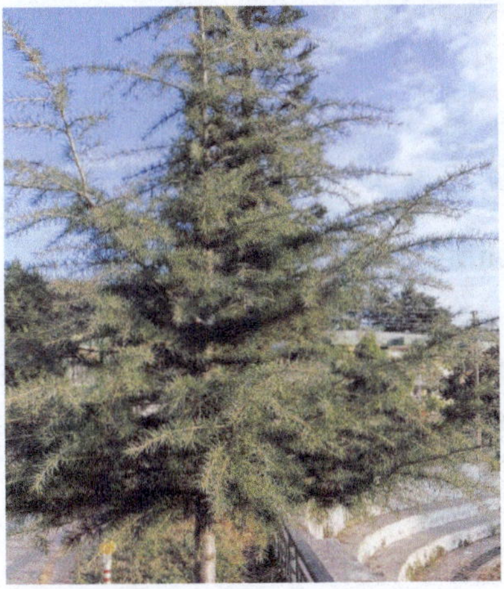

Scientific name*: Cedrus deodara*

Common name: Deodar cedar

Distribution: Himachal Pradesh, Uttarakhand

Parts used: wood and oil

Bioactive principles: alpha pinene, cisocimene, limonene, and deodarone, gallic acid, shikimic acid, ferulic acid, protocatechuic acid, Matairesinol, myricetin,and polysaccharides.

Remarks: Has anti-inflammatory and analgesic properties, and may be effective in treating arthritis

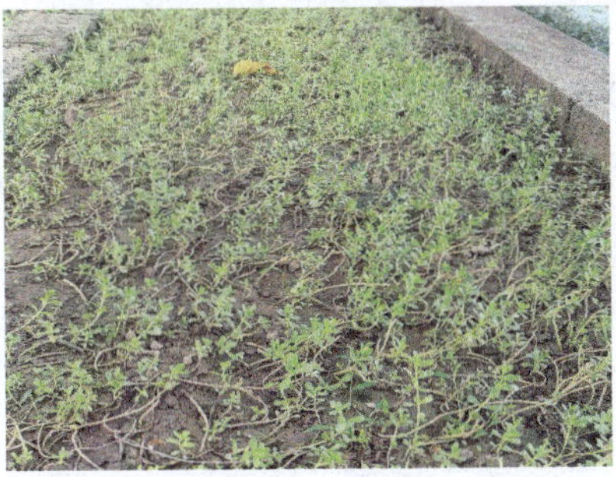

Scientific name: *Bacopa monnieri*

Common name: Brahmi, Water hyssop, Indian pennywort, and Herb of grace

Distribution: Andaman & Nicobar, Assam, Punjab, Andhra Pradesh, Delhi, Kerala, Gujarat, Karnataka, Manipur, Goa, Odisha, Tamil Nadu, Rajasthan, Bihar and West Bengal .

Parts used: leaves

Bioactive principles: Serine and pseudojujubogenin glycoside, β-sitosterol, D-mannitol, stigmastanol, betulinic acid, stigmasterol, α-alanine, aspartic acid, glutamic acid, alkaloid brahmine, bacosides, herpestine, saponins, nicotinine, and triterpenoid saponins.

Remarks: It reduces the swelling present over the ankle joint in patient with arthritis.

Scientific name: ***Paederia foetida***

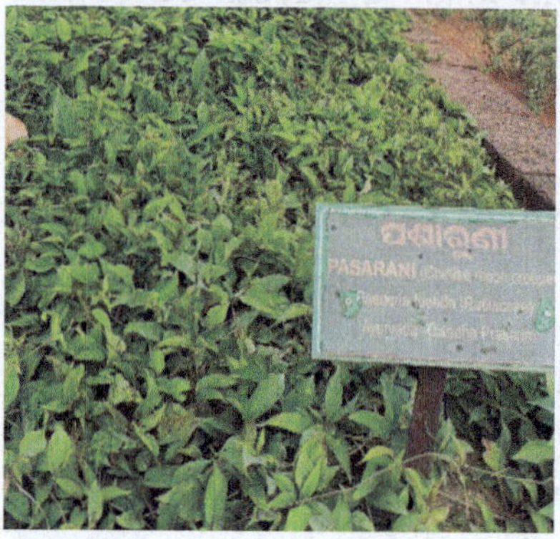

Common name: Pasarani, Skunk Vine, Gandhali Paduri lata

Distribution: Manipur, Andhra Pradesh, Assam, Meghalaya,

Nagaland, Odisha, Mizoram, Sikkim, Arunachal Pradesh and Telangana

Parts used: leaves, roots, barks

Bioactive principles: stigmasterol, sitosterol, iridoid glycosides, alkaloids, volatile oil, carbs, protein, and amino acids.

Remarks: prevent arthritis by inhibiting COX-2 and PGE (2) expression through nuclear factor-κB.

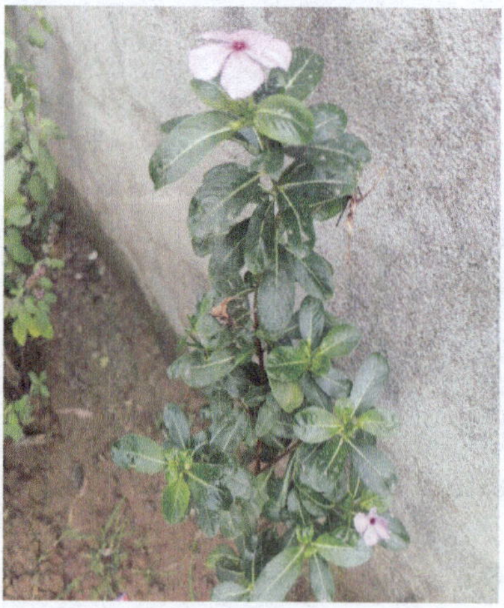

Scientific name: *Canthranthus roseus*

Common name: Sadabihari

Distribution: Tamil Nadu, Karnataka, Madhya Pradesh, assam, bihar , maharasthra , uttar Pradesh

Parts used: leaves, stems, flowers, roots

Bioactive principles: ajmalicine and serpentine

Remarks: has anti-arthritic and anti-inflammatory properties.

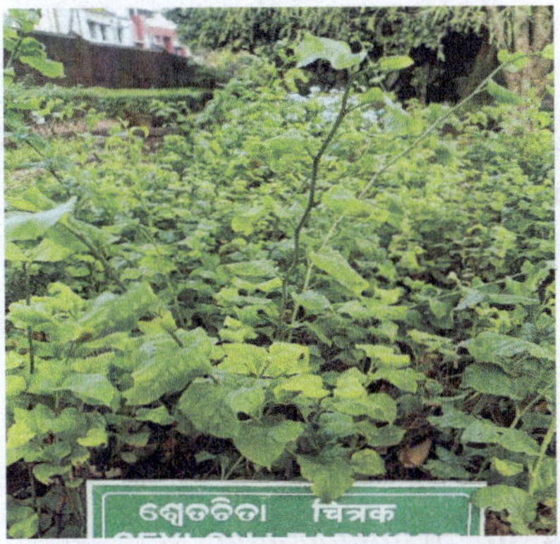

Scientific name: ***Plumbago zeylanica***

Common name: Ceylon Leadwort

Distribution: Tamil Nadu, maharasthra, rajasthan, assam, Madhya Pradesh, bihar, uttar Pradesh, chattisgarh ,West Bengal.

Parts used: leaves, bark, roots

Bioactive principles: plumbagin, napthoquinones, coumarins

Remarks: It has anti-inflammatory properties and can be used to treat chronic rheumatoid arthritis.

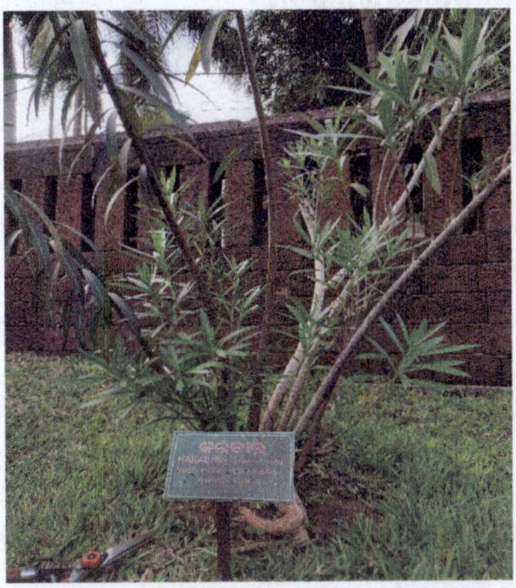

Scientific name: ***Indian Oleander/ Nerium Oleander***

Common name: Karabira

Distribution: Gujarat, Jharkand, Karnataka, Kerala, Maharashtra, Odisha, Uttar Pradesh, Bihar, Andhra Pradesh, and Assam

Parts used: leaves, bark

Bioactive principles: oleandrin, α tocopherol, digitoxingenin, urosolic acid, quercetin , odorosidesa

Remarks: has anti-inflammatory and anti bacterial properties

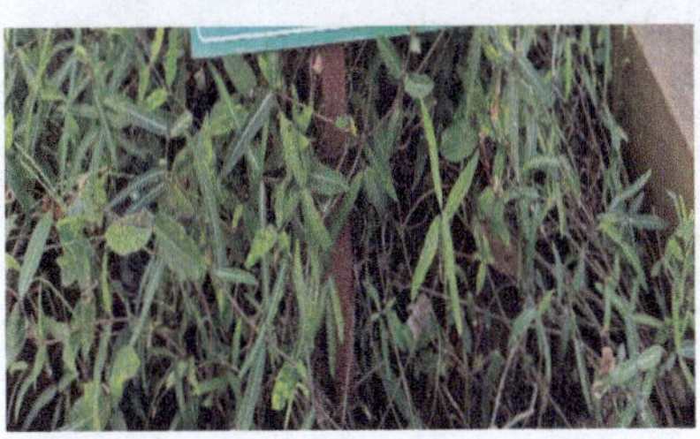

Scientific name: ***Tylphora indica***

Common name: Antamula

Distribution: Tamil Nadu, Karnataka, Odisha, Kerela, Assam, Bihar ,West Bengal

Parts used: leaves, roots

Bioactive principles: alkaloids(Tylophorine), flavonoids(Kaemferol and quercetin), terpenoids (αAmyrin, β-Amyrin), sterols (β sitosterol)

Remarks: has anti-neuroinflammatory properties and can be used to treat chronic rheumatoid arthritis.

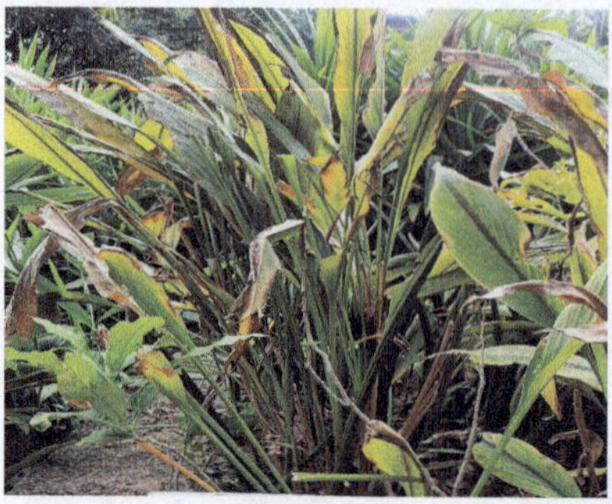

Scientific name: *Curcuma Caesia*

Common name: Nilakantha Kedar

Distribution: Madhya Pradesh, uttar Pradesh, Odisha chattisgarh , west Bengal

Parts used: leaves, rhizomes

Bioactive principles: curcuminoids, tumerone, curcumene, β -ocimene.

Remarks: reduces inflammation and pain in people with arthritis.

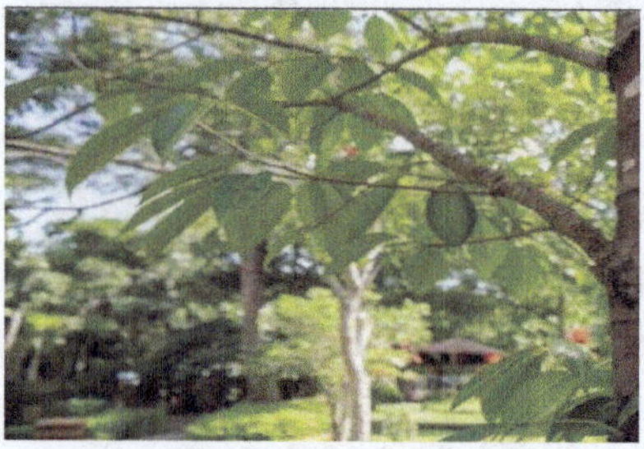

Scientific name*:* *Cinnamomum verum*

Common name: Dalchini

Distribution: Tamil Nadu, kerela

Parts used: leaves, bark

Bioactive principles: Cinnamaldehyde, eugenol, procyanidins, linalool, coumarins, cinnamic acid.

Remarks: has anti-inflammatory and anti arthritic properties and helps to reduce joint pain.

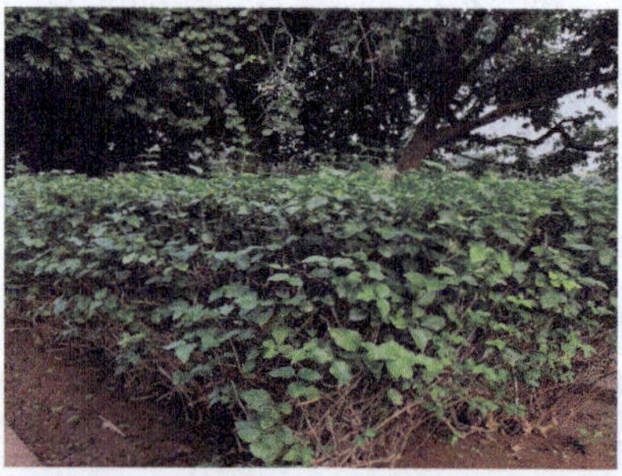

Scientific name: *Gelsemium sempervirens*

Common name: Jui, Yellow jasmine

Distribution: Tamil Nadu, andra Pradesh, Punjab, Karnataka

Parts used: leaves, bark, roots, stem

Bioactive principles: phenols, alkaloids, saponins, terpenoids, quinines, sambacosides.

Remarks: has anti-inflammatory properties.

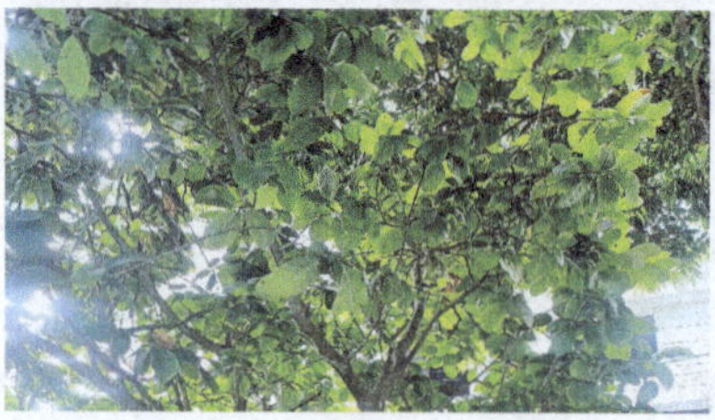

Scientific name*:* *Ferula assafoetida*

Common name: Hengu

Distribution: Himachal Pradesh Uttarakhand, jammu & Kashmir.

Parts used: rhizome, roots

Bioactive principles: β- pinene, ferulic acid , γ- elemene, coumarins, β-maaliene, α-pinene, α/β-eudesmol.

Remarks: has anti-inflammatory properties and reduces inflammation.

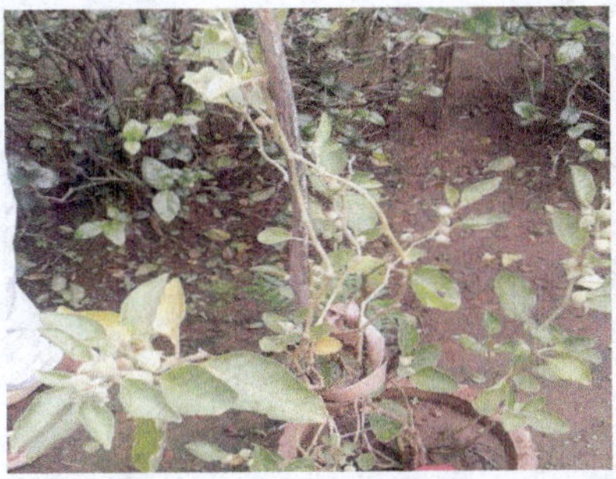

Scientific Name: *Withania somnifera*

Common Name: Ashwagandha

Distribution: Found in Rajasthan, Madhya Pradesh, Punjab, and Uttar Pradesh, commonly in drier regions.

Part Used: Roots and leaves

Bioactive Principles: Withanolides, alkaloids, and steroidal lactones

Remark: Ashwagandha is widely used in Ayurveda for its anti-inflammatory and pain-relieving properties. It helps in reducing joint pain and stiffness, improving mobility, and addressing symptoms of arthritis.

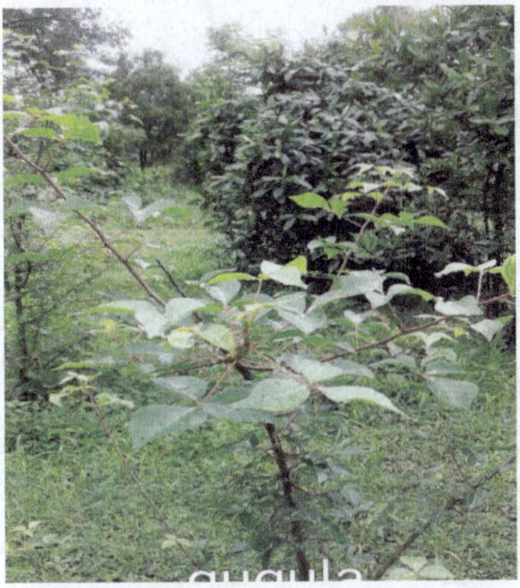

Scientific Name: Commiphora wightii

Common Name: Guggul

Distribution: Found in Rajasthan, Gujarat, and Karnataka, in arid and semi-arid regions.

Part Used: Gum resin

Bioactive Principles: Guggulsterones, essential oils, and flavonoids

Remark: Guggul is known for its anti-inflammatory and analgesic properties, making it effective in managing arthritis symptoms. It reduces swelling, improves joint mobility, and alleviates pain.

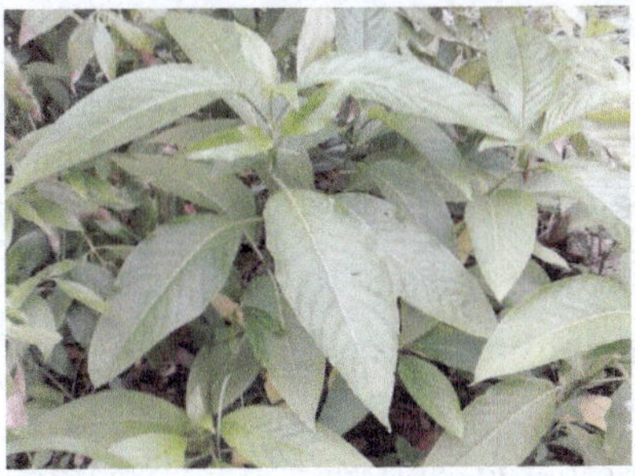

Scientific Name: *Adhatoda vasica*

Common Name: Malabar Nut

Distribution: Commonly found in Odisha, West Bengal, Assam, and southern India, in moist and forested areas.

Part Used: Leaves, roots, and flowers

Bioactive Principles: Vasicine, vasicinone, and alkaloids

Remark: *Adhatoda vasica* is known for its anti-inflammatory properties and is used in managing joint inflammation and mild arthritis symptoms in traditional medicine.

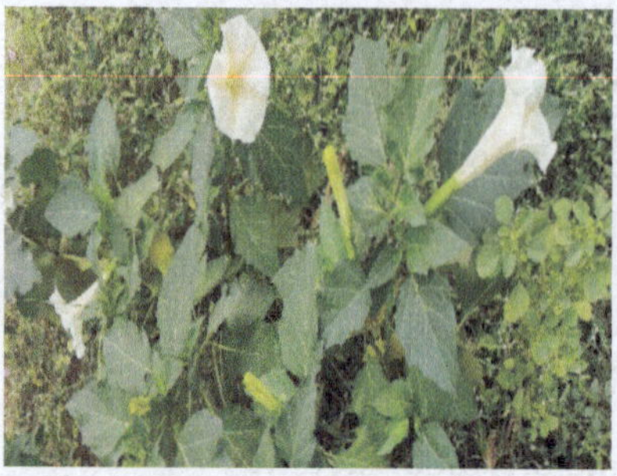

Scientific Name: *Datura stramonium*

Common Name: Thorn Apple, Dhatura

Distribution: Found in Uttar Pradesh, Odisha, Maharashtra, and across India in wild and semi-wild regions.

Part Used: Seeds and leaves

Bioactive Principles: Scopolamine, atropine, and hyoscyamine

Remark: The leaves and seeds of *Datura* are used topically in traditional remedies for pain relief in arthritis. Due to its potent properties, it is often applied with caution under expert guidance.

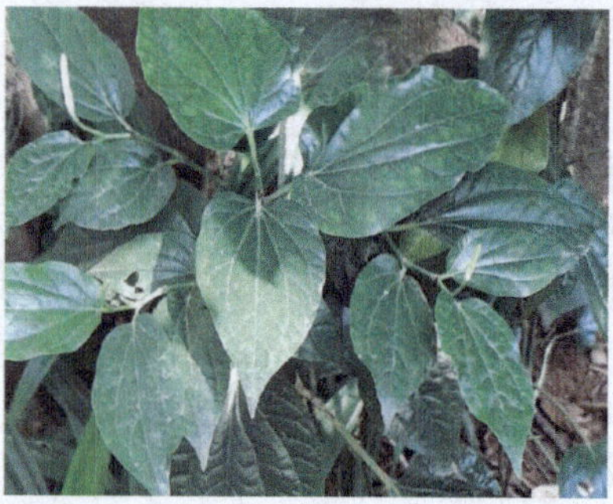

Scientific Name: *Piper longum*

Common Name: Long Pepper, Pipali

Distribution: Found in West Bengal, Assam, Odisha, and southern India, in moist forests and cultivated areas.

Part Used: Fruits and roots

Bioactive Principles: Piperine, alkaloids, and volatile oils

Remark: *Piper longum* is traditionally used in Ayurveda for its anti-inflammatory effects. It helps reduce swelling, alleviate joint pain, and improve circulation in arthritic conditions.

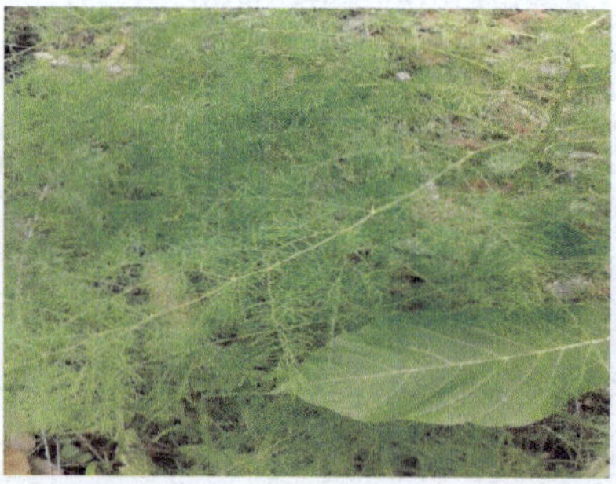

Scientific Name: Asparagus racemosus

Common Name: Shatavari

Distribution: Found in Odisha, West Bengal, and southern India, in forested and hilly regions.

Part Used: Roots and shoots

Bioactive Principles: Saponins, flavonoids, and alkaloids

Remark: Shatavari is known for its adaptogenic and anti-inflammatory properties. It is used in traditional medicine to support joint health and reduce inflammation associated with arthritis.

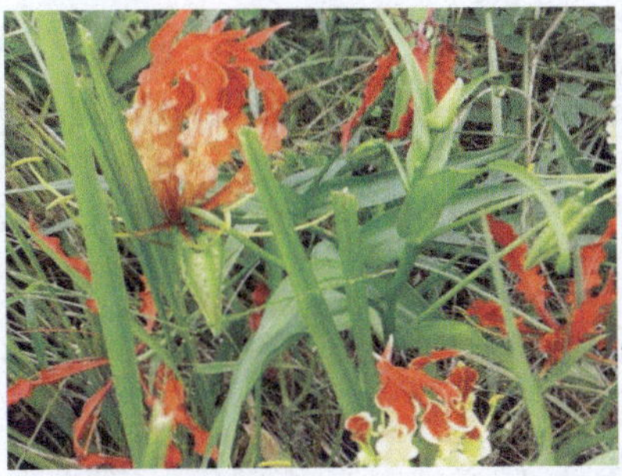

Scientific Name: *Gloriosa superba*

Common Name: Glory Lily, Langali

Distribution: Found in Odisha, Tamil Nadu, Kerala, and West Bengal, in wild forested areas.

Part Used: Tubers and seeds

Bioactive Principles: Colchicine, alkaloids, and flavonoids

Remark: *Gloriosa superba* has been used in traditional remedies for its anti-inflammatory and analgesic properties. It helps alleviate arthritis symptoms, but its use requires caution due to its toxicity.

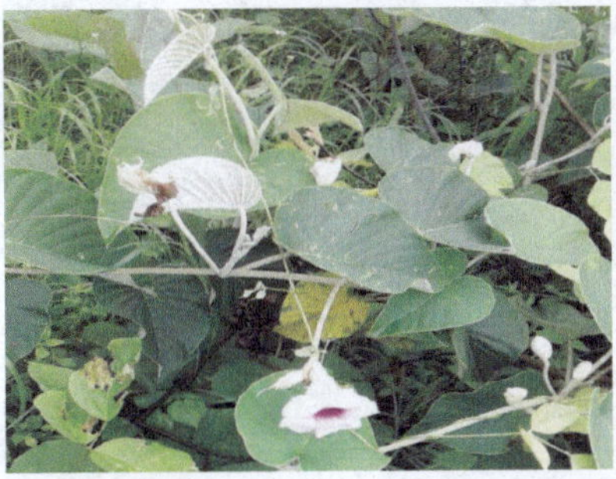

Scientific Name: *Argyreia nervosa*

Common Name: Hawaiian Baby Woodrose

Distribution: Found in Odisha, West Bengal, and southern India, in forested and semi-arid regions.

Part Used: Roots and seeds

Bioactive Principles: Lysergic acid derivatives, alkaloids, and flavonoids

Remark: Traditionally used for its anti-inflammatory properties, it helps in managing joint pain and stiffness associated with arthritis.

Conclusion

Medicinal plants offer promising alternatives to conventional pharmacological treatments for arthritis in livestock. The anti-inflammatory, analgesic, and antioxidative properties of the above herbs have provided effective management options for arthritis. For animals with arthritis, adding these herbs to their diet or applying them topically can help lessen pain, increase movement, and improve their general quality of life. However, proper veterinary guidance is essential for ensuring safe and effective use, particularly regarding dosage and potential interactions with other treatments.

References

Duan SJ, Zhang L, Li HY. Effects of Curcumin on Proinflammatory Cytokines in Dairy Cattle with Arthritis. J Vet Sci. 2017;18(3):333-339.

Gibson S, Brown J, Richardson J. Efficacy of Willow Bark (Salix alba) in Reducing Pain and Swelling in Swine with Arthritis. Anim Health Stud. 2015;25(4):95-101.

Jagetia GC, D'Souza S, Rao SG. Efficacy of Boswellia serrata Extract in the Treatment of Arthritis in Horses. Vet Res J. 2019;32(2):56-62.

Khanna D, Manjunatha K, Bhaskar D. Ginger (Zingiber officinale) in the Treatment of Arthritis in Goats. J Anim Physiol. 2019;28(3):123-128.

Thyagarajan M, Pandey M, Ghosh A. Clinical Study on the Effectiveness of Arnica in Managing Joint Inflammation in Horses. Altern Vet Med. 2018;12(1):45-49.

Van der Merwe D. The Use of Harpagophytum procumbens (Devil's Claw) in Cattle with Osteoarthritis. Vet J Tradit Med. 2016;20(1):75-80.

5

Medicinal Plants Effective Against Bacterial Diseases in Animals

Priyadarshini Sahoo[1*] and Sonali Sahoo[2]

[1]Department of Veterinary Epidemiology and Preventive Medicine, College of Veterinary Science and Animal Husbandry, Odisha University of Agriculture and Technology, Bhubaneswar, Odisha

[2]Department of Veterinary Medicine, Institute of Veterinary Science and Animal Husbandry, Siksha 'O' Anusandhan Deemed to be University Bhubaneswar, Odisha

The therapeutic potential of plants and its parts has been explored since ancient times and has been used for the well being of humans as well as animals. In the era of emergence of multi drug resistant bacteria modern research aims to find out alternative therapeutic approaches preferably from herbal source to combat the infection. Medicinal plants owing to their antibacterial, antioxidant, anti inflammatory capabilities have been used against many bacterial infections in livestock and companion animals. Ethnoveterinary practices have been documented against bacterial diseases in animals like mastitis, colibacillosis, Salmonellosis, pyoderma, otitis externa, gastrointestinal infection, pneumonia and many others, some of which are enlisted below.

Bovine mastitis, predominantly a bacterial disease continues to threaten the dairy sector as it inflicts great economic losses to the dairy farmers. The disease caused by more than 200 species of bacteria is characterized by inflammation of the mammary gland with physical and chemical changes in the milk and pathological changes in the glandular tissue. There is a significant reduction in the milk yield and many times it's accompanied with abnormalities in the udder, milk and the cow. In addition to this, milk from affected animals may harbor the organisms which are potentially pathogenic to humans. Use of antibiotics is a common practice to cure mastitis. However, their use is not free from hazards due to unwanted antibiotic residues in milk as well as development of variable degree of antibiotic resistance. Traditional healers use a number of plants for the treatment of bovine mastitis. Essential oils (EO) of *Thymus vulgaris* and *Lavandula angustifolia* exhibit strong antibacterial activity against the predominant mastitogens i.e. *Staphylococcus* sp. and *Streptococcus* sp. Herbs like *Berberis lycium*, *Curcuma longa, Eucalyptus globulus, Azadirachta indica* has been used as post milking teat dips to reduce the new intramammary infections in dairy cows. Topical application of a water based preparation composed of aloe vera (250 mg), turmeric powder (50 mg) and calcium hydroxide or lime (15 mg) ten times a day followed by application of the same ingredients mixed with mustard oil (200 ml) three times a day on the udder for five days along with feeding two lemons thrice daily for three days has a curative effect in bovine mastitis.

Avian colibacillosis, an economically devastating disease of poultry, caused by *Escherichia coli* is a principal cause of morbidity and mortality. The organism is also a potential pathogen in animals and human beings. The infection in birds results in a variety of syndromes including acute fatal septicemia, pericarditis, perihepatitis, air sacculitis, peritonitis. Treatment of colibacillosis with antimicrobials is problematic due to widespread multidrug resistance among Avian pathogenic *E. coli* (APEC) isolates and also restrictions on their use in poultry imposed by regulation and public health concern. So, use of plant derived drugs will be helpful in this aspect. Cinnamon (*Cinnamomum zeylanicum*) and clove (*Syzygium aromaticum*) essential oils possessing antibacterial activity, when used alone or in combination, are effective against *E. coli* strains isolated from poultry with colibacillosis. Antibacterial effects of *Cymbopogon citratus, Ocimum basilicum* and *Mentha piperita* EO against *E. coli* has also been demonstrated through *in vitro* studies.

Pyoderma, a common dermatological problem encountered frequently in dogs refers to bacterial infections of the skin and results in accumulation of neutrophilic exudates. The infection is limited to the epidermis and hair follicles (superficial pyoderma) or may involve the dermis (deep pyoderma). The primary pathogen of dogs is *Staphylococcus pseudintermedius*, although many other species of bacteria may also be associated with pyoderma. Many a times it is triggered by an overgrowth or overcolonization of normal resident flora of the skin. A variety of clinical signs and lesions i.e. alopecia, pruritus, erythematous papules, pustules, crusts, scales, exudation of pus may be exhibited by the affected dogs. The treatment of pyoderma has become more challenging with the spread on methicillin-resistant and multidrug-resistant *Staphylococcus* (MDRS).Topical preparations containing *Cedrus deodara, Pongamia glabra, Azadirachta indica* extract, *Eucalyptus globulus* and *Acorus calamus* are helpful in alleviating the clinical signs of pyoderma due to their antibacterial and anti-inflammatory properties. Bactericidal effects of Chamomile (*Matricaria chamomilla*) against *Proteus mirabilis, Proteus vulgaris, S. aureus, S. epidermidis* and other Staphylococci renders it as an alternative approach for treatment of pyoderma in dogs.

Otitis externa is a frequently presented problem in dogs and cats. It is the inflammation of the ear canal and also sometimes involving the ear pinna. It is predominantly caused by bacteria like *Staphylococcus, Streptococcus, Enterococcus, Pseudomonas, Proteus*, etc. The animal exhibits varying degrees of head shaking, pruritus, pain, erythema, malodor, swelling and purulent or waxy discharges from the affected ear canals. Successful treatment depends on use of topical antibiotics based on the culture and sensitivity reports. Despite advances in therapeutic approaches, dogs refractory to treatment cannot be ruled out due to the complexity of etiology and emergence of resistance to antibiotics. Phytotherapy thus proves beneficial in this context. Essential oils from cinnamon (cinnamaldehyde), clove (*Syzygium aromaticum*) and oregano (*Origanum vulgare*) show *in vitro* efficacy against bacterial isolates recovered from dogs with otitis externa. The antibacterial properties of the essential oils of *Lavandula angustifolia, Melaleuca alternifolia* help in resolution of clinical signs in dogs suffering from otitis externa.

Medicinal plants used in bacterial infections

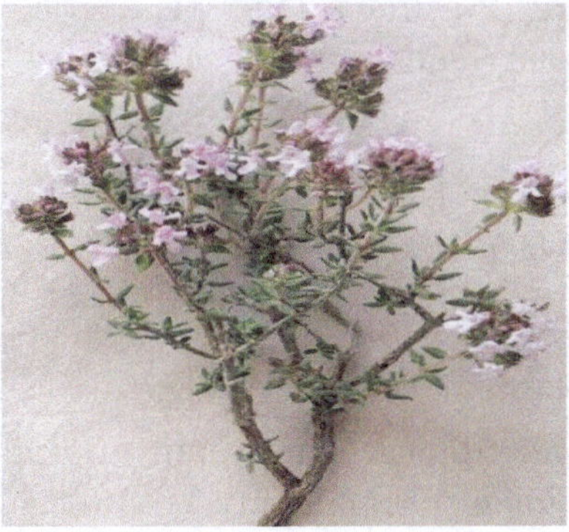

Scientific Name: *Thymus vulgaris*

Common Name: Thyme

Distribution: Southern Europe Mediterranean and neighboring countries Northern Africa, and parts of Asia

Plant part used: Essential oil

Active principle: Thymol, p-cymene

Remarks: Mastitis

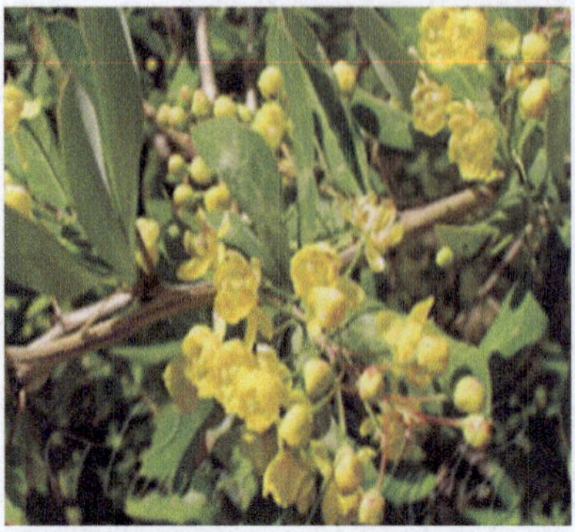

Scientific Name: *Berberis lyceum*

Common Name: Indian barberry

Distribution: Himachal Pradesh, Jammu & Kashmir, Madhya Pradesh, Tamil Nadu, Uttar Pradesh, Uttarakhand

Plant part used: Root-bark extract

Active principle: Berberine

Remarks: Mastitis

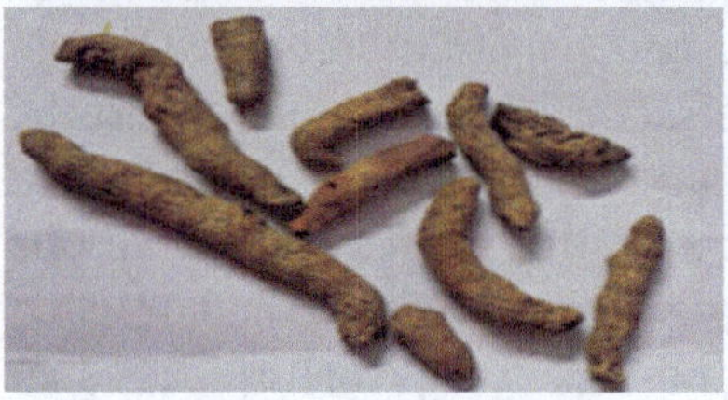

Scientific Name: *Curcuma longa*

Common Name: Turmeric

Distribution: India, China, Indonesia, tropical and sub tropical regions of South and South-east Asia

Plant part used: Rhizome

Active principle: Curcumin

Remarks: Mastitis

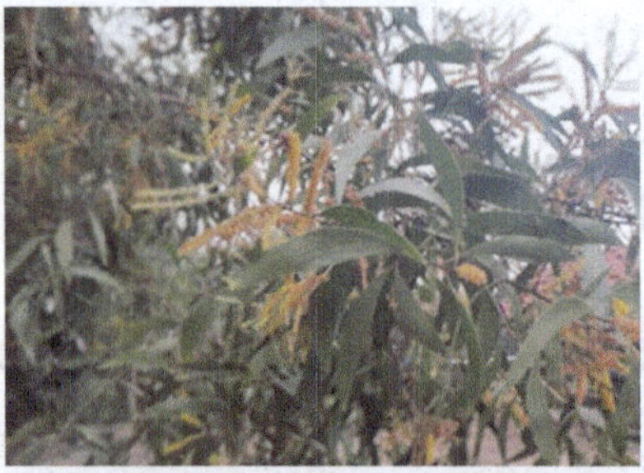

Scientific Name: *Eucalyptus globulus*

Common Name: Southern blue gum

Distribution: Australia, Europe, Africa, western United States

Plant part used: Leaf extract, essential oil

Active principle: Eucalyptol (1,8-cineole)

Remarks: Mastitis, pyoderma

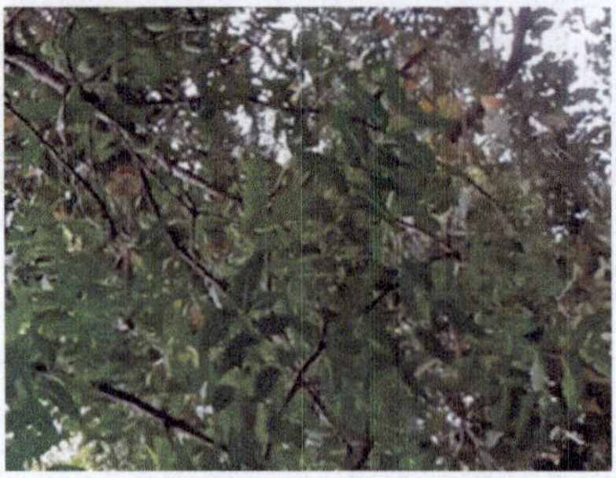

Scientific Name: *Azadirachta indica*

Common Name: Neem

Distribution: tropical and semi tropical regions of Indian subcontinent

Plant part used: Leaf extract

Active principle: Azadirachtin

Remarks: Mastitis

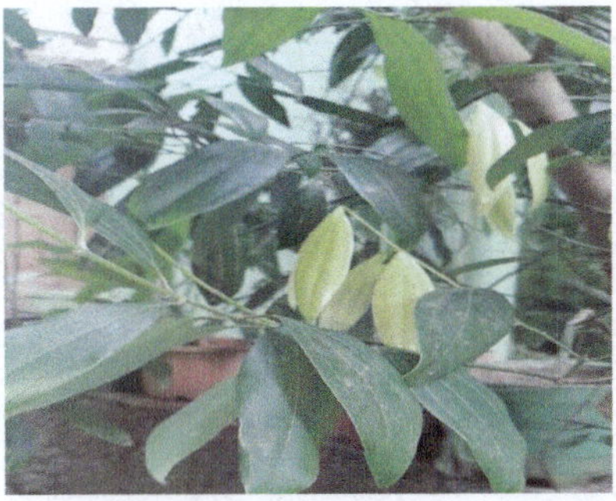

Scientific Name: *Cinnamomum zeylanicumi*
Common Name: Cinnamon
Distribution: India (Kerala, Tamil Nadu), Sri Lanka , Myanmmar
Plant part used: Essential oil
Active principle: Eugenol, trans-cinnamaldehyde
Remarks: Colibacillosis, Otitis externa

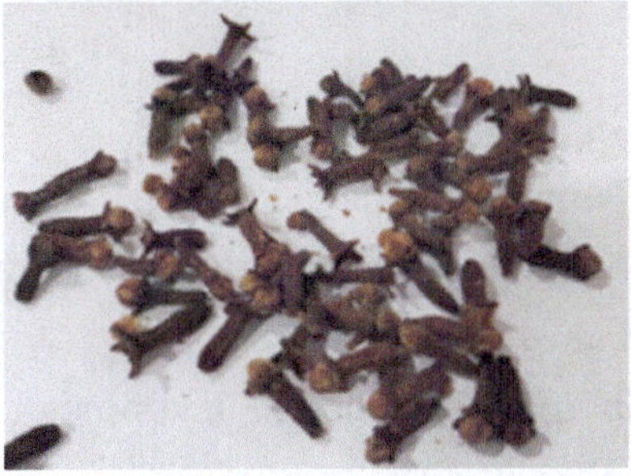

Scientific Name: *Syzygium aromaticum*
Common Name: Clove
Distribution: Indonesia, India, Sri Lanka, Madagascar and Tanzania
Plant part used: Essential oil
Active principle: Eugenol
Remarks: Colibacillosis, Otitis externa

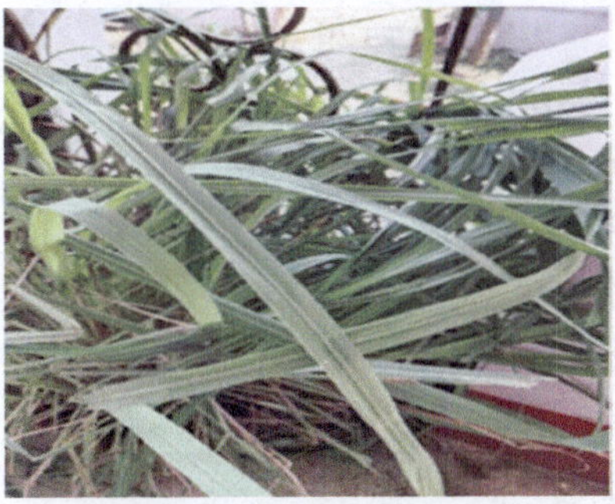

Scientific Name: *Cymbopogon citratus*
Common Name: Lemon grass
Distribution: India and Sri Lanka
Plant part used: Essential oil
Active principle: Citral, geranial, neral
Remarks: Colibacillosis

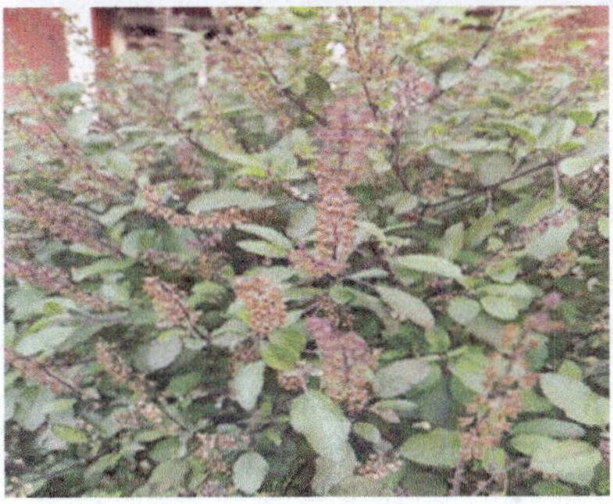

Scientific Name: *Ocimum basilicum*
Common Name: Basil
Distribution: Assam, Meghalaya, Odisha
Plant part used: Essential oil
Active principle: Linalool
Remarks: Colibacillosis

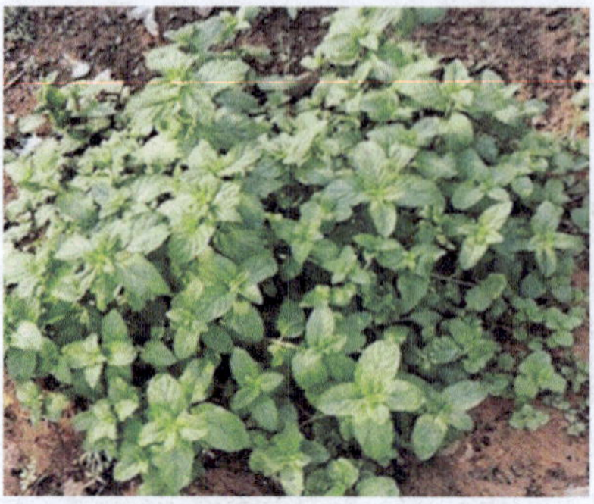

Scientific Name: *Mentha piperita*

Common Name: Peppermint

Distribution: Asia, Europe, North America, Australia

Plant part used: Essential oil

Active principle: Menthol, menthone

Remarks: Colibacillosis

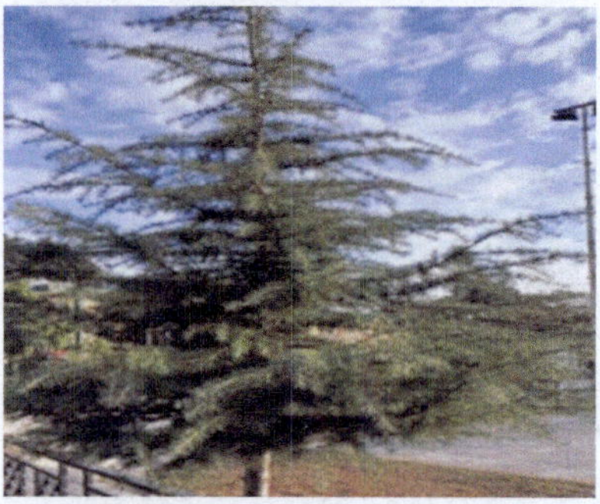

Scientific Name: *Cedrus deodara*

Common Name: Himalayan cedar

Distribution: India, Nepal, China, Pakistan

Plant part used: Plant extract

Active principle: Terpenoids, flavonoids

Remarks: Pyoderma

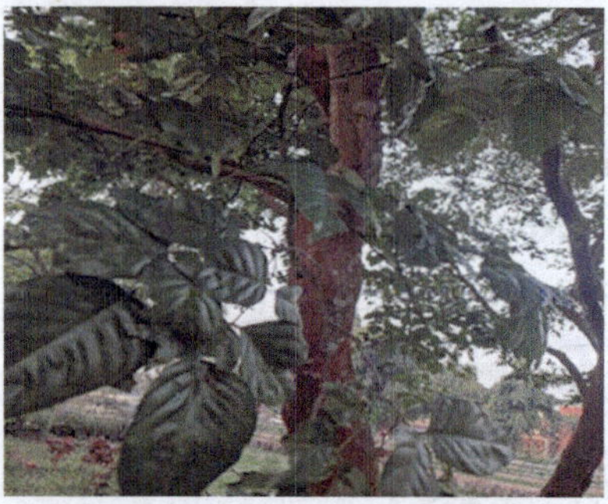

Scientific Name: *Pongamia glabra*

Common Name: Karanja

Distibution: Southeastern Asia, Sri Lanka, Burma, Malaya, Australia

Plant part used: Plant extract

Active principle: Karanjin

Remarks: Pyoderma

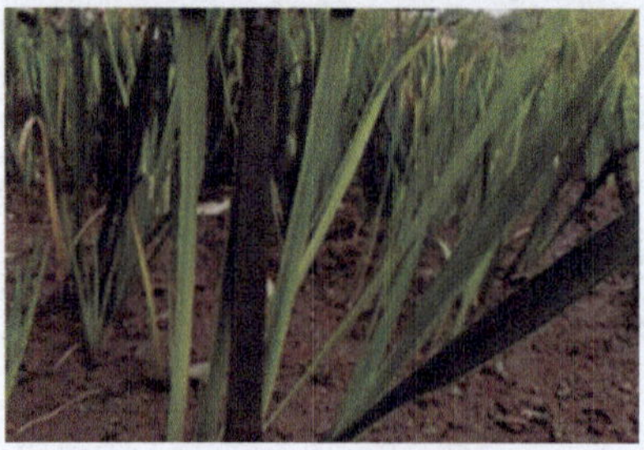

Scientific Name: *Acorus calamus*

Common Name: Sweet flag

Distribution: India (Kashmir, Manipur, Sikkim), Ceylon

Plant part used: Essential oil, plant extract

Active principle: Asarone

Remarks: Pyoderma

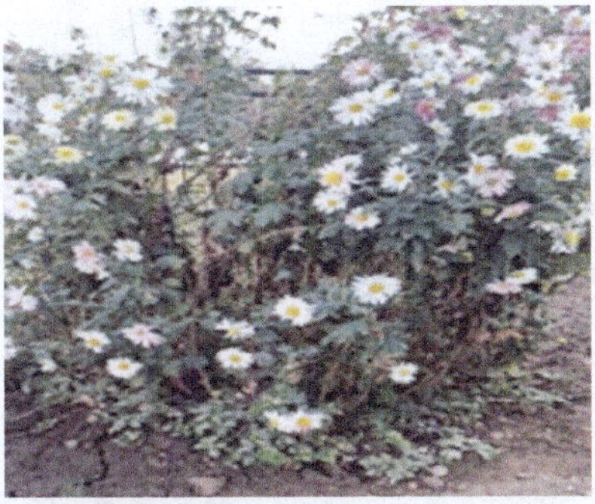

Scientific Name: *Matricaria chamomilla*

Common Name: Chamomile

Distribution: Southern and eastern Europe and northern and western Asia

Plant part used: Plant extract, essential oil

Active principle: Coumarins, flavonoids

Remarks: Pyoderma

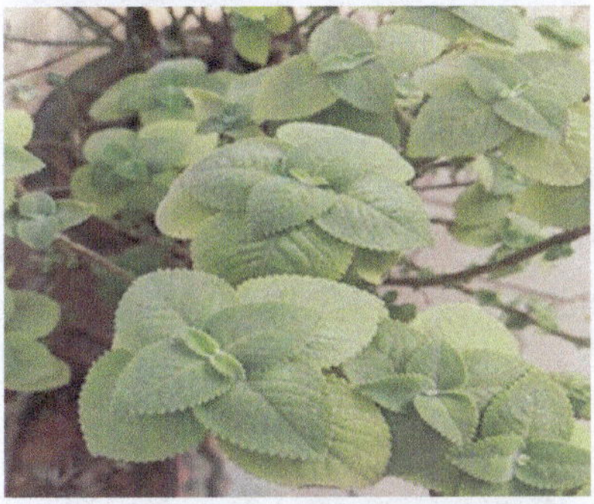

Scientific Name: *Origanum vulgare*

Common Name: Oregano

Distribution: Mediterranean region

Plant part used: Essential oil

Active principle: Carvacol, thymol, p-cymene

Remarks: Otitis externa

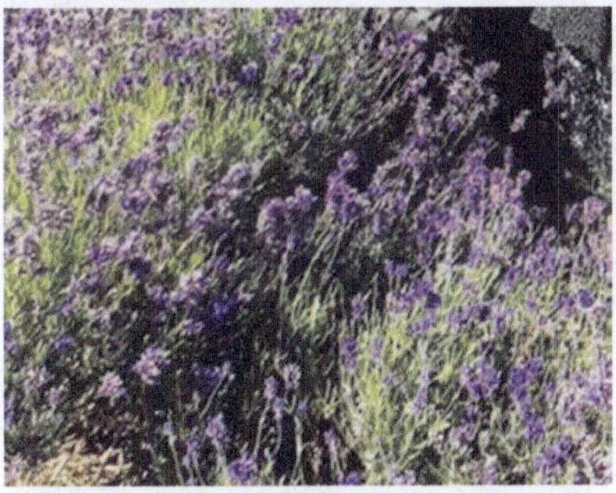

Scientific Name: *Lavandula angustifolia*

Common Name: Lavender

Distribution: Spain, France, Italy, Croatia

Plant part used: Essential oil

Active principle: Linalool, linalyl acetate

Remarks: Mastitis, Otitis externa

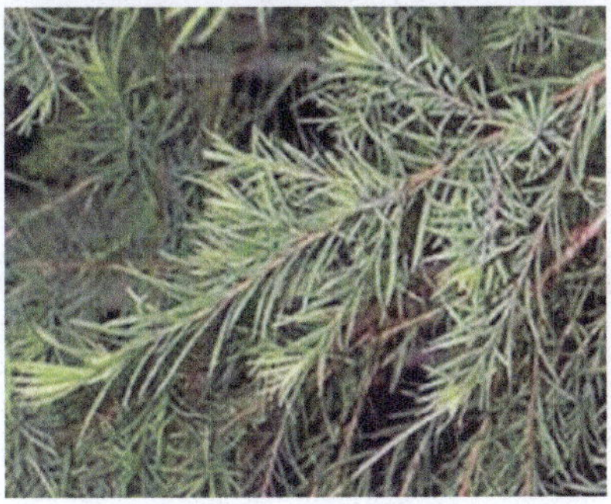

Scientific Name: *Melaleuca alternifolia*

Common Name: Tea tree

Distribution: Australia, India (Karnataka)

Plant part used: Essential oil

Active principle: Terpinen-4-ol, 1,8-cineole

Remarks: Otitis externa

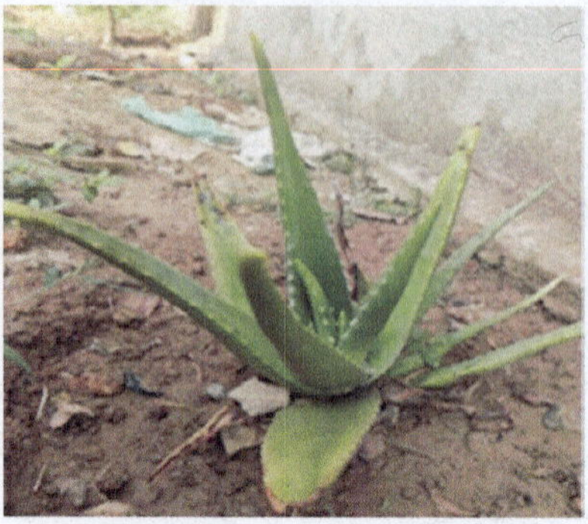

Scientific Name: *Aloe vera*

Distribution: Africa, Asia, Europe, America

Plant part used: stem after removing thorns, plant extract

Active principle: Emodin

Remarks: Mastitis

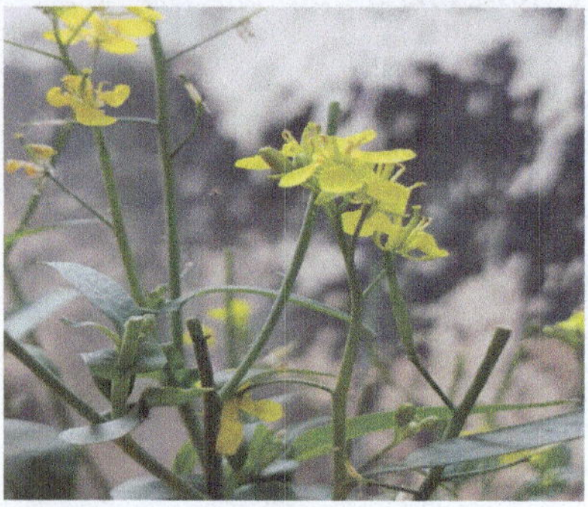

Scientific Name: *Brassica nigra* (Black Mustard)

Distribution: Europe, Africa, Asia

Plant part used: Seeds, oil

Active principle: Allyl isothiocyanate

Remarks: Mastitis

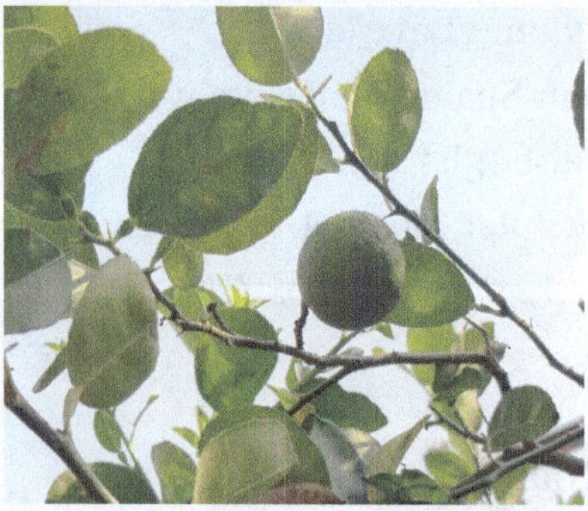

Scientific Name: *Citrus limon*

Distribution: South east Asia, China

Plant part used: Fruits, fruit peels

Active principle: limonene, citric acid, vitamin C

Remarks: Mastitis

References

Ebani, V. V. and Mancianti, F. 2020. Use of Essential Oils in Veterinary Medicine to Combat Bacterial and Fungal Infections. Vet. Sci. 7, 193; doi:10.3390/vetsci7040193

https://www.nddb.coop/farmer/health/evm

Kim, Sang-Hun , Kim, Suk , Jun, Hyung-Kyou and Kim, Duck-Hwan. 2009. Efficacy of aromatherapy for the treatment of otitis externa in dogs. Korean Journal of Veterinary Research. 49(1): 85-89.

Li, X., Xu, C., Liang, B., Kastelic, J.P., Han, B., Tong, X. and Gao, J. 2023. Alternatives to antibiotics for treatment of mastitis in dairy cows. Front. Vet. Sci. 10:1160350. doi: 10.3389/fvets.2023.1160350

Ramprabhu, R., Jairam, Karthik, A., Ravikanth, K., Maini, S. and Adarsh. 2014. Evaluation of regular teat sanitization control measures for prevention of subclinical mastitis in cattle. American Journal of Phytomedicine and Clinical Therapeutics, 2(10): 1212-1216.

Saritha, G., Haritha, G. S. and Nalini Kumari, K. 2023. Application of Ayurvedic Medicine as an Alternative in Certain Skin Disorders in Dogs. Int.J.Curr.Microbiol.App.Sci 12(01): 283-289.

Sim, J.X.F., Khazandi, M., Pi, H., Venter, H., Trott, D.J. and Deo, P. 2019. Antimicrobial effects of cinnamon essential oil and cinnamaldehyde combined with EDTA against canine otitis externa pathogens. Journal of Applied Microbiology. 127(1): 99–108

Tresch, M., Mevissen, M., Ayrle, H., Melzig, M., Roosje, P. and Walkenhorst, M. 2019. Medicinal plants as therapeutic options for topical treatment in canine dermatology? A systematic review. BMC Vet Res. 15(1):174.

Vercelli, C., Pasquetti, M., Giovannetti, G., Visioni, S., Re, G., Giorgi, M., Gambino, G. and Peano, A. 2021. In vitro and in vivo evaluation of a new phytotherapic blend to treat acute externa otitis in dogs. J Vet Pharmacol Ther. 44(6):910-918.

6

Medicinal Plants Effective Against Viral Diseases in Animals

P. Mekala

Professor and Head, Department of Veterinary Pharmacology and Toxicology
Veterinary College and Research Institute, Udumalpet – 642 205
Tamil Nadu Veterinary and Animal Sciences University

Viral Diseases in Domestic Animals

Viral diseases significantly impact the health and productivity of domestic animals, including livestock and companion animals, leading to substantial economic and emotional costs. In livestock, diseases like *Foot-and-Mouth Disease (FMD)* and *Peste des Petits Ruminants (PPR)* cause severe production losses in terms of milk, meat, and wool. Similarly, in poultry, *Newcastle disease* and *Avian Influenza* outbreaks result in high mortality and disruptions to egg production. Among companion animals, viruses such as *Canine Distemper* and *Feline Leukemia Virus (FeLV)* lead to serious morbidity and reduced quality of life. Current control measures rely heavily on vaccination and biosecurity practices, but the lack of effective antiviral treatments, coupled with the emergence of drug-resistant strains, underscores the need for novel therapeutic approaches. Medicinal plants with antiviral properties have garnered significant interest as sustainable and holistic solutions. Plant-derived bioactive compounds offer a dual advantage of modulating immune responses and directly targeting viral pathogens, making them a promising area of research for the management of viral diseases in both livestock and pet animals.

Treatment Modalities for Viral Diseases

The treatment of viral diseases primarily relies on antiviral drugs, immunotherapies, vaccines, and supportive care. Direct-acting antivirals target specific viral components, while broad-spectrum agents like remdesivir address multiple viruses. Immunotherapies, including monoclonal antibodies and interferons, enhance the host's antiviral response. Vaccination remains the most effective preventive tool, with technologies ranging from traditional inactivated vaccines to advanced mRNA platforms. Supportive therapies, such as fluid management or oxygen therapy, are crucial for diseases lacking specific treatments. However, significant gaps persist, including the limited availability of broad-spectrum antivirals, resistance development, inadequate vaccine coverage, high treatment costs, and emerging pathogens. Bridging these gaps requires innovation, equitable access, and exploration of alternative therapies like medicinal plants.

Herbal Treatment in Viral Diseases

Herbal treatments have been a cornerstone of traditional medicine for centuries, offering relief and protection against viral infections, particularly in times when modern treatment options were unavailable. Plants like turmeric, neem, garlic, and onion have long been utilized for their antiviral properties. Turmeric, with its active compound curcumin, has been shown in scientific studies to possess anti-inflammatory and antiviral effects, particularly against respiratory viruses like influenza and coronaviruses. Neem contains azadirachtin, which has demonstrated the ability to inhibit viral replication and boost immune responses, especially in the case of hepatitis B and dengue. Garlic, rich in allicin, exhibits broad-spectrum antiviral activity, with research supporting its effectiveness against herpes simplex, influenza, and other viral infections. Similarly, onion has compounds like quercetin that support immune function and have antiviral properties. Studies on *Andrographis paniculata* and *Phyllanthus niruri* have revealed their potential in reducing viral load in conditions like the common cold and hepatitis B. The growing body of scientific evidence validates these time-tested herbal remedies, showcasing their ability to alleviate symptoms and provide a natural defense against viral infections. While modern pharmaceutical therapies continue to evolve, these herbal treatments remain valuable, particularly in regions with limited access to conventional medicines. Furthermore, combinations of these plant-based remedies have proven effective in controlling viral diseases in livestock and poultry, further emphasizing their potential as holistic approaches in veterinary care.

The traditional system of animal healthcare has long been based on indigenous knowledge and practices, passed down through generations. These methods utilized locally available materials and natural resources to treat various ailments in livestock and poultry. Over time, this approach has evolved into what is now known as ethnoveterinary medicine.

Many of these traditional practices have undergone scientific evaluation, resulting in the development of formulations designed to address common viral diseases in animals. These formulations have been tested and proven effective under field conditions, offering practical solutions for the farming community. This chapter aims to highlight such formulations, with the intention of supporting the agricultural sector in enhancing animal health care using time-honored, yet scientifically validated methods.

Proven Ethno Veterinary Formulations for Viral Diseases of Livestock and Poultry

a) Foot and Mouth Disease

Etiology: Aphthovirus of Picornaviridae family

Symptoms: Pyrexia, anorexia, profuse salivation, blisters on the nose, tongue, lips, mouth, between the toes and around hooves.

General treatment: No specific treatment, only Symptomatic

Ethnoveterinary Formulation for oral administration:

Cumin : 10g

Pepper : 10g

Fenugreek : 10g

Turmeric :10g

Garlic : 4 cloves

Coconut : 1 number (make into Grated)

Jaggery : 100g

Grind all the ingredients, mix with grated coconut and jaggery and administer orally three times daily for three to five days

External application / Wound dressing

Clean the wound with lukewarm water containing turmeric or with 1% potassium permanganate solution and apply the following oil and cover with a bandage

Gingelly oil/ Coconut oil : 1 litre

Garlic clove : 10 Nos.

Turmeric : 10g

Grind the following leaves

Acalypha indica : 1 handful

Lawsonia inermis: 1 handful

Ocimum sanctum: 1 handful

Azadirachta indica: 1 handful

Heat gingelly oil / coconut oil, add garlic cloves, turmeric and add the ground leaves, boil and cool down.

Apply the above oil two times daily externally on the hoof and apply a bandage.

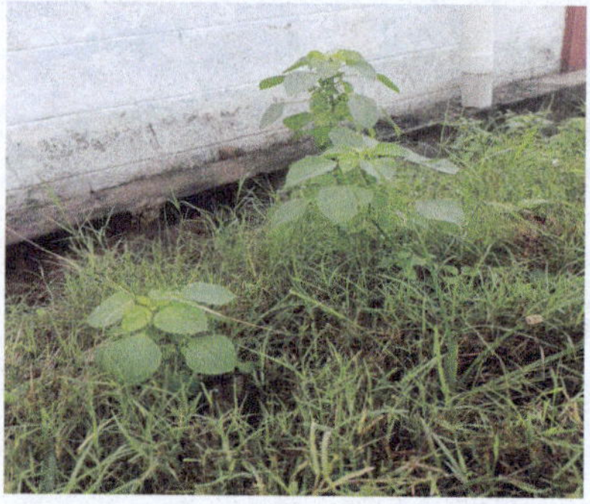

Scientific Name: *Acalypha indica*

Common Name: Indian Copperleaf, Cat's Tail, Chili Plant.

Distribution: Native to tropical and subtropical regions of Asia, widely distributed in Africa and America.

Parts Used: Leaves, roots, stems, seeds, and flowers.

Active Principle: Triterpenoids, flavonoids, alkaloids, phenolic compounds, saponins.

Remarks: Used in traditional medicine in treatment of inflammation, skin diseases, digestive disorders, and as an antimicrobial and antidiabetic agent.

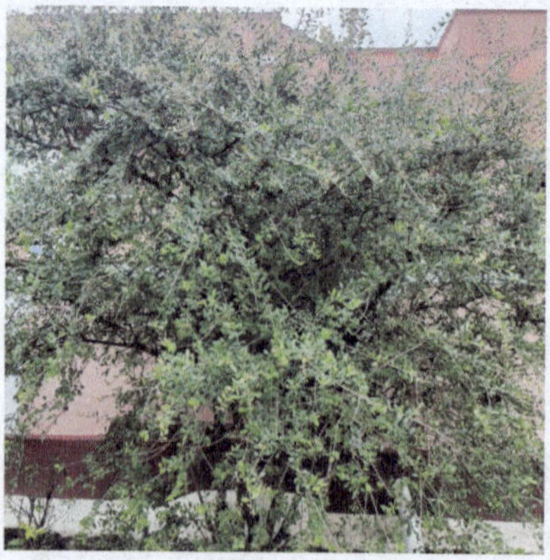

Scientific Name: *Lawsonia inermis*

Common Name: Henna, Mehndi.

Distribution: Native to North Africa, South Asia, and the Middle East, widely cultivated in tropical and subtropical regions.

Parts Used: Leaves, flowers, seeds, and stems.

Active Principle: Lawson (lawsone), flavonoids, tannins, glycosides.

Remarks: Antimicrobial, anti-inflammatory, and antioxidant properties, used in traditional medicine for wound healing and skin disorders.

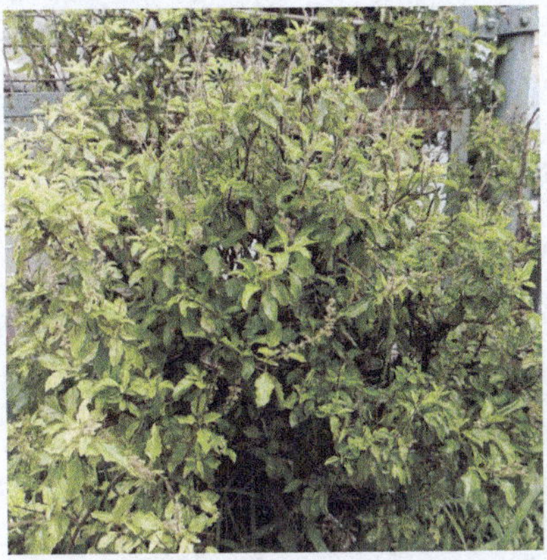

Scientific Name: *Ocimum sanctum*

Common Name: Tulsi, Holy Basil.

Distribution: Native to India, widely cultivated in subtropical and tropical areas of Asia and beyond.

Parts Used: Leaves, seeds, stems, and roots.

Active Principle: Eugenol, ursolic acid, rosmarinic acid, flavonoids, phenolic compounds.

Remarks: Revered in Ayurveda for its adaptogenic, anti-inflammatory, antioxidant, and antimicrobial properties, used to support immunity, relieve stress, and treat respiratory and digestive ailments.

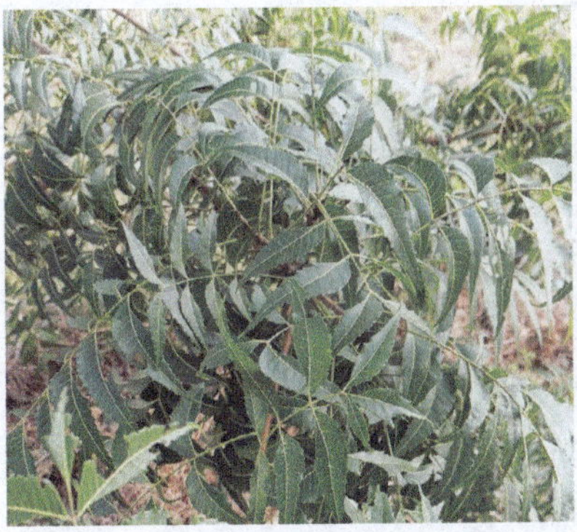

Scientific Name: *Azadirachta indica*

Common Name: Neem, Indian Lilac.

Distribution: Native to Southeast Asia and the Indian subcontinent, widely cultivated in subtropical and tropical regions globally.

Parts Used: Leaves, bark, seeds, flowers, fruit, and roots.

Active Principle: Azadirachtin, nimbin, nimbidin, salannin, quercetin.

Remarks: Known for its antimicrobial, anti-inflammatory, antifungal, and antiviral properties, used in traditional medicine for treating skin conditions, dental health, fever, and as a pesticide.

b) Peste des Petits Ruminants in Goat

Etiology: Morbilivirus family Paramixoviridae

Symptoms: Fever, sores in the mouth, discharges from the eyes and nose, foul-smelling diarrhoea disturbed breathing and cough, and death.

General treatment: No specific treatment, only Symptomatic

Ethnoveterinary Formulation for Oral Administration

Cumin seeds : 15g

Fenugreek : 15 g

Turmeric : 5g

Pepper : 5g

Garlic : 5 nos.

Cissus quadrangularis: 5 nodes

Moringa oleifera: 50 g

Jaggery : 500g

Grind the above ingredients, mix with jaggery and administer orally three times a day

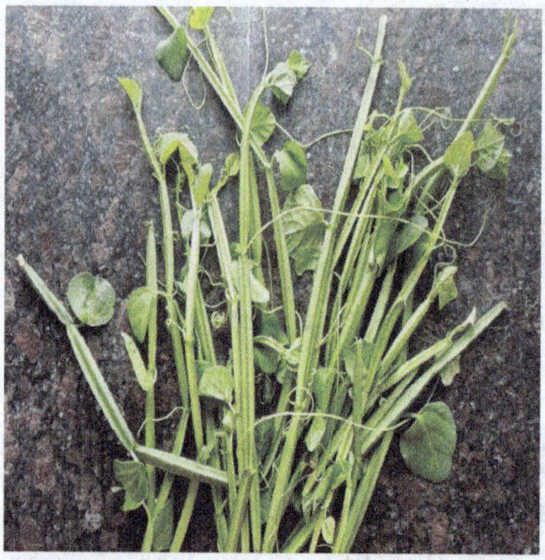

Scientific name: *Cissus quadrangularis*

Common name: Veldt Grape, Bone Setter, Devil's Backbone

Distribution: Subtropical and tropical regions of Asia and Africa, including India, Sri Lanka, Pakistan, some parts of Southeast Asia.

Parts used: Stem

Active principle: Polyphenols, Quercetin, Kaempferol, Oleanolic acid

Remarks: Healing of fracture and bone injuries by increasing collagen production, appetite stimulant, healing of ulcer, improves gut health and protects liver

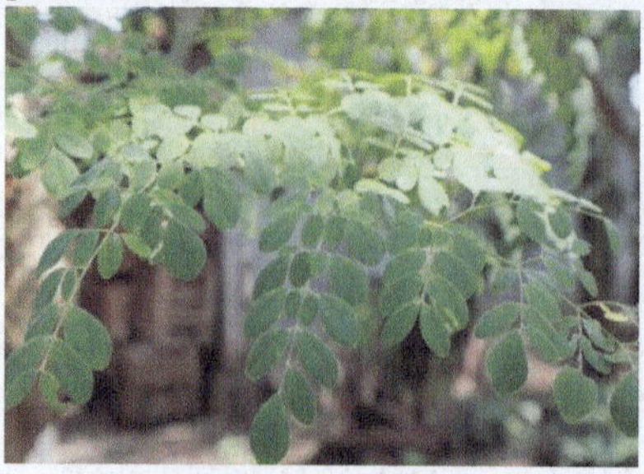

Scientific name: *Moringa oleifera*

Common Name: Miracle tree, Drumstick tree, Moringa.

Distribution: Native to Northwestern India, widely cultivated in subtropical and tropical areas.

Parts Used: Leaves, seeds, pods, roots, bark, and flowers.

Active Principle: Moringin, Flavonoids, Vitamins (C, A), Minerals (Calcium, Potassium), Alkaloids.

Remarks: Known for its nutritional value, antioxidant, anti-inflammatory, and antimicrobial properties, and widely used as a supplement for general health and in traditional medicine.

c) Ranikhet Disease in Poultry

Etiology: Avian Paramyxo virus type 1

Symptoms: Drooping wings, circling, coughing and gasping, twisting of the head and neck, depression, dragging legs, inappetence

General treatment: No specific treatment, only Symptomatic

Ethnoveterinary Formulation for 10 birds

Cumin seeds	: 10 g
Pepper	: 5 g
Turmeric	: 5g
Small Onion	: 5 nos.
Garlic cloves	: 5 nos.
Phyllanthus amarus	: 50 gram

Grind all the ingredients and mix with rice and feed if the birds are taking feed. If not make into small balls and administer orally for 5 days. Birds shall be given water mixed with jaggery or water boiled with cumin seeds.

Apart from this few more formulations are being evolved based on the clinical result for the betterment of the farming community.

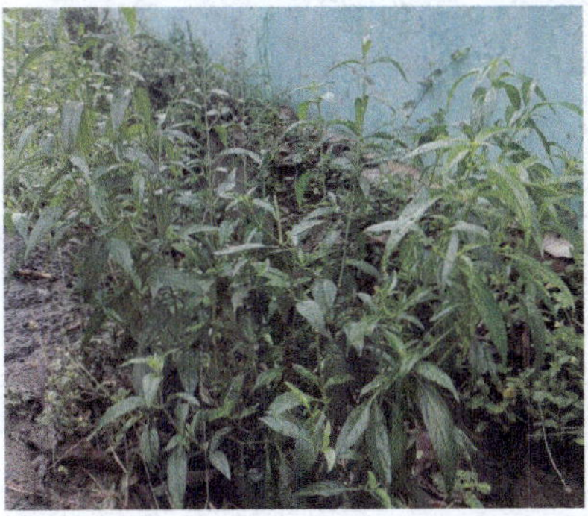

Medicinal Plants and Spices Possessing Antiviral Activity

Scientific name: *Andrographis paniculata*

Common name: Andrographis, King of Bitters

Distribution: Native to Southeast Asia and India

Parts used: Whole plant

Active principle: Andrographolide

Remarks: Effective against common cold (rhinovirus), influenza virus, **dengue virus**; boosts immunity and has antiviral properties

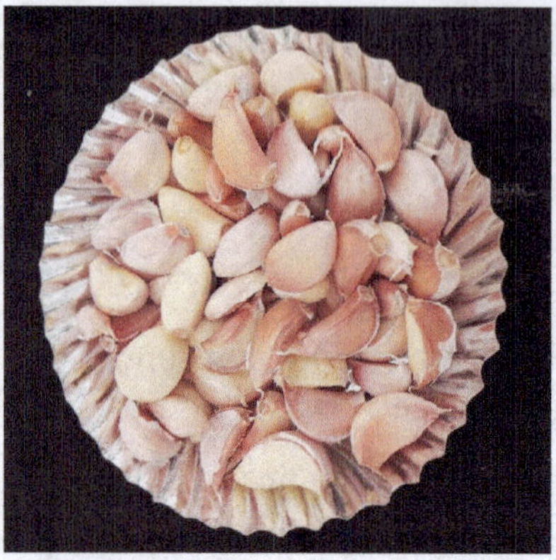

Scientific name: *Allium sativum*

Common name: Garlic

Distribution: Native to Central Asia, cultivated worldwide.

Parts used: Bulb.

Active principle: Allicin, ajoene.

Remarks: Effective against influenza virus, common cold viruses, and herpes simplex virus (HSV); allicin, helps inhibit viral replication and strengthens the body's immune response.

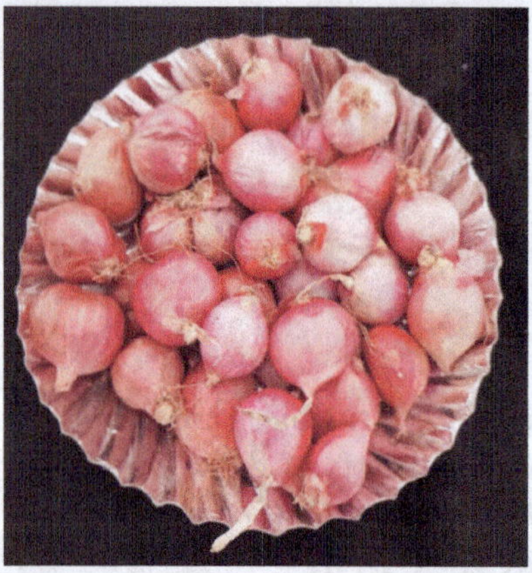

Scientific name: ***Allium cepa***

Common name: Onion

Distribution: Native to Central Asia, widely cultivated worldwide.

Parts used: Bulb.

Active principle: Quercetin, Sulfur compounds (allyl propyl disulfide).

Remarks: Effective against influenza virus, common cold viruses, and respiratory viruses; quercetin and sulfur compounds help boost the immune system and fight viral infections

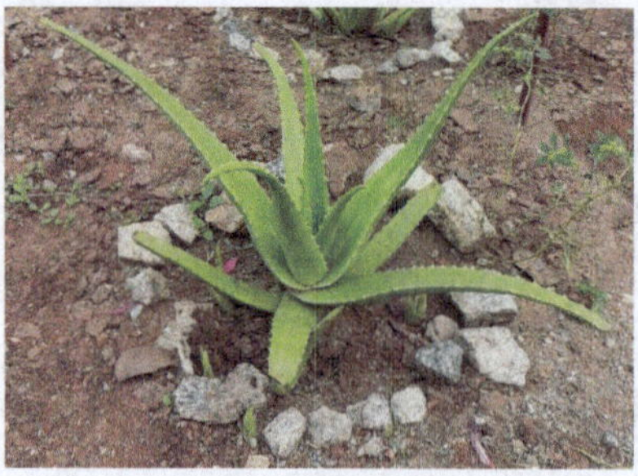

Scientific name: ***Aloe vera***

Common name: Aloe

Distribution: Native to Arabian Peninsula, now widely cultivated in tropical and subtropical regions.

Parts used: Leaves (gel and latex).

Active principle: Acemannan, Aloins, Anthraquinones.

Remarks: Aloe vera has antiviral properties, especially against herpes simplex virus (HSV) and HIV, and is also used for skin infections

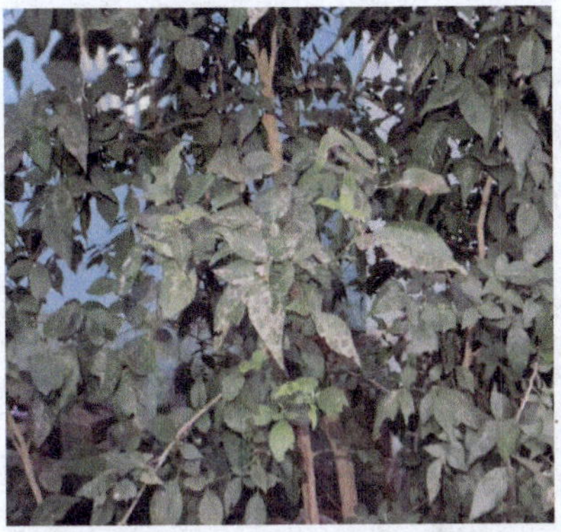

Scientific name: *Aegle marmelos*

Common name: Bael

Distribution: Native to India and Southeast Asia.

Parts used: Fruit, leaves, bark.

Active principle: Marmelosin, coumarins, alkaloids.

Remarks: Effective against influenza virus, hepatitis virus, and herpes simplex virus (HSV); especially in the treatment of gastrointestinal viral infections and respiratory conditions.

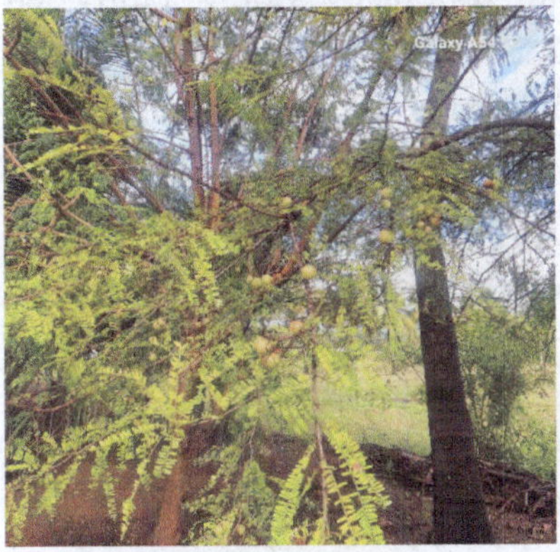

Scientific name: *Phyllanthus emblica*

Common name: Indian Gooseberry

Distribution: Native to India, widely distributed in Asia.

Parts used: Fruit, leaves.

Active principle: Vitamin C, flavonoids, tannins.

Remarks: Effective against HSV, influenza virus; boosts immunity and acts as an antioxidant.

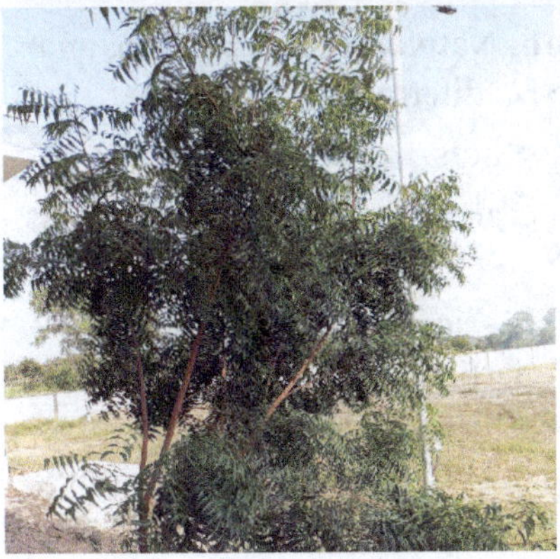

Scientific name: *Azadirachta indica*

Common name: Neem

Distribution: Native to India, widely found in tropical regions.

Parts used: Leaves, bark, seeds, flowers.

Active principle: Azadirachtin, nimbin, nimbidin.

Remarks: Potent antiviral, antibacterial, and antifungal properties, effective against various viral infections, including herpes and chickenpox.

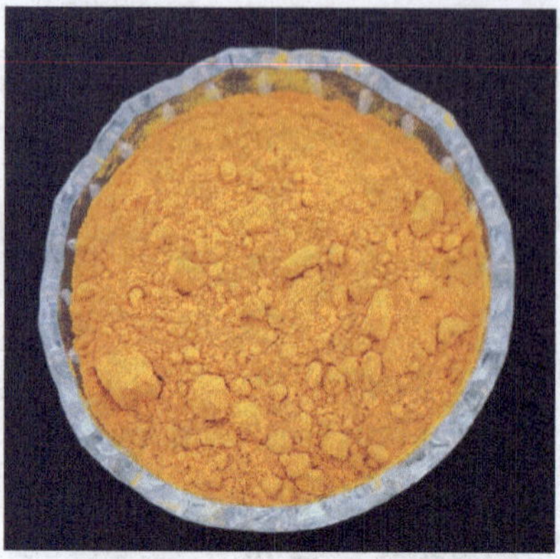

Scientific name: *Curcuma longa*

Common name: Turmeric

Distribution: Native to Southeast Asia, particularly India.

Parts used: Rhizomes.

Active principle: Curcumin.

Remarks: Known for its anti-inflammatory and antiviral properties, turmeric can treat numerous viral infections, like hepatitis and flu.

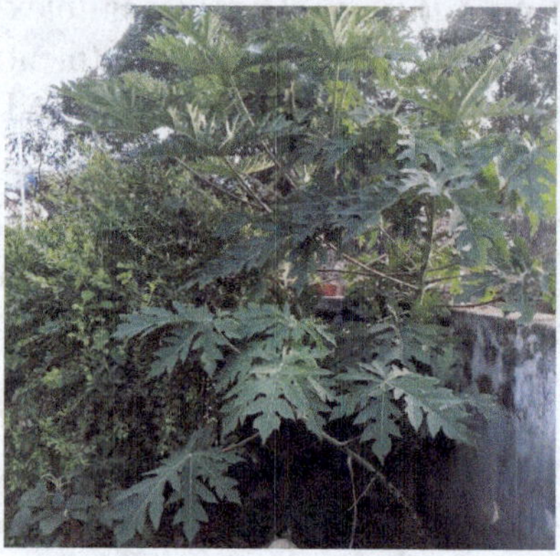

Scientific name: ***Carica papaya***

Common name: Papaya

Distribution: Native to southern Mexico and Central America, widely cultivated worldwide.

Parts used: Fruit, leaves, seeds.

Active principle: Papain, flavonoids, alkaloids.

Remarks: Known for its antiviral properties, especially against the dengue virus and other tropical viral infections. It also has immune-boosting and digestive properties.

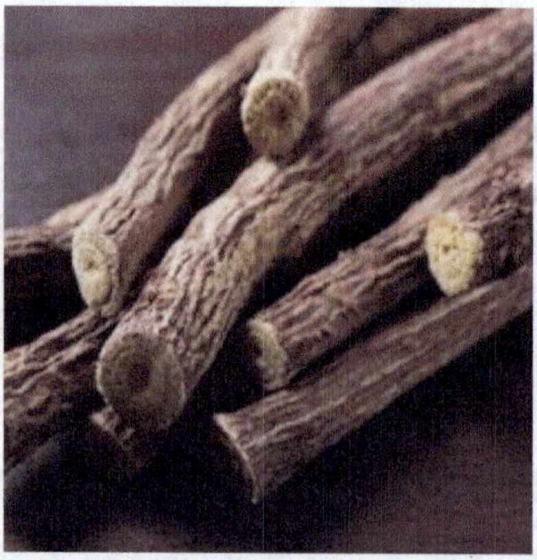

Scientific name: *Glycyrrhiza glabra L.*

Common name: Licorice

Distribution: Native to Asia, Europe, and parts of the Mediterranean region.

Parts used: Roots.

Active principle: Glycyrrhizin, flavonoids, saponins.

Remarks: Licorice is widely used for its antiviral properties, particularly against the hepatitis C virus and herpes simplex virus (HSV). It also helps in boosting immunity.

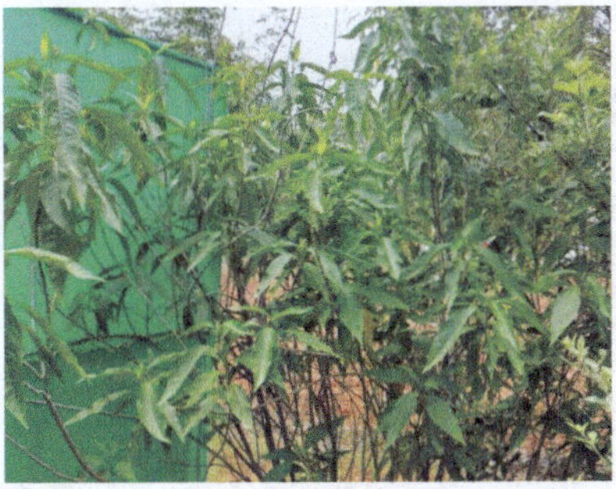

Scientific name: *Justicia adhatoda L.*

Common name: Malabar Nut

Distribution: Native to India and Southeast Asia.

Parts used: Leaves, roots.

Active principle: Vasicine, alkaloids, flavonoids.

Remarks: Widely used in Ayurvedic medicine, it has antiviral properties, especially against respiratory viruses, and is used to treat coughs, colds, and bronchitis.

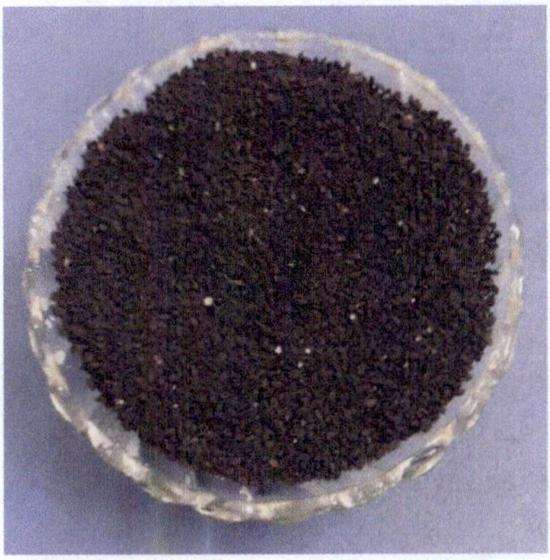

Scientific name: *Nigella sativa*

Common name: Kalonji, Black Cumin,

Distribution: Native to South and Southwest Asia.

Parts used: Seeds.

Active principle: Thymoquinone, nigellone.

Remarks: Exhibits antiviral activity, particularly against respiratory viruses and the hepatitis C virus. It also has anti-inflammatory and immune-boosting properties.

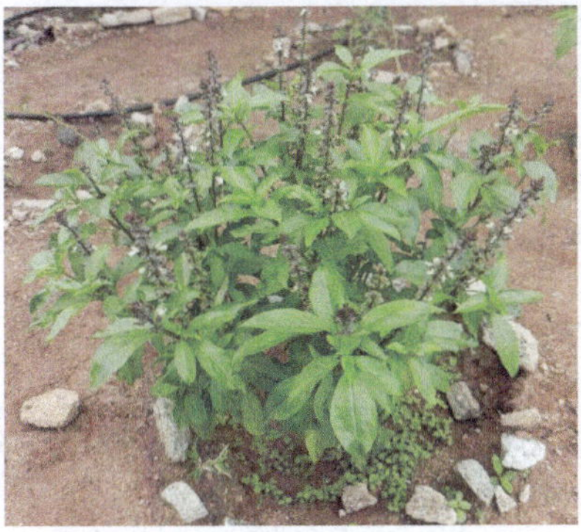

Scientific name: *Ocimum basilicum*

Common name: Tulsi, Sweet Basil

Distribution: Native to India and Southeast Asia.

Parts used: Leaves, stems.

Active principle: Eugenol, ursolic acid, flavonoids.

Remarks: Effective against HSV, influenza virus, HIV; has antiviral, antibacterial, and immune-modulating properties.

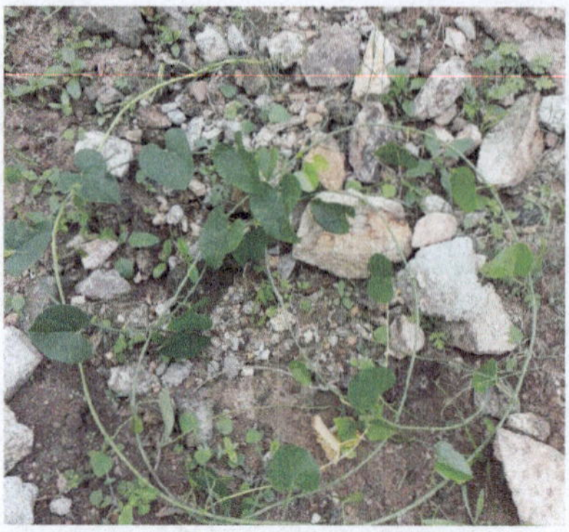

Scientific name: *Tinospora cordifolia*

Common name Giloy,: Guduchi, Amrita

Distribution: Native to India, found in tropical regions.

Parts used: Whole plant, roots.

Active principle: Tinosporide, alkaloids, glycosides.

Remarks: Effective against dengue virus, Hepatitis B; boosts immune function and fights viral infections.

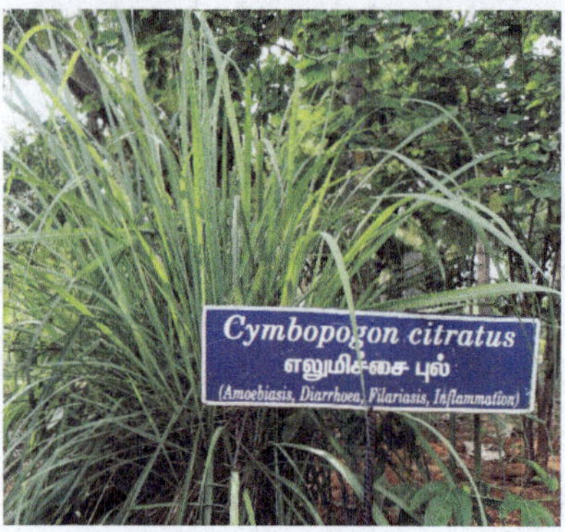

Scientific name: *Cymbopogon citratus*

Common name: Lemongrass

Distribution: Native to Southeast Asia, including India, Africa, and parts of Central and South America.

Parts used: Leaves, essential oil.

Active principle: Citral, geraniol, limonene, myrcene

Remarks: Effective against influenza virus, dengue virus, and herpes simplex virus (HSV), inhibit viral replication and support immune function.

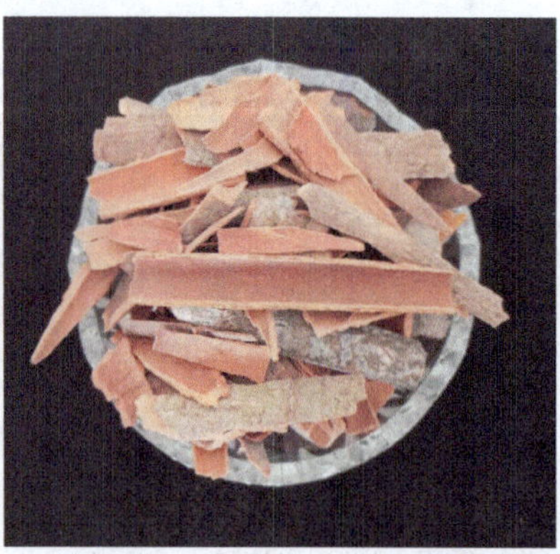

Scientific name: *Cinnamomum verum*

Common name: Cinnamon

Distribution: Native to Sri Lanka, India, and other parts of Southeast Asia.

Parts used: Bark, leaves, essential oil

Active principle: Cinnamaldehyde, eugenol, coumarin

Remarks: Effective against hepatitis C virus, herpes simplex virus (HSV), and influenza virus; inhibits viral replication and supports immune health

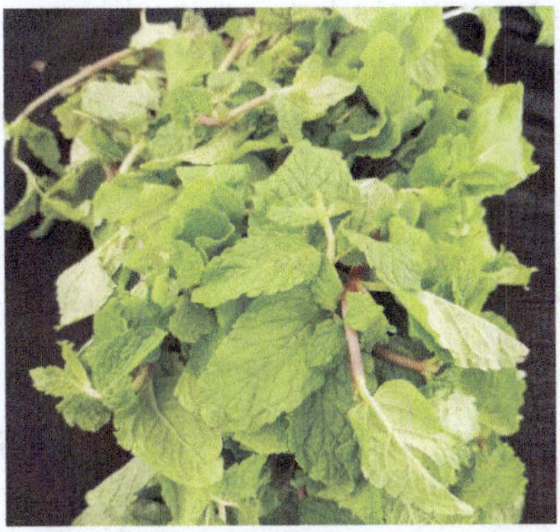

Scientific name: *Mentha piperita*

Common Name: Peppermint

Distribution: Native to Europe and Asia; now widely cultivated around the world, including in North America and parts of India.

Parts Used: Leaves, essential oil.

Active Principle: Menthol, menthone, flavonoids, rosmarinic acid.

Remarks: Effective against influenza virus, common cold viruses, and respiratory viruses, primarily by inhibiting viral replication and supporting immune response.

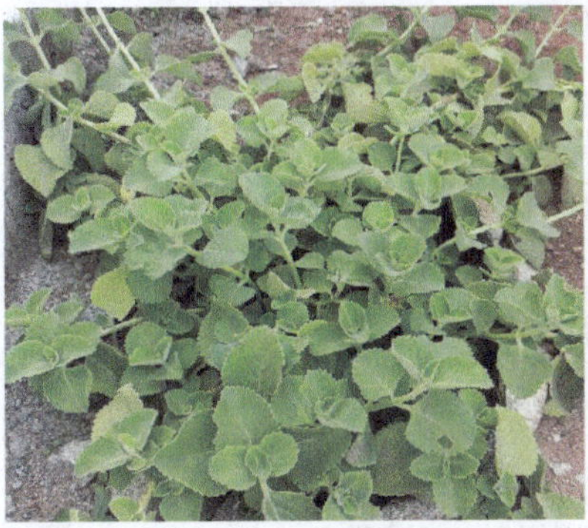

Scientific name: *Coleus amboinicus*

Common Name: Indian Coleus, Oregano,

Distribution: Native to Southeast Asia, particularly India, and found in subtropical and tropical regions worldwide.

Parts Used: Leaves, stems.

Active Principle: Volatile oils (carvacrol, thymol), flavonoids, terpenes.

Remarks: Effective against influenza virus, common cold viruses, and respiratory infections.

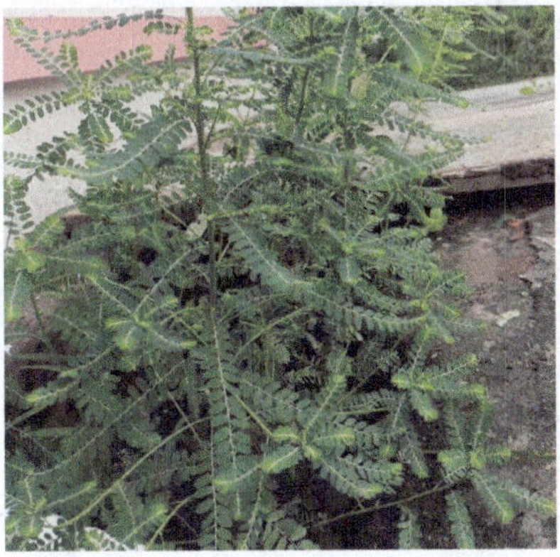

Scientific name: *Phyllanthus amarus*

Common name: Stonebreaker, Gale of the wind

Distribution: Native to tropical regions of India and Africa.

Parts used: Leaves, stems.

Active principle: Phyllanthin, hypophyllanthin, flavonoids.

Remarks: Strong activity against hepatitis B and C viruses, also used in treating liver infections and promoting liver health.

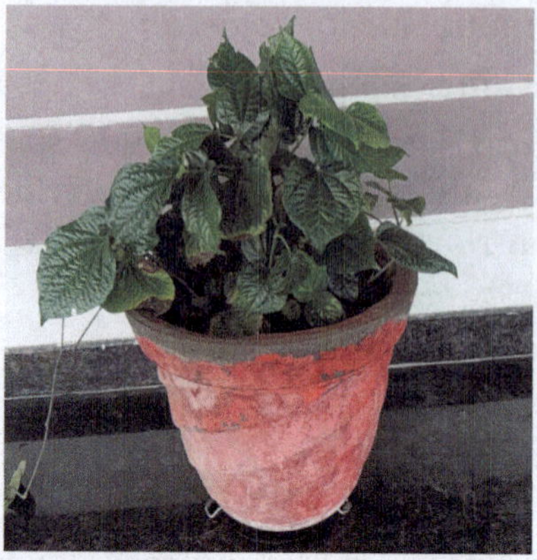

Scientific name: *Piper longum L.*

Common name: Long Pepper

Distribution: Native to the Southeast Asia and Indian subcontinent.

Parts used: Fruit, root.

Active principle: Piperine, piperlongumine.

Remarks: Antiviral and anti-inflammatory properties, especially in treating respiratory viral infections like colds and coughs.

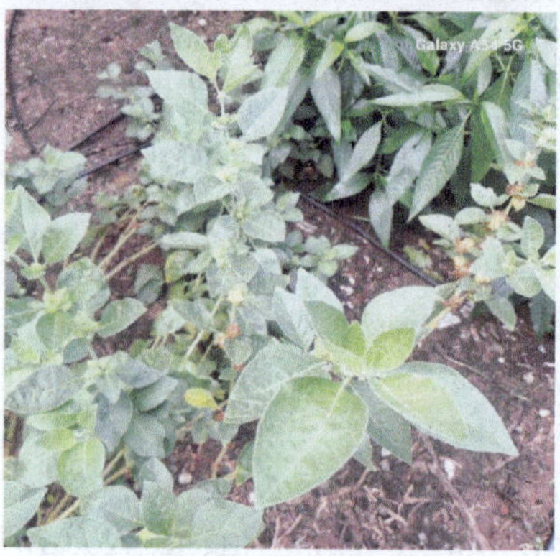

Scientific name: *Withania somnifera*

Common name: Indian Ginseng, Ashwagandha

Distribution: Native to India and parts of Africa.

Parts used: Roots, leaves.

Active principle: Withanolides

Remarks: Effective against HSV, influenza, HIV; has adaptogenic properties and boosts immune defence

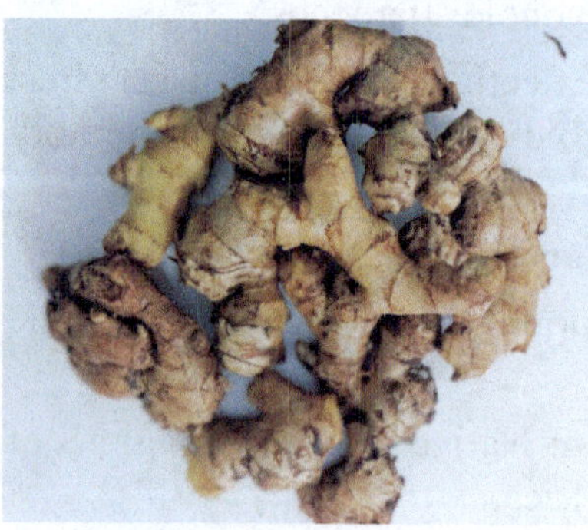

Scientific name: *Zingiber officinale*

Common name: Ginger

Distribution: Native to Southeast Asia, widely cultivated worldwide.

Parts used: Rhizomes.

Active principle: Gingerol, shogaol.

Remarks: Effective against influenza virus, common cold viruses, and nausea-inducing viruses; has strong antiviral, anti-inflammatory, and antioxidant properties

Conclusion

Medicinal plants have shown substantial potential in combating viral diseases in animals, offering an alternative or complementary approach to conventional treatments. While much of the research is still in its early stages, the evidence supports their role in enhancing immune function, inhibiting viral replication, and alleviating symptoms of viral infections. As veterinary practices evolve, medicinal plants could play a crucial role in holistic treatment strategies, promoting better health outcomes for animals across the globe.

References

Choi, H. J., Song, J. H., et al. (2010). Antiviral activity of quercetin 7-rhamnoside against influenza A virus in vitro and in vivo. Antiviral Research, 83(3), 312-315

Coon, J. T., & Ernst, E. (2004). Andrographis paniculata in the treatment of upper respiratory tract infections: A systematic review of safety and efficacy. Planta Medica, 70(4), 293-298

Formulations devised and tested by Prof. Dr. N. Punniamurthy, Rtd. Professor of Veterinary Pharmacology and Toxicology, Tamil Nadu Veterinary and Animal Sciences University, Chennai -51.

https://www.nddb.coop/farmer/health/evm

Li, J., & Huang, X. (2021). Andrographolide and its derivative potassium dehydrographolide succinate inhibit porcine reproductive and respiratory syndrome virus replication in vitro. Frontiers in Veterinary Science, 8, 769

Parida, M. M., Upadhyay, C., & Pandey, V. C. (2002). Inhibitory potential of neem (Azadirachta indica) leaves on Dengue virus type-2 replication. Journal of Ethnopharmacology, 79(2), 273-278.

7

Medicinal Plants Effective in Fungal Diseases in Animals

***Vandana Singh*[1*], *Anuj Singh*[2]**

[1]*Department of Veterinary Pharmacology & Toxicology, COVAS, Kishanganj Bihar Animal Science University, Patna, Bihar*
[2]*Department of Animal Nutrition, COVAS, Kishanganj, Bihar Animal Science University, Patna, Bihar*

Introduction

The use of medicinal plants for the treatment of diseases is a practice that spans centuries. In recent years, there has been a growing interest in using herbal remedies for treating fungal infections in livestock and animals. Fungal infections, caused by pathogenic fungi such as *Aspergillus*, *Candida*, *Dermatophytes*, and *Mucor*, can lead to significant health issues in animals, affecting both domestic and wild species. These infections often manifest as skin diseases, respiratory illnesses, gastrointestinal problems, and systemic infections, and can even lead to death if left untreated. While antifungal drugs are commonly used to manage these infections, concerns about drug resistance, toxicity, and sustainability have encouraged the exploration of alternative therapeutic options, particularly herbal medicine.

This chapter explores the potential of medicinal plants used as antifungal agents in livestock and animals, highlighting their efficacy, safety, and practical applications.

Fungal Infections in Livestock and Animals

Fungal infections in livestock and animals are a growing concern, particularly in animals subjected to stress, poor living conditions, or compromised immune systems. The most common types of fungal infections in animals include:

1. **Dermatophytosis** (Ringworm): Caused by dermatophytes like *Trichophyton* and *Microsporum*, this infection affects the skin, causing hair loss, lesions, and itching.

2. **Candidiasis**: Caused by *Candida* species, this infection often affects the gastrointestinal tract, urinary system, and mucous membranes.
3. **Aspergillosis**: Primarily caused by *Aspergillus* species, this fungal infection affects the respiratory system and can lead to severe lung damage in animals.
4. **Mucormycosis**: Caused by fungi in the order Mucorales, this infection can result in systemic disease and is particularly dangerous in immunocompromised animals.

The symptoms of fungal infections can range from mild skin irritations to severe systemic involvement, posing challenges for animal health and productivity. Traditional antifungal treatments, such as synthetic drugs (e.g., azoles, polyenes, and allylamines), are widely used. However, concerns about side effects, drug resistance, and environmental impact have led to the search for safer, more sustainable alternatives—many of which can be found in herbal medicine.

Diagnosis of Fungal Diseases

There is no single test that is the most reliable way to diagnose fungal infections. Cases (like, bacterial pyoderma) are often misdiagnosed as Dermatophytosis. Still, direct examination of hairs or scales, skin biopsy, dermoscopy, fungal culture, or PCR testing—which is unable to distinguish between viable and nonviable spores—can all be used to reach a confirmatory diagnosis of fungal infections. A handheld device called a Dermoscope is used to find aberrant hairs for direct inspection and/or culture, enabling a comprehensive skin examination. Infections can be confirmed in over 85% of cases by examining hair and scales scraped and plucked from lesions and mounted in mineral oil. Wood's lamp is used to detect M.canis-infected hairs, which light or fluoresce apple green. Hair spores can be found using Fungal culture, although it's advisable to sample just the lesions and not the full hair coat. A skin biopsy is advised for nodular lesions or atypical skin disease presentation, but not for normal cases of fungal infection. The presence or absence of fungal DNA on the hair coat can be confirmed by PCR testing.

Treatment of Fungal Disease

Treatment for animals can expedite the disease's progression and lessen the likelihood that it will spread to other vulnerable animals or people.Oral anti-fungal medication is commonly used to treat skin lesions involving scales, crusts, and hair loss. These medications must be taken for three to four weeks following remission and are usually recommended across several months.

Topical therapy, which disinfects the hair coat, is necessary in conjunction with systemic treatment. Contagion and transmission are caused by infectious spores, and disinfection reduces environmental contamination. Infectious materials are eliminated from the environment through environmental cleaning. Treatment outcomes include both mycologic and clinical cure. The resolution of every lesion and the absence of any new ones is known as clinical cure. A fungal culture or PCR can be used to check for mycologic cure after lesions have healed and a clinical cure is evident. Some popular Antifungal drugs include Amphotericin B, Griseofulvin, Ketoconazole, Itraconazole etc.

Herbal Plants with Antifungal Properties

Herbal plants contain a wide range of bioactive compounds, including alkaloids, flavonoids, terpenoids, phenolic compounds, and essential oils, which have demonstrated antifungal properties. These compounds can inhibit the growth of fungi through various mechanisms, such as disrupting cell wall synthesis, interfering with fungal enzyme activity, and altering the permeability of fungal cell membranes.

Herbal Treatment of Fungal Diseases

Several medicinal plants have shown potential in the treatment of fungal infections in animals. Some of these plants include:

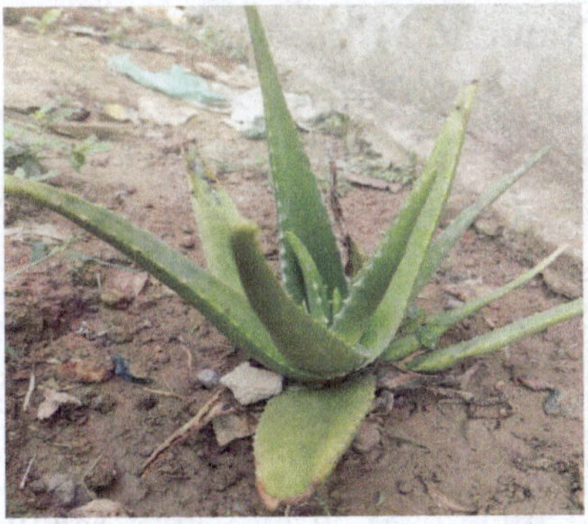

Scientific Name: *Aloe vera*

Common Name: Aloe vera, Ghritkumari

Distribution: Tropical and subtropical regions of India.

Part Used: Leaves (gel and latex)

Bioactive Principles: Aloin, aloesin, emodin, saponins, and polysaccharides

Remark: Aloe vera gel is used for its soothing, moisturizing, and healing properties in skin infections and burns. It promotes wound healing and has antibacterial and anti-inflammatory effects.

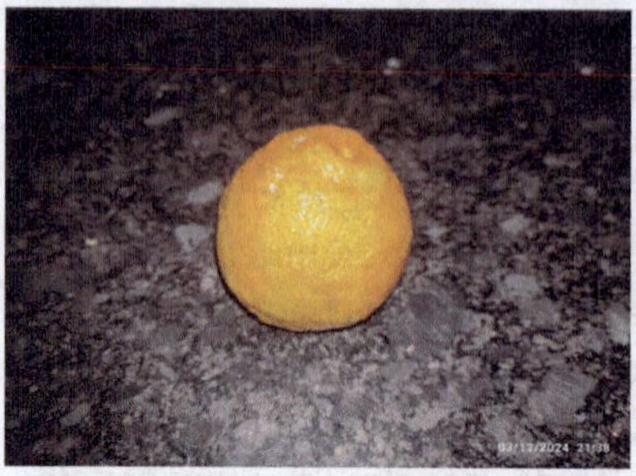

Scientific Name: *Citrus aurantium*

Common Name: Bitter Orange

Distribution: Mediterranean regions, Southeast Asia, and North America.

Part Used: Peel and oil

Bioactive Principles: Flavonoids (hesperidin, naringin), synephrine, and essential oils

Remark: The essential oil from the peel is antimicrobial and is often used in treating skin conditions. It also has astringent and rejuvenating properties.

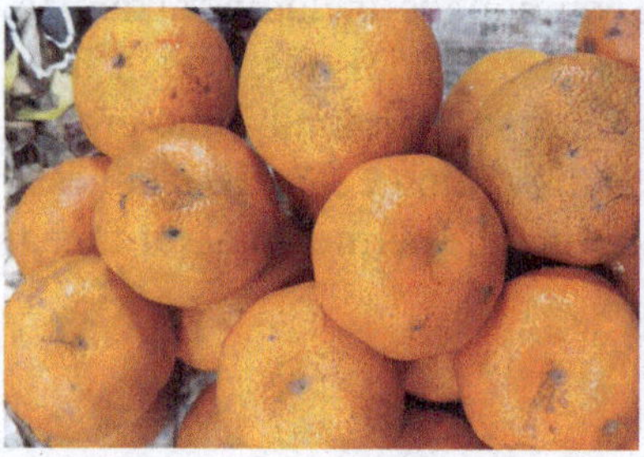

Scientific Name: *Citrus sinensis*

Common Name: Sweet Orange

Distribution: Brazil, United States, India, and China

Part Used: Peel and juice

Bioactive Principles: Limonene, flavonoids, and vitamin C

Remark: The peel oil is used for its antimicrobial and antioxidant properties. It aids in skin rejuvenation and protects against oxidative stress.

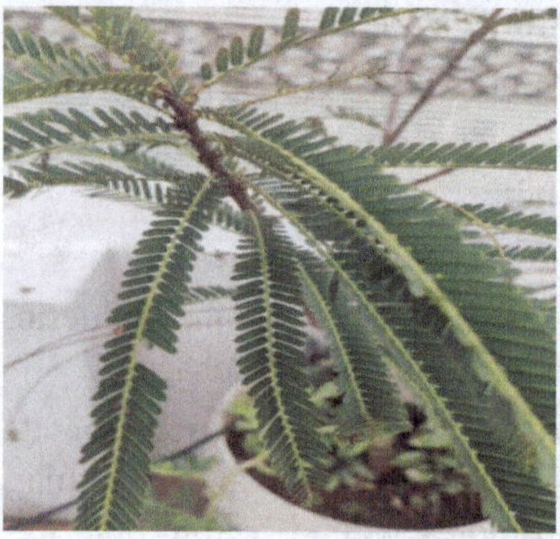

Scientific Name: *Emblica officinalis* (Syn. Phyllanthus emblica)

Common Name: Amla, Indian Gooseberry

Distribution: India, Southeast Asia, and the Middle East

Part Used: Fruits

Bioactive Principles: Vitamin C, gallic acid, ellagic acid, and tannins

Remark: Amla has strong antioxidant properties, enhances collagen production, and is used in treating acne and pigmentation issues. It also improves skin elasticity.

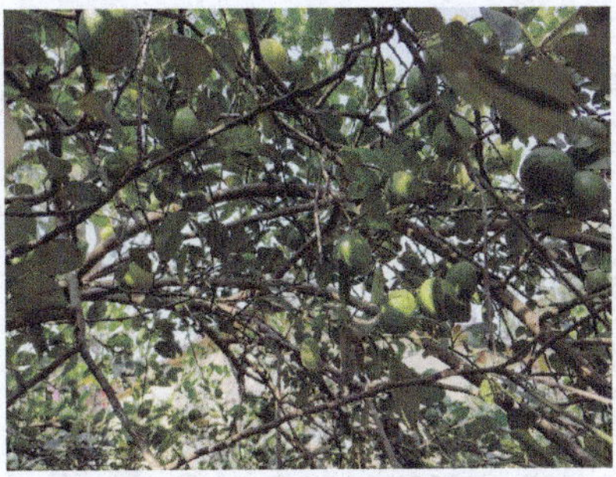

Scientific Name: *Citrus limon*

Common Name: Lemon

Distribution: India, Mexico, Argentina, and the Mediterranean

Part Used: Peel and juice

Bioactive Principles: Citric acid, limonene, and flavonoids

Remark: Lemon juice is widely used for its astringent, antibacterial, and skin-lightening properties. It is effective in treating acne and hyperpigmentation.

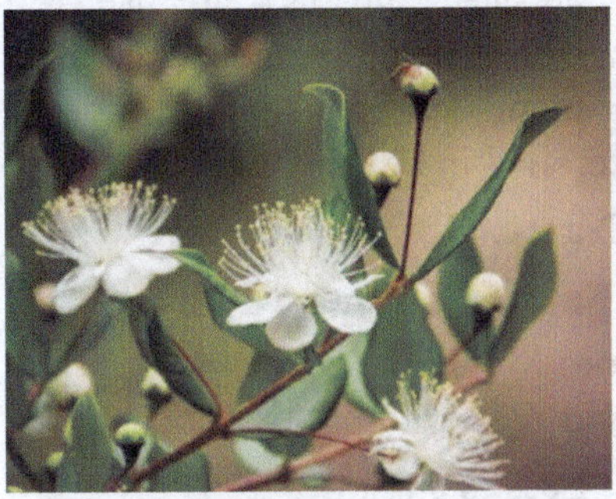

Scientific Name: *Myrtus communis*

Common Name: Myrtle, fox tail myrtle

Distribution: Mediterranean region and North Africa

Part Used: Leaves and berries

Bioactive Principles: Myrtucommulone, flavonoids, tannins, and essential oils (myrtenol)

Remark: Myrtle oil is known for its antimicrobial and anti-inflammatory effects. It helps in treating skin infections and soothing irritated skin.

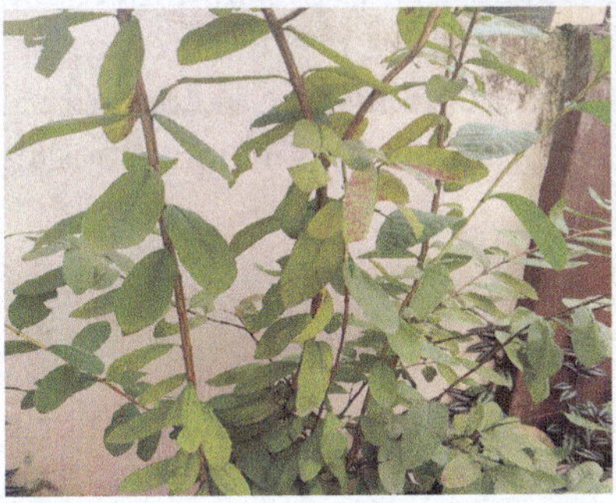

Scientific Name: *Psidium guajava*

Common Name: Guava

Distribution: Tropical and subtropical regions, particularly in India, Southeast Asia, Central and South America

Part Used: Leaves and fruits

Bioactive Principles: Flavonoids (quercetin), tannins, carotenoids, and vitamin C

Remark: Guava leaves are used for their antimicrobial and anti-inflammatory properties to treat skin infections, acne, and blemishes. The antioxidants in guava also protect against oxidative damage and promote healthy skin.

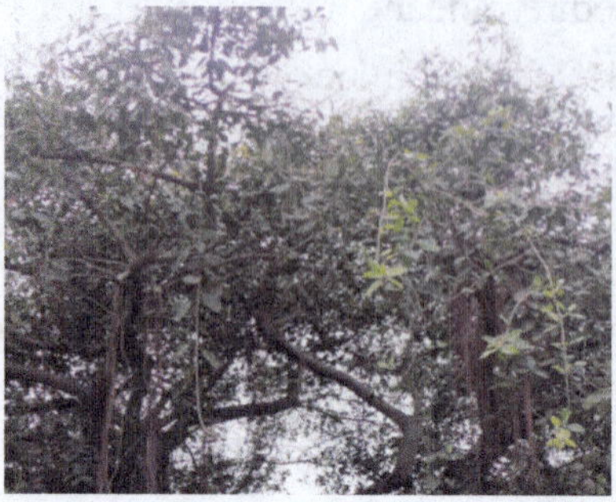

Scientific Name: *Ficus benghalensis*

Common Name: Banyan Tree

Distribution: India, Southeast Asia, and tropical Africa

Part Used: Bark, leaves, and latex

Bioactive Principles: Tannins, flavonoids, sterols, and alkaloids

Remark: The latex and bark are used for their antimicrobial and astringent properties to treat skin infections, ulcers, and acne. The plant's components also help in maintaining skin elasticity and promoting overall skin health.

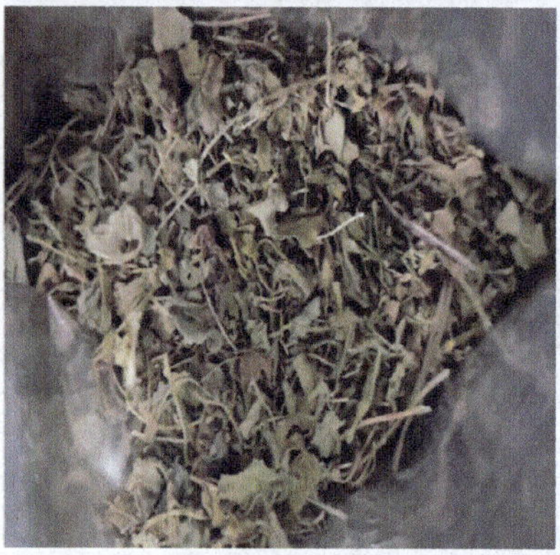

Scientific Name: *Origanum vulgare*

Common Name: Oregano

Distribution: Mediterranean regions, North America, and Western Asia

Part Used: Leaves and oil

Bioactive Principles: Carvacrol, thymol, rosmarinic acid, and terpenes

Remark: Oregano oil is highly antimicrobial and antifungal, making it effective against skin infections, including fungal conditions. It also reduces inflammation and soothes irritated skin.

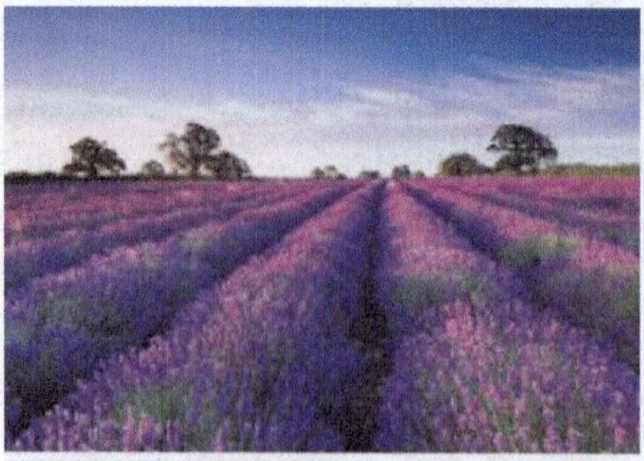

Scientific Name: *Lavandula angustifolia*

Common Name: Lavender

Distribution: Mediterranean regions, Europe, and North America

Part Used: Flowers and essential oil

Bioactive Principles: Linalool, linalyl acetate, and terpenoids

Remark: Lavender oil is known for its soothing, antimicrobial, and healing properties. It helps in treating acne, wounds, and burns and reduces skin irritation while promoting relaxation.

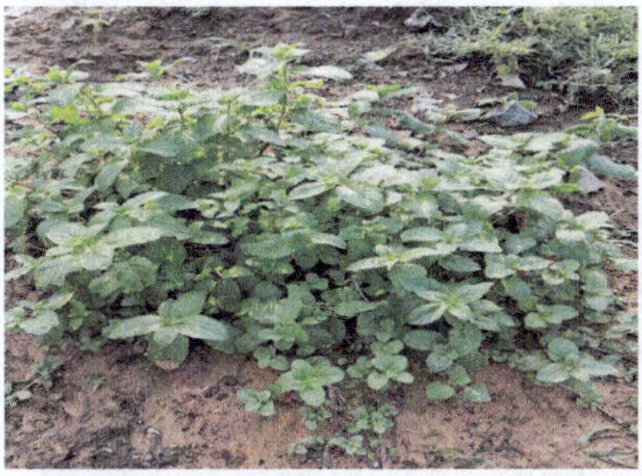

Scientific Name: *Mentha spp.* (e.g., *Mentha piperita*)

Common Name: Mint, Peppermint

Distribution: Europe, Asia, and North America

Part Used: Leaves and oil

Bioactive Principles: Menthol, menthone, and rosmarinic acid

Remark: Mint is known for its cooling, antiseptic, and anti-inflammatory properties. It is commonly used to treat acne, itching, and minor skin irritations.

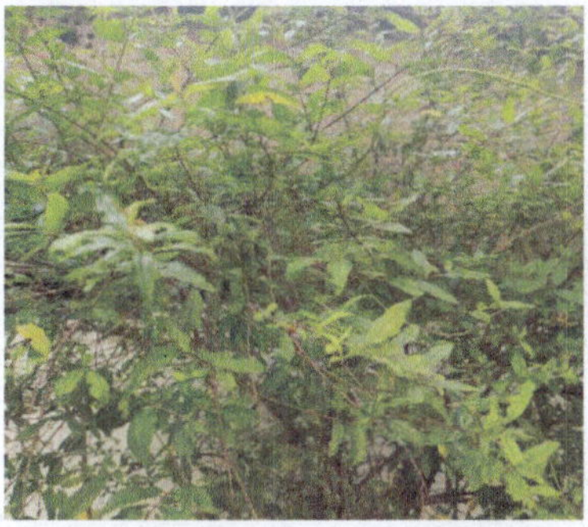

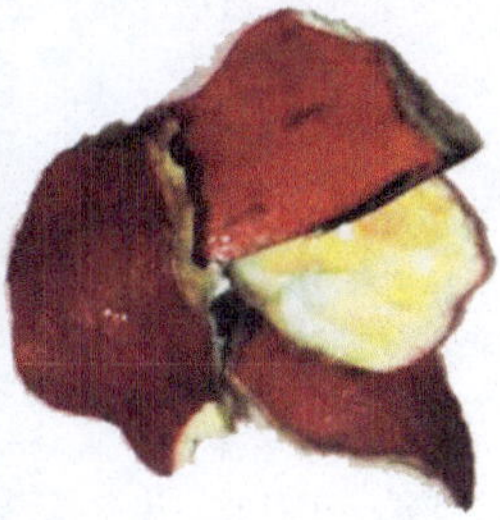

Scientific Name: *Punica granatum*

Common Name: Pomegranate

Distribution: India, Iran, Mediterranean regions, and the Middle East

Part Used: Peel

Bioactive Principles: Ellagic acid, tannins, and anthocyanins

Remark: Pomegranate peel is rich in antioxidants and anti-inflammatory compounds. It helps in healing acne, scars, and other skin conditions by promoting cell regeneration and protecting against oxidative stress.

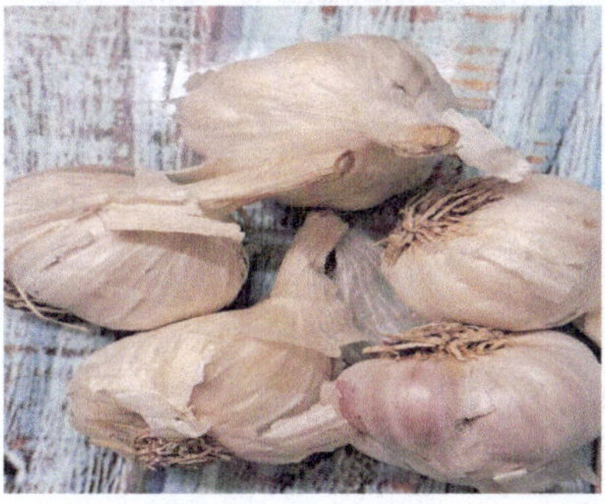

Scientific Name: *Allium sativum*

Common Name: Garlic

Distribution: Worldwide, especially in China, India, and the Mediterranean

Part Used: Bulb

Bioactive Principles: Allicin, sulfur compounds, and flavonoids

Remark: Garlic has potent antibacterial,

antifungal, and anti-inflammatory properties. It is used to treat acne, fungal infections, and other skin conditions while improving overall skin health.

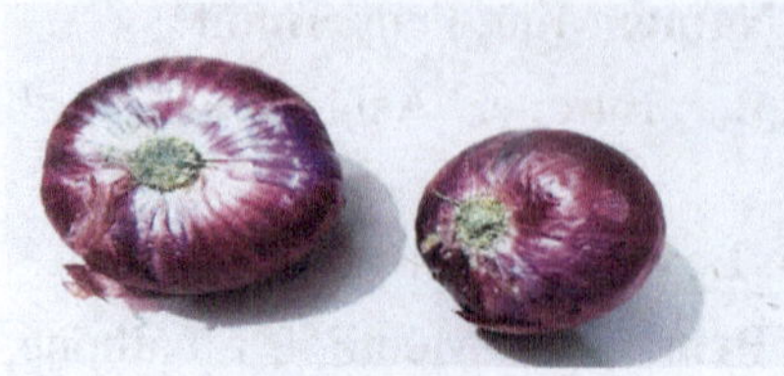

Scientific Name: *Allium cepa*

Common Name: Onion

Distribution: Worldwide, especially in India, China, and the Mediterranean

Part Used: Bulb

Bioactive Principles: Quercetin, sulfur compounds, and flavonoids

Remark: Onion extract is used for scar reduction, improving skin elasticity, and treating acne marks. It also has antibacterial and anti-inflammatory properties.

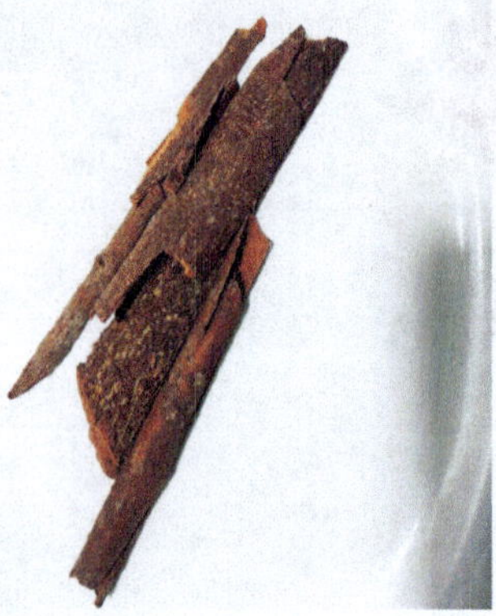

Scientific Name: *Cinnamomum verum* or *Cinnamomum cassia*

Common Name: Cinnamon

Distribution: India, Sri Lanka, and Southeast Asia

Part Used: Bark

Bioactive Principles: Cinnamaldehyde, cinnamic acid, and eugenol

Remark: Cinnamon is antimicrobial and antioxidant, making it effective for acne treatment and reducing signs of aging. It enhances skin tone and helps in wound healing.

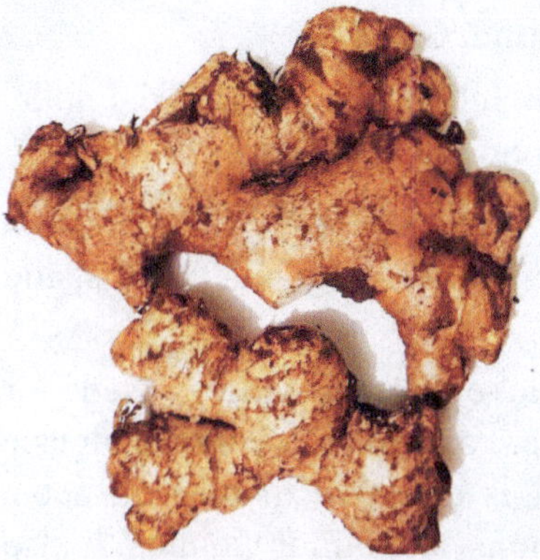

Scientific Name: *Zingiber officinale*

Common Name: Ginger

Distribution: India, China, and tropical regions worldwide

Part Used: Rhizome

Bioactive Principles: Gingerol, shogaol, and zingerone

Remark: Ginger has strong anti-inflammatory and antimicrobial properties. It is used to treat acne, scars, and skin irritation while improving circulation and skin health.

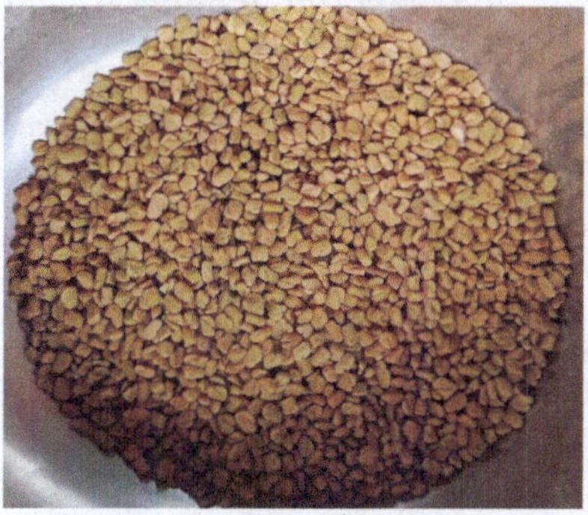

Scientific Name: *Trigonella foenum-graecum*

Common Name: Fenugreek, Methi

Distribution: India, the Middle East, and North Africa

Part Used: Seeds and leaves

Bioactive Principles: Diosgenin, trigonelline, and flavonoids

Remark: Fenugreek is used for its antimicrobial and anti-inflammatory effects to treat acne, wounds, and skin infections. It also helps in skin hydration and reduces blemishes.

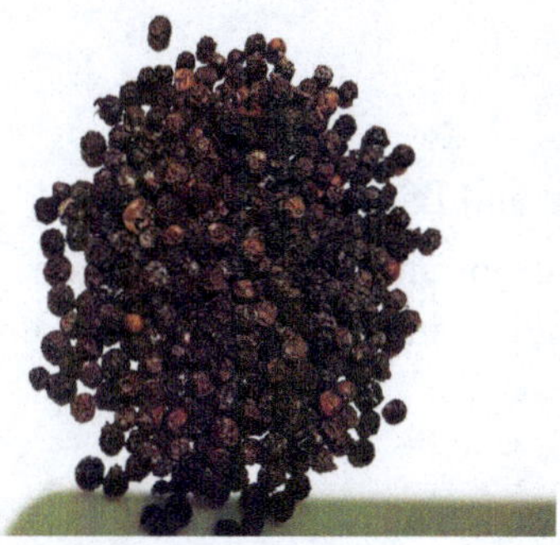

Scientific Name: *Piper nigrum*

Common Name: Black Pepper

Distribution: India, Vietnam, Indonesia, and other tropical regions

Part Used: Dried fruits (peppercorns)

Bioactive Principles: Piperine, volatile oils, and flavonoids

Remark: Black pepper is antimicrobial, anti-inflammatory, and antioxidant. It is used to treat skin infections, enhance blood circulation, and promote skin rejuvenation. Piperine also aids in the absorption of nutrients, enhancing overall skin health.

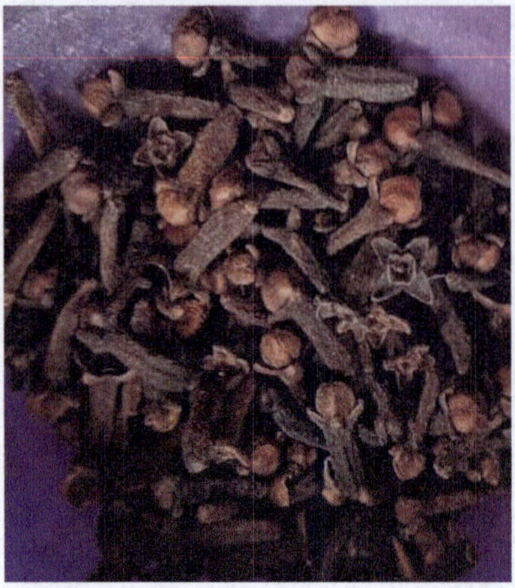

Scientific Name: Syzygium aromaticum

Common Name: Cloves

Distribution: Indonesia, India, Sri Lanka, and tropical regions

Part Used: Flower buds and essential oil

Bioactive Principles: Eugenol, tannins, and flavonoids

Remark: Clove oil is widely used for its antiseptic, antifungal, and analgesic properties. It is effective in treating acne, fungal infections, and minor wounds. It also helps in reducing skin inflammation and irritation.

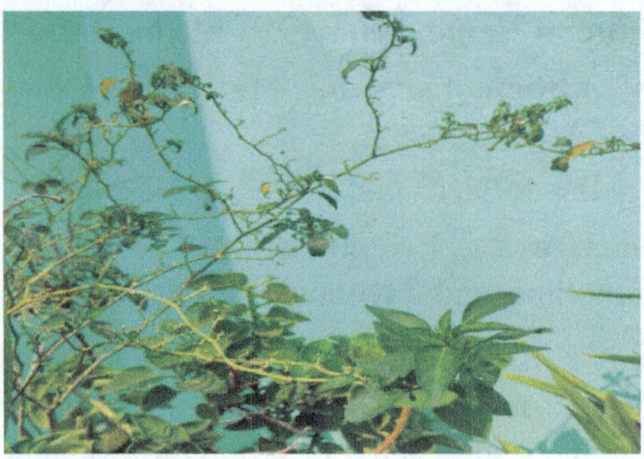

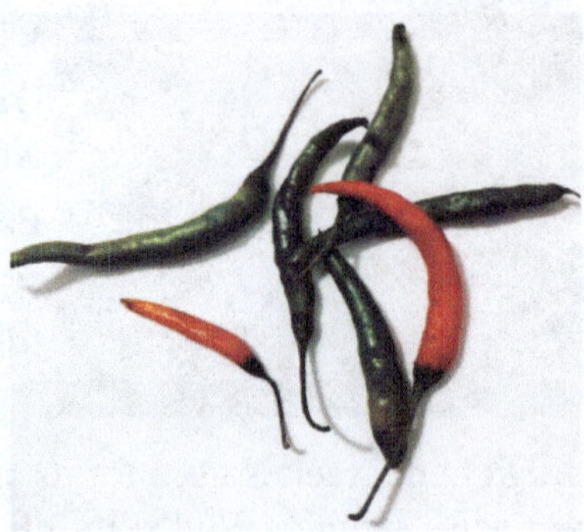

Scientific Name: Capsicum annuum or Capsicum frutescens

Common Name: Cayenne Pepper

Distribution: Americas, India, and Africa

Part Used: Fruits

Bioactive Principles: Capsaicin, carotenoids, and flavonoids

Remark: Cayenne promotes blood circulation and is used for its anti-inflammatory and analgesic properties. It helps in skin detoxification and reduces signs of irritation and inflammation.

Conclusion

Herbal plants provide a valuable, sustainable alternative to synthetic antifungal drugs in the treatment of fungal infections in livestock and animals. Plants such as garlic, tea tree oil, neem, turmeric, thyme, and echinacea have demonstrated strong antifungal activity and offer various therapeutic applications. The growing interest in natural remedies reflects the need for safer, more eco-friendly approaches to animal health. Further research into the pharmacological properties, optimal dosages, and practical applications of these herbs will enhance their use in veterinary care, contributing to better health outcomes for animals worldwide.

References

Bouhdid, S., et al. (2010). Antifungal activity of thyme essential oil against Candida albicans and Aspergillus niger. Journal of Applied Microbiology, 109(5), 1427–1434.

Carson, C. F., et al. (2002). Antifungal activity of tea tree oil and its components. Journal of Applied Microbiology, 92(5), 778-784.

Chandra, J., et al. (2008). The antifungal activity of garlic extract against Candida albicans. Phytotherapy Research, 22(5), 745-748.

Colvin, B. A., et al. (2013). Inhibition of Candida albicans biofilm formation by garlic extract. Mycological Research, 117(12), 1481-1487.

Gazzaz, Z. J., et al. (2014). Antifungal activity of tea tree oil against Candida albicans and Aspergillus niger. Journal of Mycology and Plant Pathology, 44(4), 426-431.

Giordani, R., et al. (2017). Thyme essential oil as an antifungal agent in poultry. Poultry Science Journal, 96(8), 2897-2904.

Hughes, J., et al. (2004). Tea tree oil treatment for Trichophyton mentagrophytes infections in small mammals. Journal of Animal Research, 23(2), 175-181.

Malu, R. M., et al. (2009). Neem leaf extract's antifungal properties against Trichophyton rubrum. International Journal of Mycological Studies, 10(2), 151-156.

Matsuura, Y., et al. (2004). Antifungal activity of garlic extracts against Aspergillus fumigatus. Mycoses, 47(10), 421-428.

Raghuveer, C., et al. (2011). In vitro antifungal activity of turmeric extract against Candida albicans and Aspergillus niger. Journal of Medical Mycology, 21(1), 52-57.

Spelman, K., et al. (2001). Echinacea: Antifungal properties and its role in immune support. Journal of Clinical Herbalism, 15(3), 108-115.

Vasconcelos, T., et al. (2013). Thyme essential oil for controlling fungal infections in small animals. Veterinary Medicine Journal, 88(4), 238-245.

8

Medicinal Plants Effective Against Internal Parasites in Animals

Sujith S.

Department of Veterinary Pharmacology and Toxicology, College of Veterinary and Animal Sciences, Pookode, Wayanad, Kerala Veterinary and Animal Sciences University, India

Introduction

Helminths are a group of internal parasites of animals and human beings that usually infest gastrointestinal tract that feed from the host which provides protection to the parasite. The infestation cause loss of blood and nutrients from the host, making it weak, and vulnerable to other infections. There can be injury to other organs due to the migration of different stages of the parasite, formation of cysts or secretion of toxins that can cause damage.

The heminths belong to two phyla including nemathelminthes which are round worms and Platyhelminthes that has flukes, and tapeworms. Nematodes are round worms who have a resistant cuticle and most of them have separate sexes with direct or indirect life cycle. The major nematodes include Ascarids, Strongyles, strongyloides, Trichostrongyles, Filarids, Trichuris etc. Tape worms have a flat body with a head or scolex, neck and strobili having proglottids. They are hermaphrodites and the proglottids contain reproductive organs. They require more than one host for completion of life cycle. The flukes are ususally leaf like , unsegmented and have suckers that help them to attach to the internal organs of the host. They also have a life cycle in more than one host.

Helminthosis is usually treated using chemical anthelmintics that include benzimidazoles, macrocyclic lactones, imidazothiazoles, tetrahydropyrimidines, organophospahtes, salicylanilides, ocatdepsipeptides, aminoacetonitriles, Isoquinolines, Substituted phenols, aromatic amides etc Most of the drugs target specific proteins in the parasite. Benzimidazoles target the beta tubulin affecting the structural integrity where as macrocyclic lactones act on glutamate gated chloride ion channels specific for nematodes. These drugs may affect specific enzymes for energy metabolism in the parasite or may cause uncoupling/inhibition of oxidative phosphorylation as in salicylanilides. Imidazothiazoles act on the autonomic ganglia of the parasiteswhere as oragnophosphates act on the acetyl choline esterase.

The major problem encountered in the therapy of helminthosis is the lack of development of newer drugs with alternate mechanism of action and rapid emergence of anthelmintic resistance due to specific mutations. The major reason for the emergence of resistance is the inadvertent use of anthelmintic and pasture contamination resulting in reinfections.

Screening for anthelmintic activity utilises *invitro* and *invivo* techniques. The *invitro* techniques include egg hatch assay or ovicidal activity, larval motility inhibition assay, larvicidal activity, larval migration inhibition assay, adulticidal activity assessment in live worms collected from slaughter houses. The invivo assessment can be done in laboratory animals that can be naturally infested or artificially infected. Assessment in livestock can be done by faecal egg count reduction test.

To control gastrointestinal nematode infections and to combat with rising anthelmintic resistance, it is very much necessary to think of some alternatives. This has highlighted the advantages of herbal remedies as an alternative. The use of herbal preparations and plants as anthelmintics is prevalent in many parts of the world, mainly developing countries. The plant derived natural substances have been used since past as such anthelmintic agents have been reported to be cheaper, more reliable and less toxic. More over, the farmers have more access for the plants which makes the use more economical, environment friendly and reducing the chances of drug resistance.

Few Medicinal Plants that Have Anthelmintic Activity Include

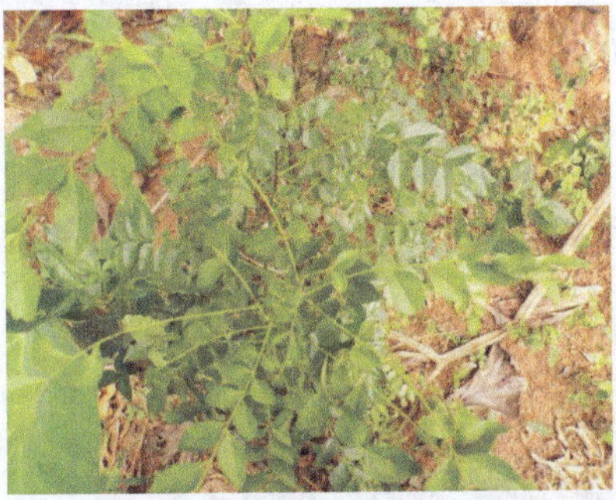

Scientific name : *Murraya Koenigii*

Common name: Curry leaf

Distribution : Asia and Indian Sub continent

Part used : Leaf, Seed

Bioactive principles: Carbazole alkaloids, O-methylmahanine, O-methylmurrayamine, Bismahanine, Isomahanine, Bispyrayafolin, Mahanimbine, Koenimbine, Koenigicine, and Murrayone

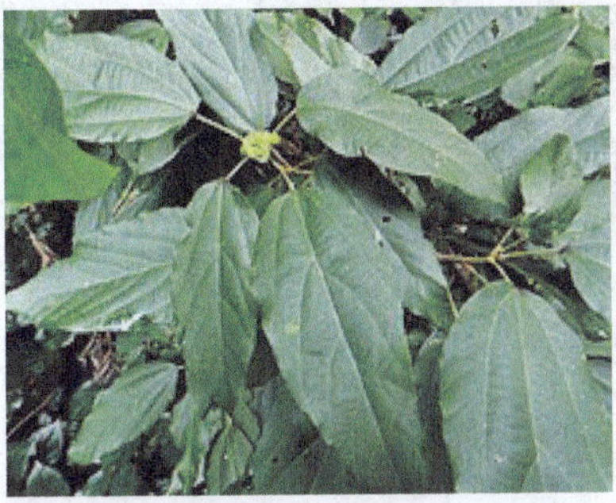

Scientific name : *Mallotus Philippensis*

Common name: Kamla

Distribution : Asia and Indian Sub continent

Part used : Fruit , leaf

Bioactive principles: Bergenin, Mallotophilippinens, Rottlerin, and Isorottlerin

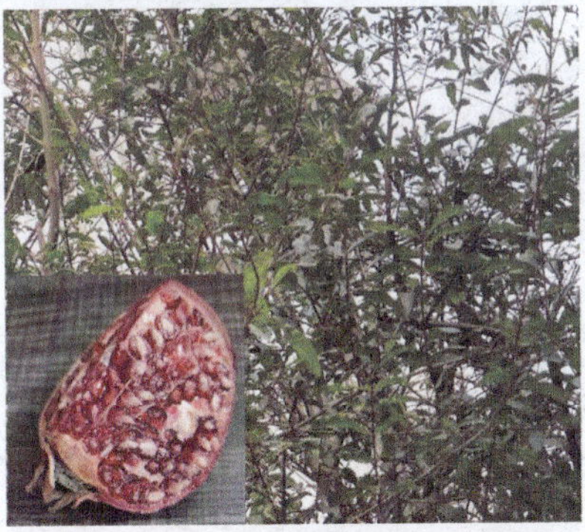

Scientific name : *Punica granatum*

Common name: Anar

Distribution : Asia and Indian Sub continent

Part used : Rind, root and stem bark

Bioactive principles: Ellagic acid, Punicalagin, Punicic acid, Pelletierine

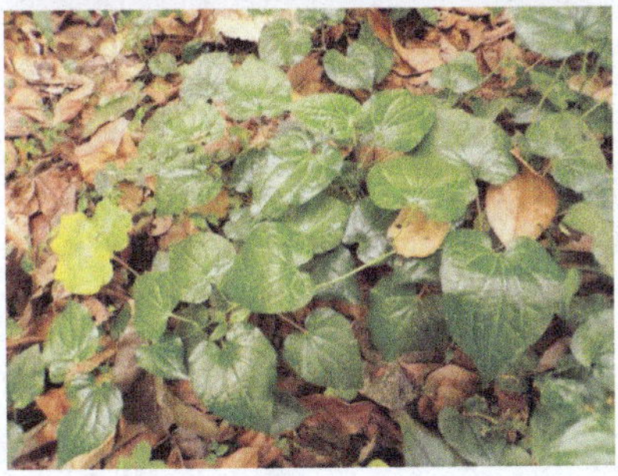

Scientific name : ***Piper longum***

Common name: Pippli, Pipali

Distribution : Asia and Indian Sub continent

Part used : Fruits

Bioactive principles: Piperine, Piper longumine, Guineensine, Chabamide, Pellitorine, Pinoresinol.

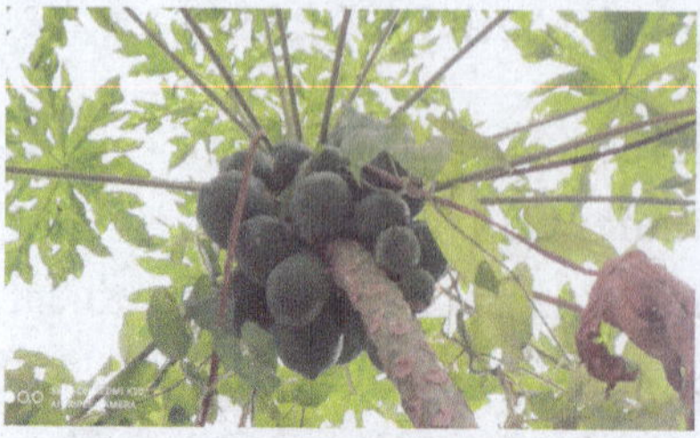

Scientific name : *Carica papaya*

Common name: Papaya

Distribution : Asia and Indian Sub continent

Part used : Seeds

Bioactive principles: Benzyl isothiocyanate, myricetin and kaempferol

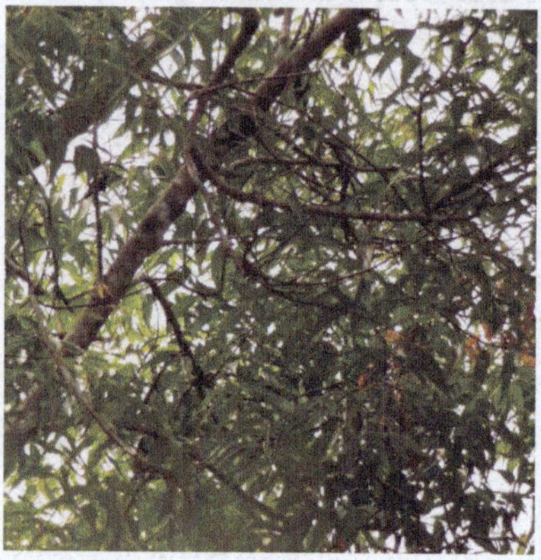

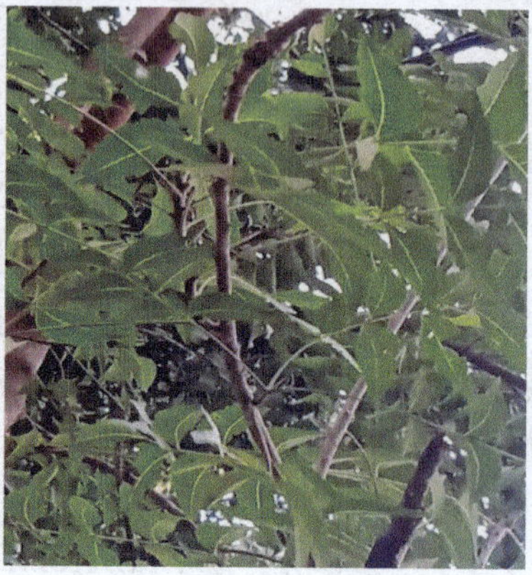

Scientific name : *Azadirachta indica*

Common name: Neem

Distribution : Asia and Indian Sub continent

Part used : Leaf, stem bark and fruits

Bioactive principles: Azadirachtin, Nimonol, Nimocinol, Nimocinolide, Gallic acid, Gallocatcchin, Epicatechin, Azadiradione, Nimbin, and Salannin.

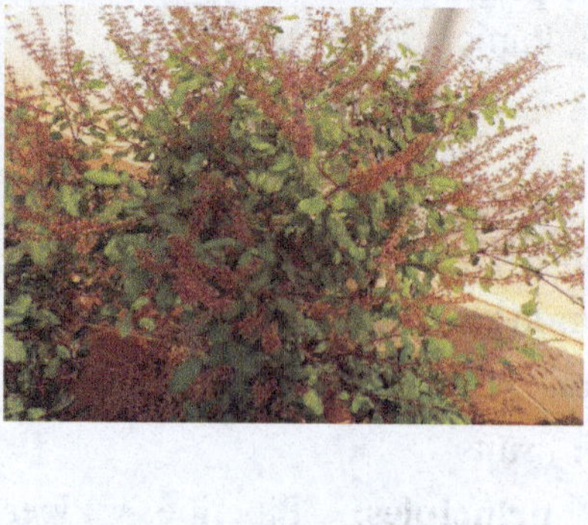

Scientific name : *Ocimum sanctum*

Common name: Tulsi, Holy basil

Distribution : Asia and Indian Sub continent

Part used : Leaves, Flowers

Bioactive principles: Oleic acid, luteolin, moludistin, carvacrol, eugenol, orientin, rosmarinic acid, and caryophyllene

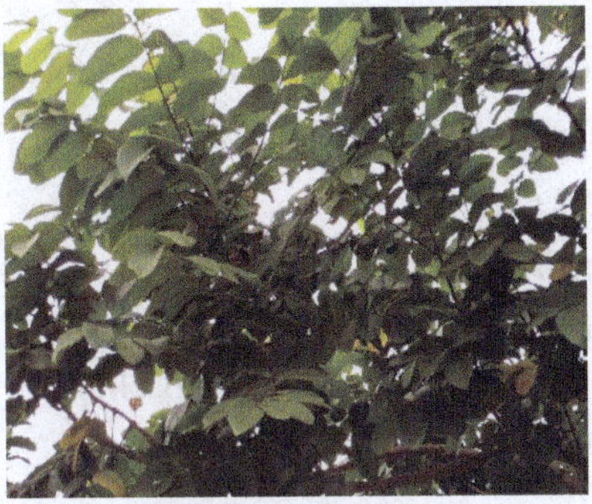

Scientific name : *Butea monosperma*

Common name: Flame of forest

Distribution : South east Asia and Indian Sub continent

Part used : Seeds

Bioactive principles: Palasonin, Butrin, butein

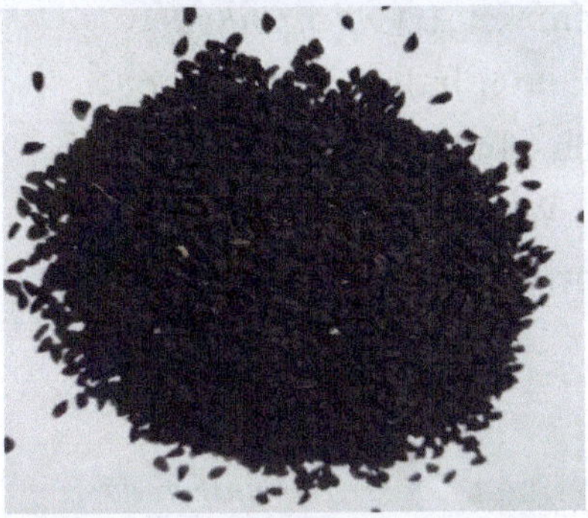

Scientific name : ***Nigella sativa***

Common name: Black cumin, Kala Jira

Distribution : Indian Sub continent

Part used : Essential oil

Bioactive principles: Thymoquinone, dithymoquinone, cymene, α-pinene

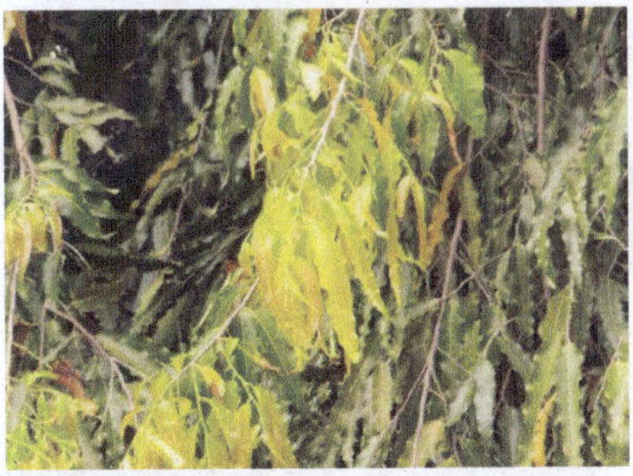

Scientific name : *Polyalthia longifolia*

Common name: Indian mast tree

Distribution : Indian Sub continent

Part used : Seeds

Bioactive principles: Diterpenes, flavonoids, phytosterols

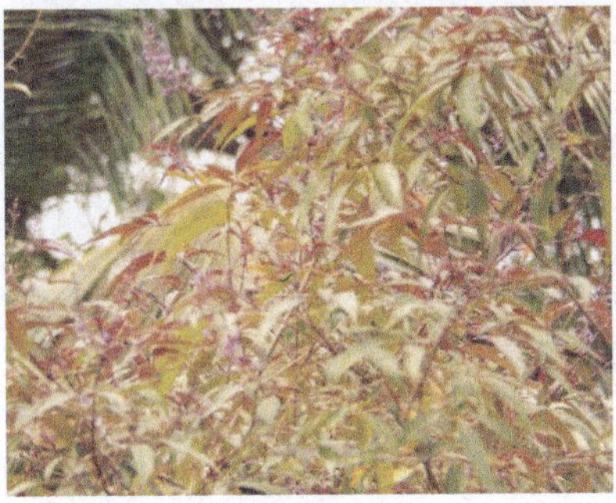

Scientific name : ***Vitex negundo***

Common name: Indian Privet

Distribution : India, South East Asia

Part used : Leaves

Bioactive principles: Terpenoids, flavonoids, Phenolics

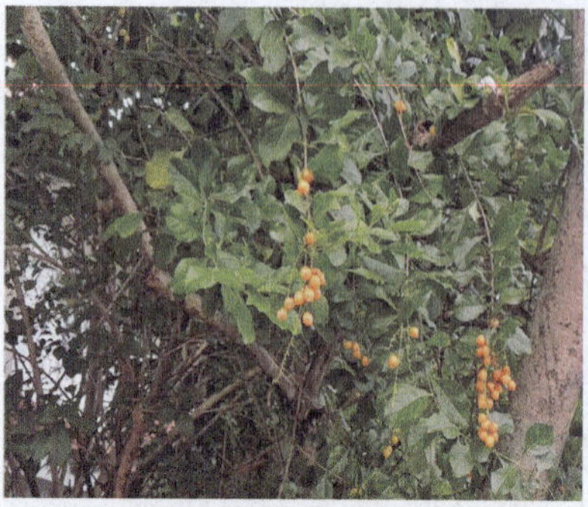

Scientific name : ***Duranta erecta***

Common name: Golden dewdrop

Distribution : India

Part used : Fruit

Bioactive principles: Acteoside, durantol, pectolinaringenin, repenins, scutellarein, and repennoside

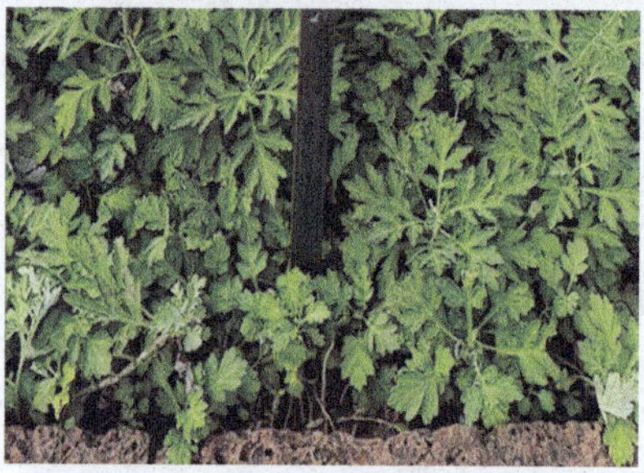

Scientific name : *Artemisia vulgaris*

Common name: Indian Worm Wood

Distribution : India

Part used : Whole Plant

Bioactive principles: Vulgarin, Artemisinin

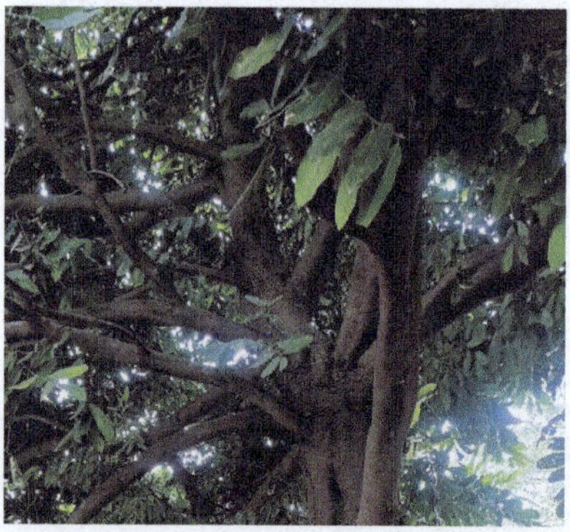

Scientific name : *Diospyros malabarica*

Common name: Indian Persimmon

Distribution : India

Part used : Seed, Bark

Bioactive principles: Betulinic acid

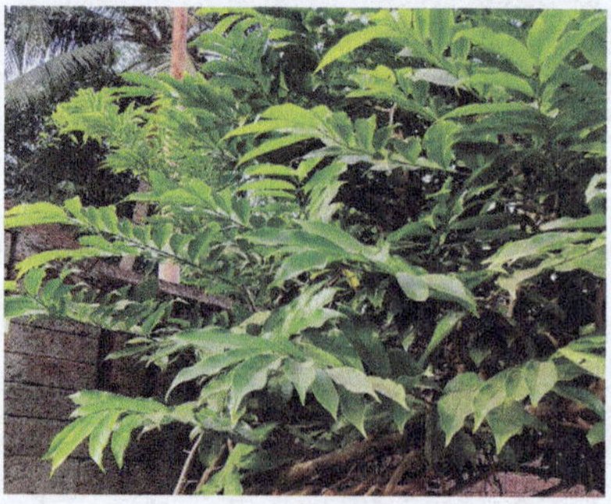

Scientific name : ***Artabotrys hexapetalus***

Common name: Chini Champa

Distribution : India

Part used : Roots,Stem

Bioactive principles: Artabotrine

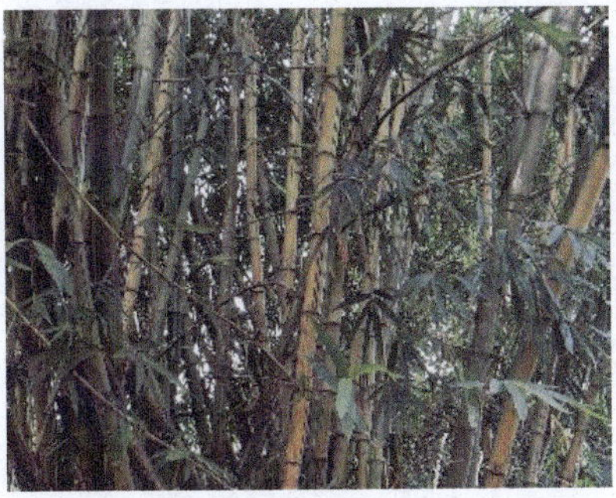

Scientific name : *Bambusa tulda*

Common name: Bamboo

Distribution: India

Part used: Shoot and leaves

Bioactive principles: Orientin

References

Deepa, C.K., Darsana, U., Sujith, S., Priya, M.N. and Juliet, S. 2015. Effect of Mallotus phillipensis flower extracts against the third stage larvae of Haemochus contortus. Int. J. Applied Pure Sci. Agri.1(3): 19-23.

Krishnaprasad , G.K., Sujith, S., John, P., Priya, M. N., Devi, S.S., Usha , P.T.A Surya, S. and Gleeja, V.L. 2018. Anthelmintic activity of fruit extract and fractions of Piper longum L. in vitro Pharmacognosy .J. 10: 333-340.

Krishnaprasad, G.K., Surya, S., Sujith, S., Preethy, J., Priya, M.N., Devi, S.S. and Usha, P.T A. 2018. In-vitro efficacy of various fruit extracts of Duranta erecta and Piper longum against adult amphistomes. Int. J. Pharmacognosy Phytochem. 10: 165-169.

Mali, R.G. and Mehta, A.A. 2008. A review on anthelmintic plants. Nat. Prod. Rad. 7(5): 466-475.

Priya, M.N., Darsana, U., Sujith S., Deepa, C.K. and Lucy, K.M. 2015. Effect of various extracts of Ocimum sanctum and Vitex negundo on Gastrothylax crumenifer. Int. J.Toxicol. Pharmacol. Res. 7(4): 180-184

Sujith, S., Priya, M.N., Deepa, C.K. and Usha, P.T.A. 2018. Characterization of the anthelmintic activity of Murraya koenigii (Linn.). Pharmacognosy J. 10:6s : 100-103.

Sujith S, Deepa CK, Priya M N Darsana U, Sreedevi R and Lucy KM 2015. Anthelmintic activity of Vitex Negundo leaf extracts against ova and third Stage larvae of Haemonchus Contortus. Int. J. Pharmacognosy Phytochem.30 (1): 1329-1334.

Sujith S, Sreedevi, R., Priya M N, Deepa C K, Darsana U., Sreeshitha S G, Suja R S and Juliet S. 2015. Anthelmintic activity of three Indian medicinal plants. Int. J. Pharmacognosy Phytochem Res. 7(2) : 361-364.

9

Medicinal Plants Effective Against External Parasites in Animals

Suja Rani S, Vadlakunata Chetana, Pooja Krishna, Sona Shaji

Department of Veterinary Pharmacology and Toxicology, College of Veterinary and Animal Sciences, Mannuthy, Thrissur-680 651, Kerala

The control of external parasites and the pertinent disease vectors using chemicals is riddled with various issues and hence there is a huge demand for alternative approaches. Natural products, being a prominent resource for poor farmers, can majorly serve as a cheaper, environment friendly and sustainable alternative. Further, ethno-veterinary and traditional knowledge has provided a diverse array of plants, which need to be validated for their repellent, insecticidal and acaricidal activities to claim their effect against external parasites. Besides, phytochemical study of these therapeutic plants has progressively revealed the existence of a variety of bioactive components in these plant derived extracts, catering to their efficacy against external parasites.

External Parasites in Domestic Animals

External parasites, also known as ectoparasites are organisms that live on the surface of domestic animals, feeding on their blood or skin. Fleas, ticks, mites, lice and flies are among the most common external parasites. These parasites can cause significant health issues in animals including discomfort, skin irritation and even severe diseases. Infestations can lead to conditions such as dermatitis, anemia and secondary infections. Moreover, many external parasites are vectors for serious diseases that can affect both animals and humans. Hence, effective management of these parasites is essential to ensure the health and well-being of domestic animals.

Experimental Infestation of External Parasites in Lab Animals

In laboratory settings, external parasites are often induced in animal models to study their life cycles, pathogenicity and potential treatments. Commonly used lab animals include mice, rats and rabbits, which can be infested with parasites such as fleas (Ctenocephalides spp.), ticks (Ixodes spp.), and mites (Sarcoptes spp.). These studies allow researchers to understand the host-parasite renowned interactions more thoroughly and also to test the efficacy of various antiparasitic drugs. Laboratory-induced infestations help in evaluating new treatment protocols and preventive measures that can be translated into effective strategies for managing external parasites in domestic animals.

Normal Treatment Drugs for External Parasites in Domestic Animals

The treatment of external parasites in domestic animals typically involves a range of pharmaceutical products designed to eliminate or control infestations. Topical treatments such as spot-on solutions (e.g., fipronil and imidacloprid) are commonly used for their ease of application and effectiveness against fleas and ticks. Oral medications like fluralaner (Bravecto) and afoxolaner (NexGard) provide systemic protection by entering the bloodstream and killing parasites upon feeding. Additionally, collars containing insecticides offer prolonged protection by releasing active ingredients over time. Regular use of these treatments is crucial for preventing infestations and managing existing ones effectively.

Herbal Treatment for External Parasites in Domestic Animals

The herbal remedies for external parasites are on huge demand as they are considered as safer and less harmful as compared to the conventional drugs. Many owners prefer natural remedies to avoid the possible side effects associated with synthetic chemicals. Herbal medicine often utilizes plant extracts known for their insecticidal properties. For example, neem oil when used correctly, apart from being effective against fleas and ticks, it's also safer for pets. Other herbs like garlic and lemongrass also serve as natural repellents against various external parasites. Few of the other herbs that act as natural repellents against a variety of external parasites include lemongrass and garlic.

Furthermore, natural organic compounds produced by plants serve various purposes in pest management, with varied degrees of use in domestic animals. Azadirachtin act as an insecticide and acaricide, though it finds little utility in domestic animals. Carvacrol, which is effective as an insecticide is not been used directly in veterinary products. Citronellal and citronellol are repellents with limited application in domestic animals, whilst D-limonene serve as an insecticide, acaricide and repellent and has been used sparingly. Eucalyptol and geraniol, both repellents, are very rarely used, as are eugenol, linalool and thymol, to act as insecticides, acaricides and repellents. Rotenone is an insecticide with limited application, while pyrethrins, which operate as insecticides, acaricides, and repellents, are widely utilized among domestic animals. Nevertheless, herbal therapies use a holistic approach to treating parasites, which can bring extra benefits such as soothing irritated skin.

Medicinal Plants Used in External Parasites in Domestic Animals

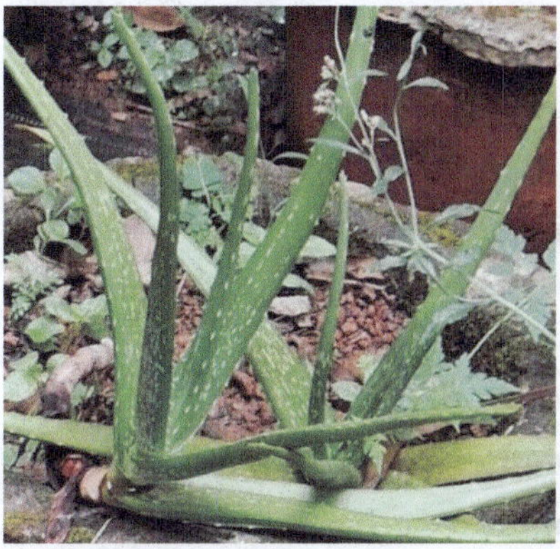

Scientific name: *Aloe vera*

Common name: Aloe

Distribution: Tropical and subtropical regions

Part used: Leaves

Bioactive principles: Anthraquinones

Remarks: Disruption of parasite membranes, leading to dehydration and death

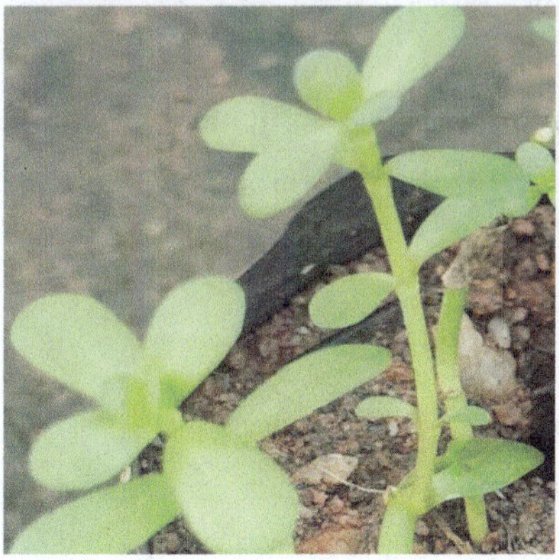

Scientific name: *Bacopa monnieri*

Common name: Brahmi

Distribution: Indian subcontinent

Part used: Leaves

Bioactive principles: Bacosides

Remarks: Interfere with neurotransmission in parasites, causing paralysis

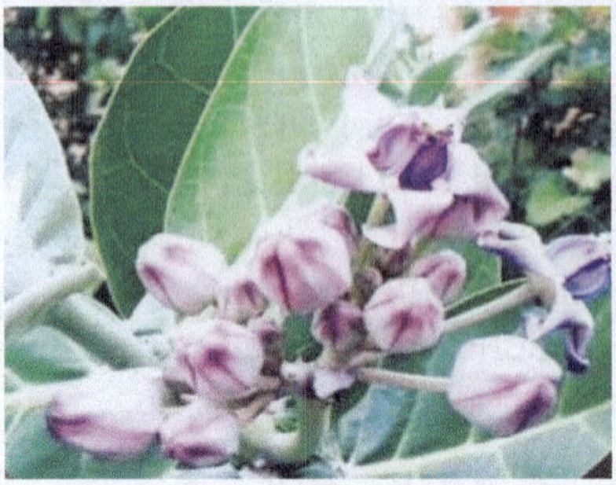

Scientific name: *Calotropis gigantea*

Common name: Crown flower

Distribution: Tropical and sub-tropical areas

Part used: Leaves, latex and flowers

Bioactive principles: Calotropin, uscharin

Remarks: Disrupt parasite ion transport and enzymatic activity, causing paralysis and death.

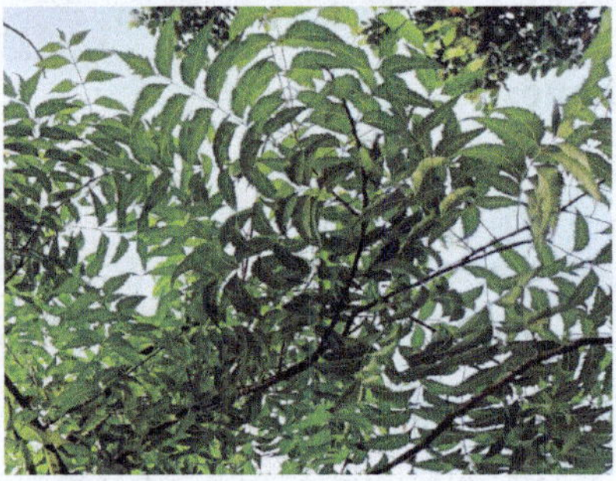

Scientific name: *Azadirachta indica*

Common name: Neem

Distribution: Indian subcontinent

Part used: Leaves, seeds

Bioactive principles: Azadirachtin

Remarks: Inhibits parasite growth and molting by disrupting hormonal pathways, while limonoids act as neurotoxins.

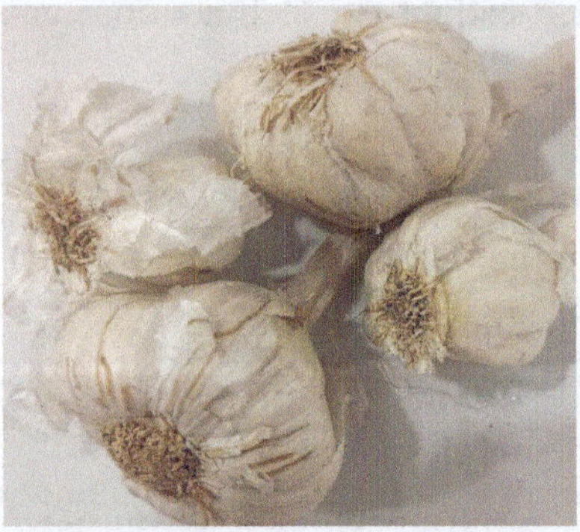

Scientific name: Allium sativum

Common name: Garlic

Distribution: Worldwide

Part used: Bulbs

Bioactive principles: Allicin

Remarks: Inhibits parasite energy metabolism by disrupting thiol-dependent enzymes

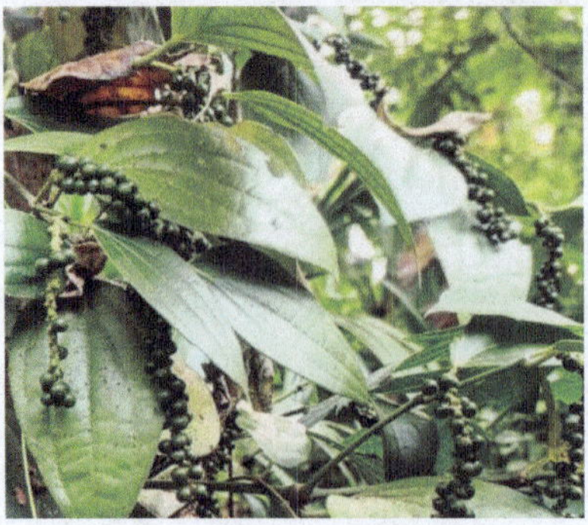

Scientific name: ***Piper nigrum***

Common name: Black Pepper

Distribution: Tropical regions

Part used: Fruits

Bioactive principles: Piperine

Remarks: Interferes with parasite neuronal transmission and acts as an insect repellent.

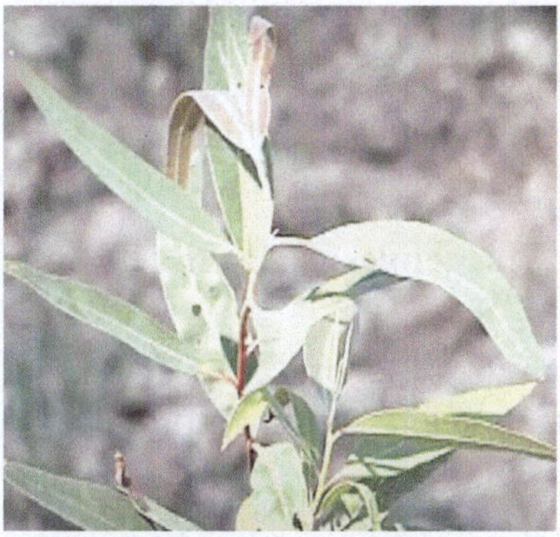

Scientific name: *Eucalyptus globulus*

Common name: Eucalyptus

Distribution: Australia, worldwide

Part used: Leaves

Bioactive principles: Eucalyptol

Remarks: Disrupts the respiratory and nervous systems of parasites by binding to GABA receptors.

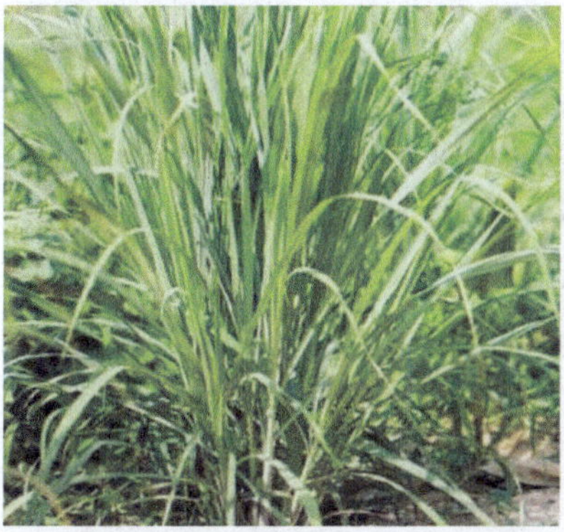

Scientific name: Cymbopogon citratus

Common name: Lemongrass

Distribution: Tropical regions

Part used: Leaves

Bioactive principles: Citral

Remarks: Destabilize parasite cell membranes and inhibit acetylcholinesterase, causing paralysis.

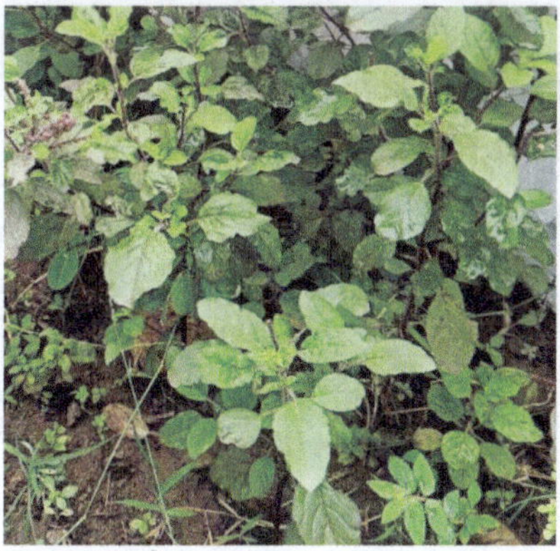

Scientific name: *Ocimum sanctum*

Common name: Holy Basil (Tulsi)

Distribution: Indian subcontinent

Part used: Leaves

Bioactive principles: Eugenol

Remarks: Disrupts membrane integrity and inhibits neurotransmitter signaling in ectoparasites.

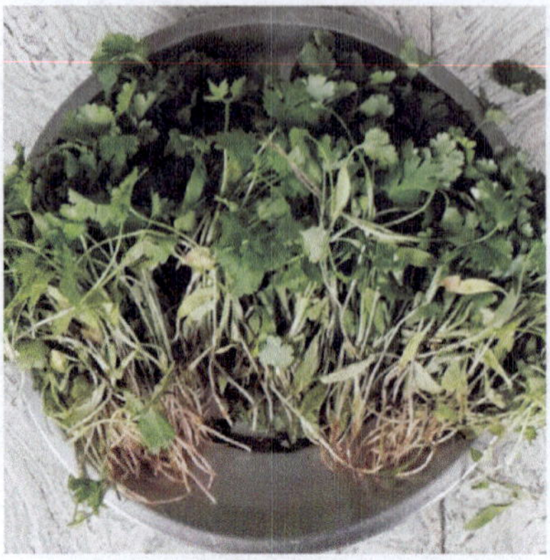

Scientific name: *Coriandrum sativum*

Common name: Coriander

Distribution: Indian subcontinent

Part used: Leaves, seeds

Bioactive principles: Essential oils (linalool)

Remarks: Act as neurotoxins, disrupting synaptic function and causing mortality.

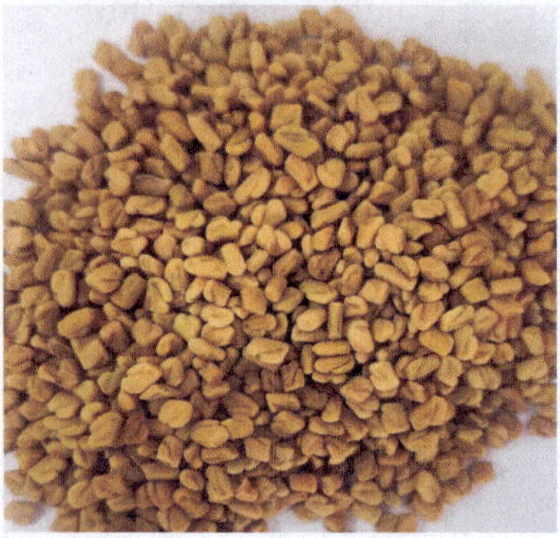

Scientific name: *Trigonella foenum-graecum*

Common name: Fenugreek

Distribution: Indian subcontinent

Part used: Seeds

Bioactive principles: Saponins, alkaloids

Remarks: Impair ectoparasite enzymatic activity, reducing viability.

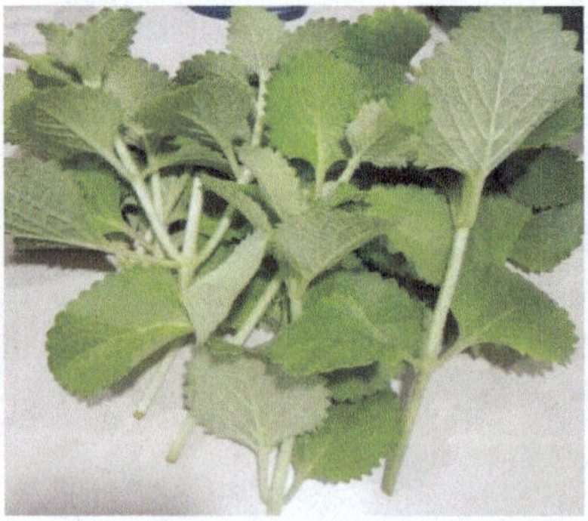

Scientific name: *Origanum vulgare*

Common name: Oregano

Distribution: Mediterranean region

Part used: Leaves

Bioactive principles: Carvacrol

Remarks: disrupt cell membranes and inhibit acetylcholinesterase, paralyzing parasites.

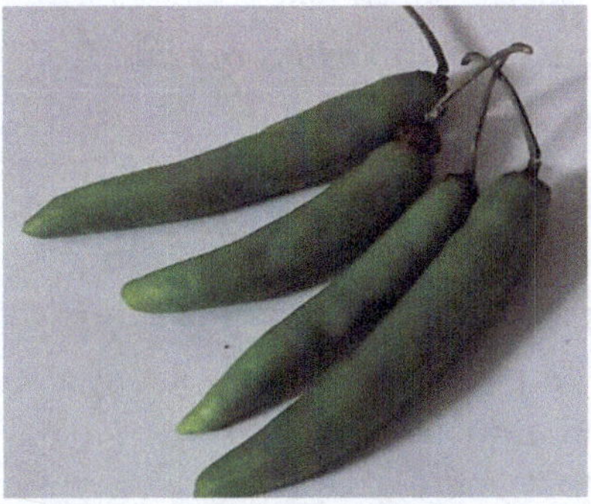

Scientific name: *Capsicum annuum*

Common name: Bell Pepper

Distribution: Americas

Part used: Fruits

Bioactive principles: Capsaicin

Remarks: Overactivation of sensory neurons, leading to paralysis and repellence.

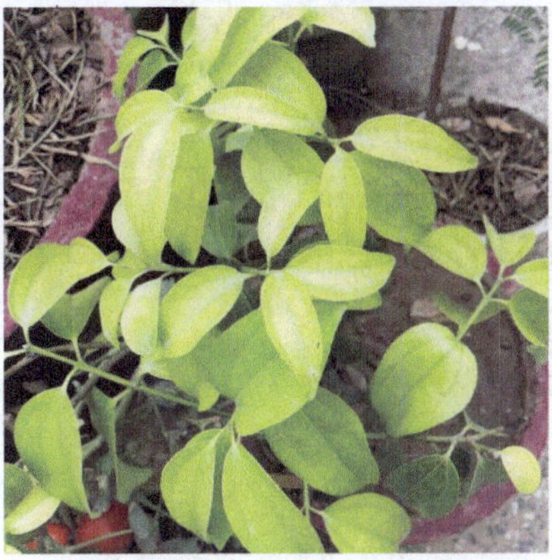

Scientific name: *Cinnamomum verum*

Common name: Cinnamon

Distribution: Southeast Asia

Part used: Bark

Bioactive principles: Cinnamaldehyde

Remarks: Disrupts membrane integrity and impairs mitochondrial function in parasites.

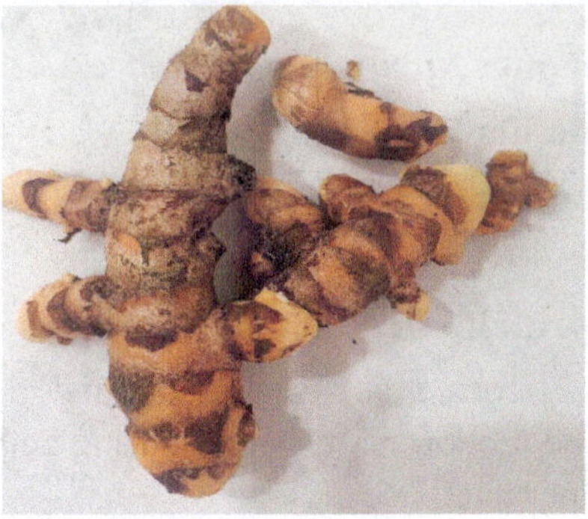

Scientific name: *Curcuma longa*

Common name: Turmeric

Distribution: South Asia

Part used: Rhizomes

Bioactive principles: Curcumin

Remarks: Inhibits parasite enzyme systems and disrupts oxidative balance, leading to cell death.

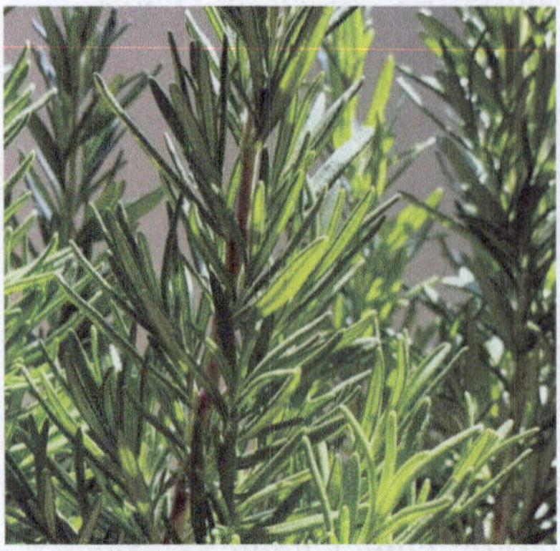

Scientific name: *Rosmarinus officinalis*

Common name: Rosemary

Distribution: Mediterranean region

Part used: Leaves

Bioactive principles: Rosmarinic acid

Remarks: Impair parasite nervous system function and mitochondrial activity.

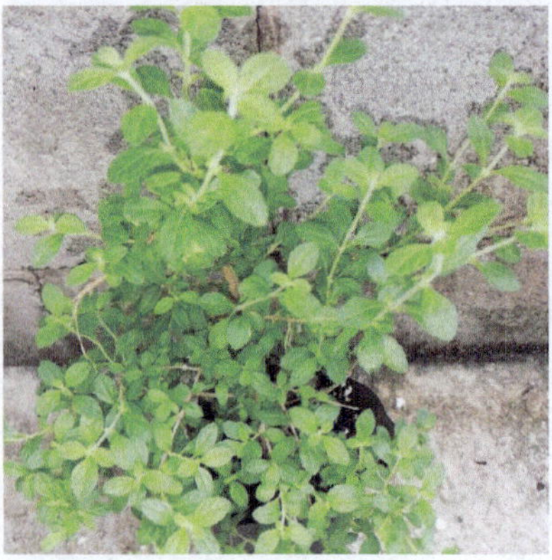

Scientific name: *Thymus vulgaris*

Common name: Thyme

Distribution: Mediterranean region

Part used: Leaves

Bioactive principles: Thymol

Remarks: Destabilize parasite membranes and inhibit neurotransmission.

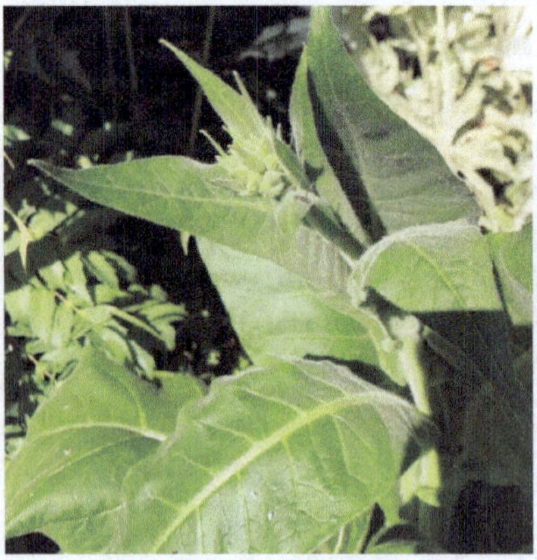

Scientific name: *Nicotiana tabacum*

Common name: Tobacco

Distribution: Americas

Part used: Leaves

Bioactive principles: Nicotine

Remarks: Nicotine acts as an agonist at acetylcholine receptors, overstimulating and paralyzing parasites.

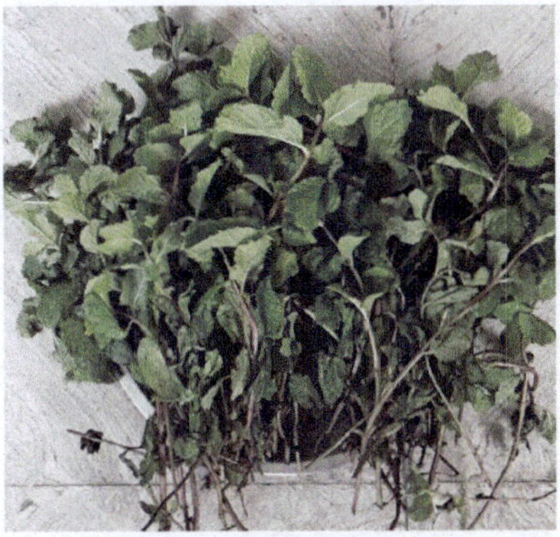

Scientific name: *Mentha piperita*

Common name: Peppermint

Distribution: Europe, North America

Part used: Leaves

Bioactive principles: Menthol

Remarks: Menthol disrupts respiratory and nervous system function in parasites.

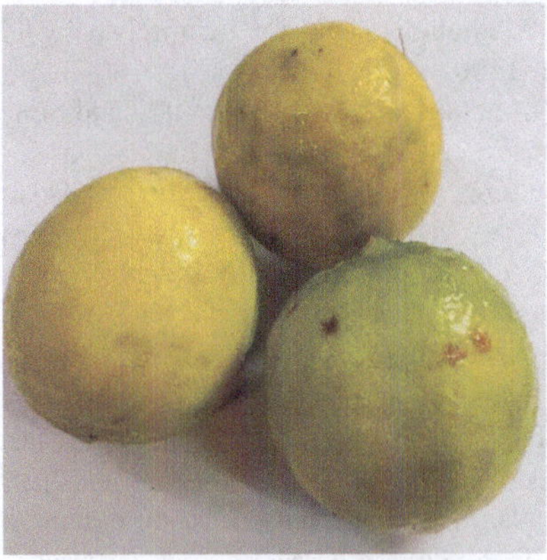

Scientific name: *Citrus limon*

Common name: Lemon

Distribution: Tropical and subtropical regions

Part used: Peels

Bioactive principles: Essential oils

Remarks: Limonene and citral interfere with parasite nervous systems, leading to paralysis and repellence.

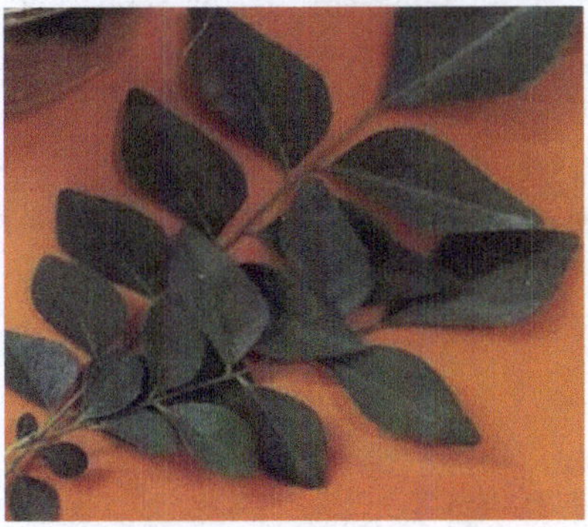

Scientific name: *Murraya koenigii*

Common name: Curry leaves

Distribution: Southeast asia

Part used: Leaves

Bioactive principles: polyphenols, alkaloids and flavonoids

Remarks: Curry leaves possess antioxidant, antimicrobial, antidiabetic, anticancer and hepatoprotective effects.

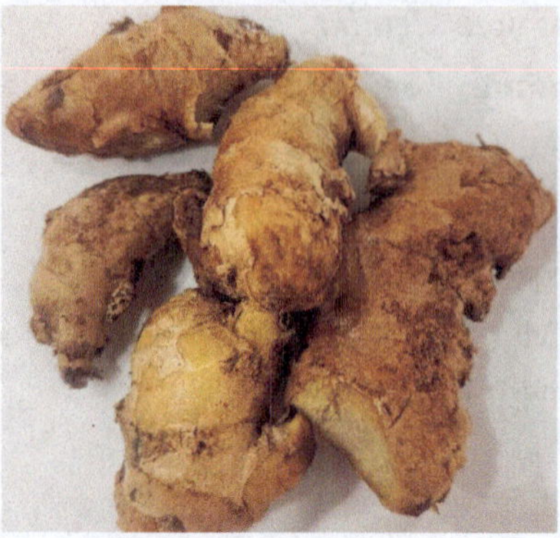

Scientific name: *Zingiber officinale*

Common name: Ginger

Distribution: Indian subcontinent

Part used: Rhizomes

Bioactive principles: Gingerol

Remarks: Gingerol and zingerone disrupt parasite energy metabolism and impair ion transport.

References

Athanasiadou, S., Githiori, J. & Kyriazakis, I., 2007. Medicinal plants for helminth parasite control: facts and fiction. Animal, 1(9), pp.1392–1400.

Cremlyn, R., 1978. Pesticides – Preparation and mode of action. New York: J. Wiley and Sons Limited.

de Silva, L.C.D., Perinotto, W.M.S., Sá, F.A., Souza, M.A.A., Bitencourt, R.O.B., Sanavria, A., Santos, H.A., Marie-Magdeleine, C. & Angelo, I.C., 2020. In vitro acaricidal activity of Cymbopogon citratus, Cymbopogon nardus, and Mentha arvensis against Rhipicephalus microplus (Acari: Ixodidae). Experimental Parasitology, 216, p.107937. Available at: https://doi.org/10.1016/j.exppara.2020.107937.

Jamil, D., Idress, A., Qadir, Z. & Imran, F., 2022. Medical and veterinary ectoparasites' importance: An insight on alternative control. Pakistan Journal of Medical and Health Sciences, 16, pp.667–673.

Ketzis, J.K., 2024. Ectoparasiticides used in large animals. MSD Veterinary Manual. Available at: https://www.msdvetmanual.com [Accessed 29 November 2024].

Mansingh, A. & Williams, L.A.D., 1998. Pesticidal potential of tropical plants: II. Acaricidal activity of crude extracts of several Jamaican plants. Insect Science and its Application, 18(2), pp.149–155.

Morton, J.F., 1981. Atlas of medicinal plants of Middle America: Bahamas to Yucatan. Springfield, IL: C.C. Thomas. Available at: https://doi.org/10.1016/0378-8741(82)90062-9.

Sanhokwe, M., Mupangwa, J., Masika, P.J., Maphosa, V. & Muchenje, V., 2016. Medicinal plants used to control internal and external parasites in goats. Onderstepoort Journal of Veterinary Research, 83(1), p.a1016. Available at: https://doi.org/10.4102/ojvr.v83i1.1016.

10

Medicinal Plants Effective in Gastrointestinal System Disorders in Animals

Jeevan Ranjan Dash

Department of Veterinary Pharmacology & Toxicology, College of Veterinary Science & Animal Husbandry, Odisha University of Agriculture & Technology Bhubaneswar-751003, Odisha

Our digestive structure is not only just a food handle centre. It's a foundation of fitness, moving everything from our immunity to mental well-being. A fit gut aids in the digesting and assimilation of nutrients supports a healthy and strong immunity, and helps in the effective elimination of waste. Asserting good gut fitness is critical because it can influence our whole body's health, prevent chronic afflictions, and develop value of growth. Plants have been second-hand for curative purposes for thousands of years, and many up-to-date cures are still coming from plant compounds. In this chapter, we will study some commonly used medicinal plants used to treat common digestive system diseases, along with associated ethnomedicinal details.

1. Diarrohea

About the condition/Definition- Loose, watery and possibly more-frequent passage of stool is called diarrohea. Feeling of urgent need of frequent bowel movement in a day.

Etiology- A few causes include infections, diseases, and food intolerances. Rotavirus, norovirus, viral gastroenteritis; salmonella, *E. coli*; giardiasis, amoebiasis and food intolerance are few important causes of diarrohea.

Symptoms- The symptoms include a strong desire to have bowel movement and frequent loose, watery feces. Occasionally linked to cramps, bloating, thirst, nausea, and abdominal pain.

Pathogenesis- Diarrhea etiology has been linked to a number of factors, including altered intestinal transit, osmotic, inflammatory, secretory, and loss of functional absorptive area.

General treatment- Most cases of sudden diarrhoea clear on their own within a couple of days without treatment.

Sufficient boiled water for rehydration.

Electrolyte or fluid replacement - oral rehydration solutions (ORS), like Pedialyte, for babies with diarrhoea. Juices made from 100% fruits and vegetables like lemon juice, sugarcane juice, coconut water etc.

Antibiotics- When the diarrohea is due to infectious origin antibiotics like loperamide (Imodium) is used.

Herbal treatment

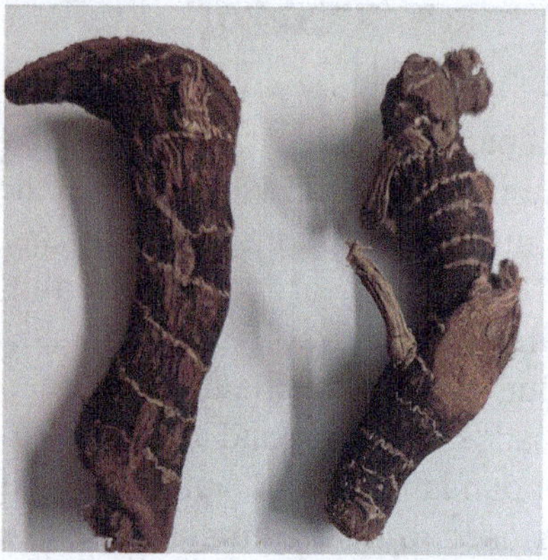

Scientific name: *Acorus calamus* L.

Common name: Sweet Flag (English), Boch (Assamese), Gorbach (Hindi)

Distribution: In India found in different parts of Assam, different parts of Kerala like Kottayam, Alappuzha, Idukki, Thiruvananthapuram, Kozhikkode, Wayanad, Thrissur, Ernakulam, Palakkad, Malappuram etc.

Part used: Rhizome

Bioactive principles: leaves and rhizomes contain a volatile oil that contain beta-asarone , methyl isoeugenol and alpha-asarone,

Remark: Root stock pounded with rock salt and mixed wit water can be used to treat diarrohea.

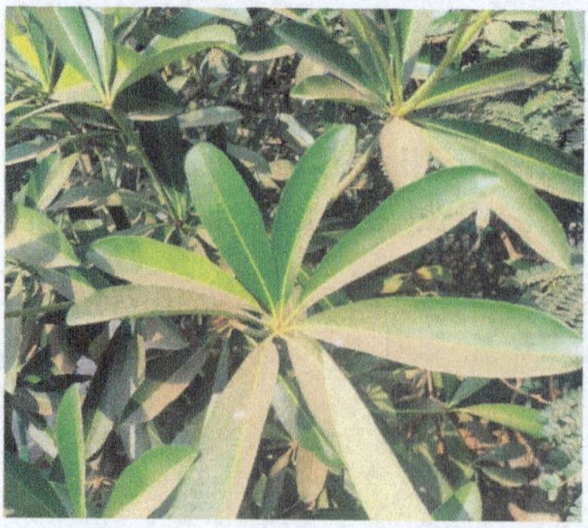

Scientific name: *Alstonia scholaris* (L.) R. Br.

Common name: Devil Tree (English), Shaitan Ka Jhar (Hindi)

Distribution: Distributed globally in South and South East Asia to Australia. In India found in Assam, Karnataka, Kerala, Tamil Nadu, Gujarat, Odisha and Uttar Pradesh

Part used: Bark and leaves.

Bioactive principles: Scholaricine, 19-epischolaricine, Picrinine and Vallesamine are some of the active principles isolated from the bark and leaves of *Alstonia scholaris* (L.) R. Br.

Remarks: Crushed stem bark can be given to cure diarrhoea.

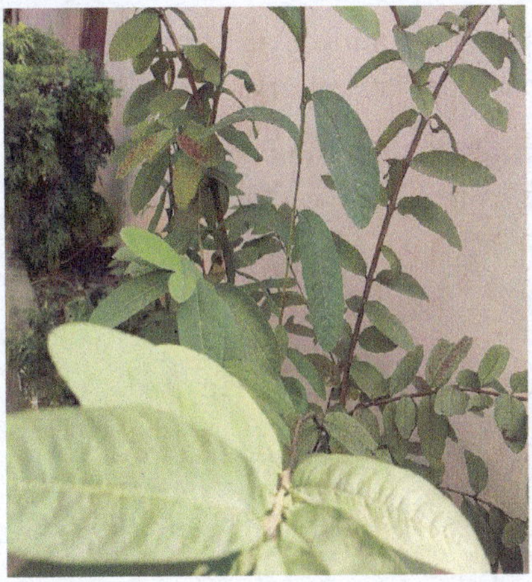

Scientific name: *Psidium guajava* L.

Common name: Guava (English), Amrood (Hindi), Pijuli (Odia)

Distribution: It is originally from South America, Central America and the Caribbean before spreading to other parts of the world including India.

Part used: Leaves, fruits and bark

Bioactive principles: lectin

Remarks: To treat diarrhoea, the bark and leaves of guava can be decocted and taken.

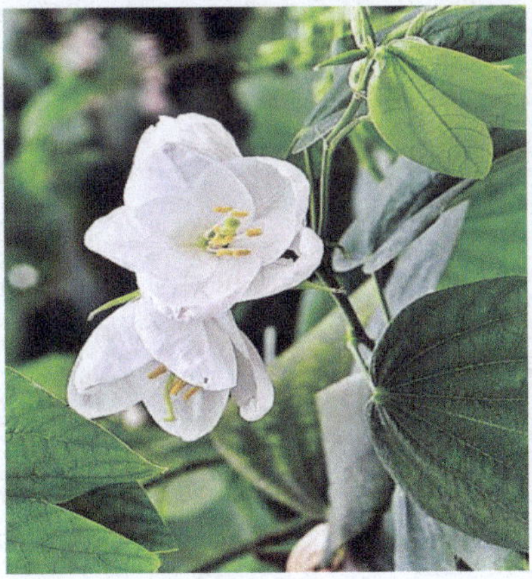

Scientific name: *Bauhinia acuminata* L.

Common name: Safed Kachnar (Hindi), Dhala Kanchan (Odia)

Distribution: mainly in the Southeast Asia such as Philippines, Indonesia, Bangladesh and Malaysia.

Part used: Leaves

Bioactive principles: Ursolic acid, Phthalic acid, Gallic acid and Palmitic acid.

Remarks: The leaves of guava can be decocted and taken to control diarrhoea.

2. Bloody Disentry

About the condition/Definition- One gastrointestinal ailment is dysentery. It results in severe bowel movements with mucus or blood in it.

Etiology- Infections with bacteria or parasites are among its causes. Two primary forms of dysentery exist: 1) Entamoeba histolytica and Balantidium coli (B. coli) are the causes of amoebic dysentery, sometimes known as amoebiasis. 2) Shigella, Salmonella, Campylobacter, and Escherichia coli are the causes of bacillary dysentery.

Symptoms- Weight loss, nausea, vomiting, diarrhea, and upset stomach are some of the mild symptoms of amoebic dysentery.

Bloody or mucus-filled diarrhea, a high temperature, nausea and vomiting, and painful stomach cramps are some signs of bacillary dysentery.

Pathogenesis- The pathogen penetrates the intestinal epithelial cells and found free in the cytoplasm, causes death of the epithelium and cause ulcerative lesion.

General Treatment

For the treatment of parasitic infections, use metronidazole (Flagyl®).

Antibiotics such as Rifaximim, Ciprofloxacin, Levofloxacin, and Azythromycin.

OTC non-steroidal anti-inflammatory drugs (NSAIDs), such as acetaminophen and ibuprofen, are used to treat fever and pain.

Suggest over-the-counter (OTC) drugs, such as bismuth subsalicylate, to alleviate nausea.

Herbal Treatment

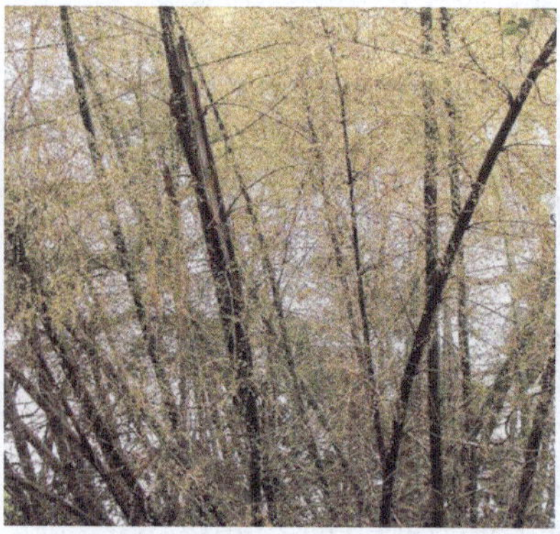

Scientific name: *Bambusa arundinacea* (Retz.) Willd.

Common name: Indian thorny bamboo (English), khare bans (Bengali), KantaBaunsa(Odia)

Distribution: It is common throughout the plains of India and in Myanmar, Bangladesh and Sri Lanka.

Part used: Leaves

Bioactive principles: Stigmast-5, 22-dien-3β-ol, Stigmast-5-en-3β-ol-β-D glucopyranoside

Remarks: Finely cut leaves are fed to the cattle to control blood dysentery.

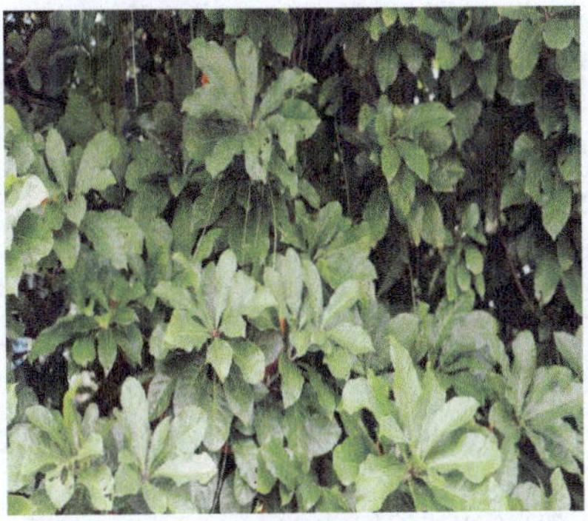

Scientific name: *Barringtonia acutangula* (L.) Gaertn.

Common name: Samudraphal/Indian Putat/ Indian Oak

Distribution: This 9–12 m tall evergreen tree is widespread in the sub-Himalayan regions from the Ganges east to Assam, as well as in Madhya Pradesh and the Indian peninsula.

Part used: Leaves

Bioactive principles: barringtogenic acid, tangulic and acutangulic acids

Remarks: Crushed leaves used to treat dysentery of cow.

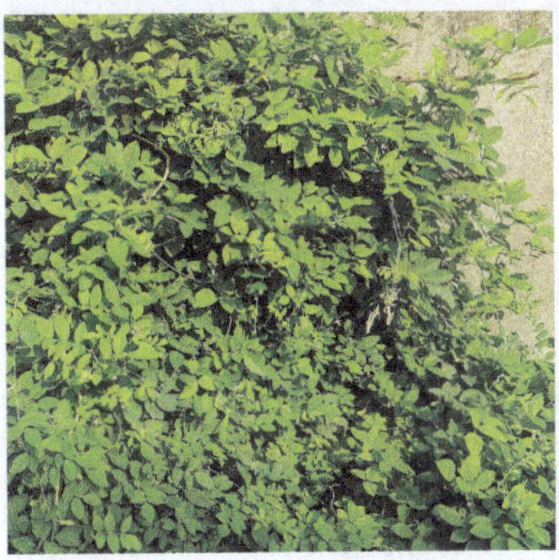

Scientific name: *Clitoria ternatea* L.

Common name: Aparajita/Asian pegionwings/Blue pea

Distribution: Global distribution. It was originated in tropical Asia and has since spread to various regions, including Africa, Asia, Australia, North America.

Part used: Leaves

Bioactive principles: Tannic acid, β-Sitosterol, p-hydroxycinnamic acid

Remarks: Leaf paste with jiggery used to treat dysentery of cow.

Reference: Manalisha Deka. International research journal of pharmacy. 2000; (12): 13c9-140.

3. Peptic Ulcer

About the condition/Definition- Peptic ulcer disease is characterized by the development of ulcers (open sores) in the gastrointestinal tract lining. “Peptic” indicates that it has to do with digestion.

Etiology- The stomach and duodenum are the most common sites of peptic ulcer disease. 2) Approximately 20% of peptic ulcers are stomach ulcers, and almost 80% are duodenal stomach ulcers. Overuse of NSAIDs and H. pylori infection are the two main causes of peptic ulcer disorders.

Symptoms- Upper abdominal pain and indigestion. Gnawing sensation (burning sensation in the stomach). If complicated black and tarry stool seen due to gastrointestinal bleeding.

Pathogenesis- Overgrowth of helicobacter infection invoke chronic inflammation in the gastrointestinal lining causing sores. Excess and unregulated use of NSAIDs inhibits prostaglandin that repairs damage to intestinal linings. Chemotherapy and radiation therapy also cause peptic ulcer.

General Treatment

Proton pump inhibitors like- Esomeprazole, Lansoprazole etc.

H2 blockers like Famotidine, Cimetidine etc.

Antibiotics like doxycycline, Clarithromycin etc. if helicobacter infection.

Cytoprotective drugs like sucralfate, bismuth subsalicylate.

Non-NSAID pain relivers like acetaminophen.

Herbal Treatment

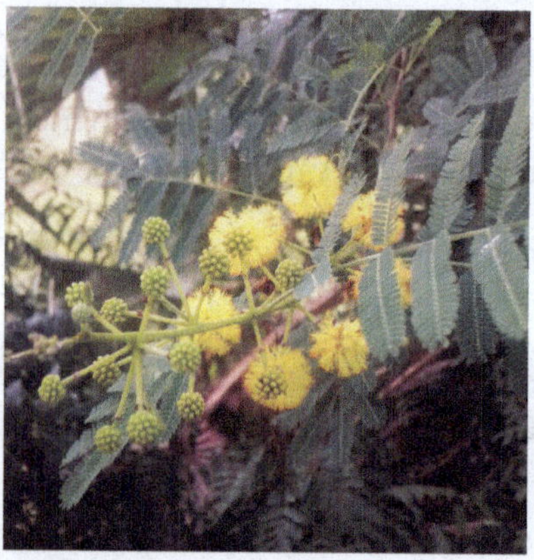

Scientific name: *Acacia arabica*

Common name: Indian gum tree, Babul

Distribution: It is native to Indian subcontinent

Part used: Leaves, Bark, Gum

Bioactive principles: Catechin, epigallocatechin, epicatechin gallate, epigallocatechin

Remarks: Bark decoction is used to treat ulcers, Gum from the bark is used as a natural astringent and antiulcer property.

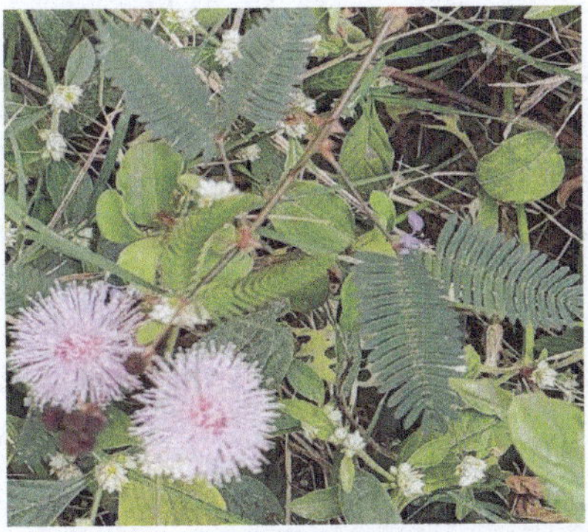

Scientific name: *Acacia catechu*

Common name: Cutch tree , Khair (Hindi)

Distribution: Found across India. Its primary habitats in the nation are the Himalayan tracts and the eastern slopes of the Western Ghats.

Part used: Bark

Bioactive principles: Catechin, epicatechin, gallate, protocatechuic acid, tannins, alkaloids quercetin and kaempferol.

Remarks: Bark decoction or dried bark powder is used for healing of wounds and ulcers.

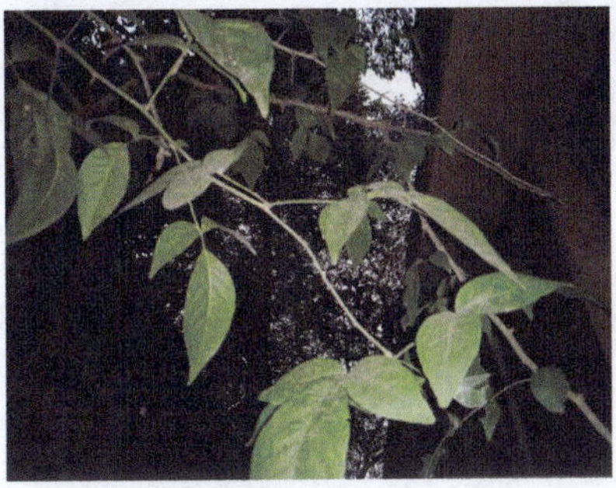

Scientific name: *Aegle marmelos*

Common name: Wood Apple, Bilva/Bael (Hindi)

Distribution: It is originally native to Western Ghats which includes parts of states like Maharashtra, Karnataka, Kerala, and Tamil Nadu. But widely cultivated across different parts of India.

Part used: Leaves, fruit

Bioactive principles: Marmelosin, luvangetin, psoralen, tannins, marmin

Remarks: Dried pulp of Bael fruit is powdered and mixed with arrowroot making it a valuable remedy for digestive issues and general health maintenance. The pale fawn flesh of Bilva fruit has astringent property due to rich tannin content.

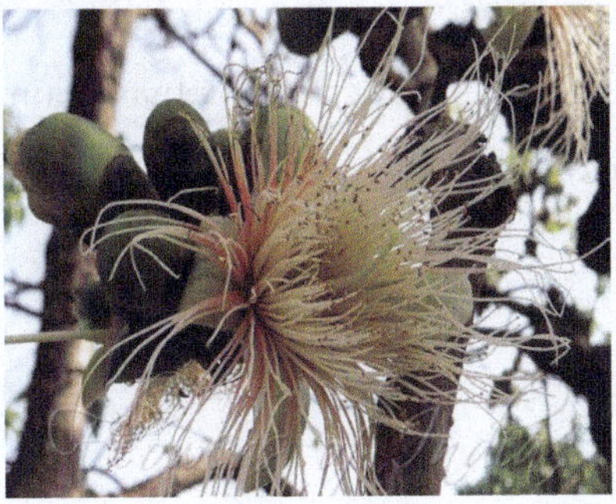

Scientific name: *Careya arborea*

Common name: Wild Guava, Kumbhi (Hindi)

Distribution: Native to the Indian subcontinent, Afghanistan and Indochina

Part used: Leaves, Bark

Bioactive principles: Bark contain Lupeol, Beutilin. Leaves contain malinic acid, 2-hydroxy ursolic acid, tannin.

Remarks: The bark of the tree are valued for their astringent and mucilaginous properties. Ethanolic extract of leaves has been said to have gastroprotective effect on different gastric ulcer models.

4. Constipation

About the condition/Definition- Dry and hard bowel movement. Passing of stool less than three times a week is constipation

Etiology- Diet with low fibre content, meat, milk, or cheese etc.

Inadequate water intake

Pregnancy

Old age

Delayed impulse to have a bowel movement may be due to medication/ change in routine /travel

Symptoms- Less than tree bowel movements in a week

Voiding of hard and dry stool

Painful bowel movement

Feeling fullness of stomach and urge for bowel movement even after having a bowel movement

Pathogenesis- Adequate water and fiber content in food keeps the stool soft. Thus low fibre dient and junk food usually cause constipation. Prolong stay of stool in the colon make it hard and difficult to pass leading to constipation.

General Treatment

Drink hot water upon awakening and consistently between meals

Avoid consumption of alcohol and caffeinated drinks that causes dehydration

Increase fiber in diet like fruits and vegetables

Avoid processed food

At least 150 minutes of exercise in a week.

Herbal Treatment

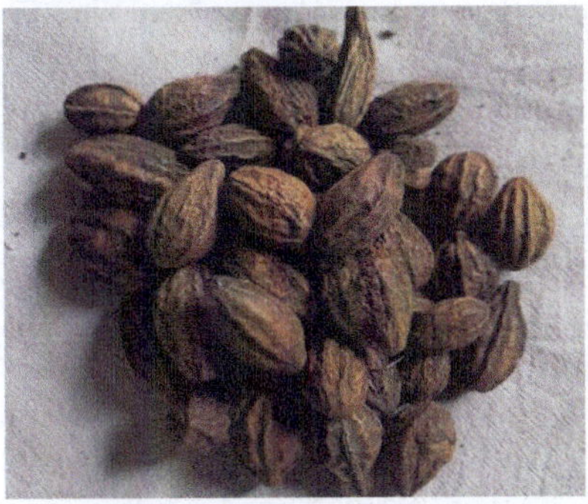

Scientific name: *Terminalia chebula*

Common name: Haritaki, Harad (Hindi)

Distribution: It grows in the deciduous backwoods of Himachal. Pradesh, Tamil Nadu, Kerala, Karnataka, Bihar, Orissa, Maharashtra, Uttar Pradesh, Madhya Pradesh, and West Bengal

Part used: Fruit

Bioactive principles: Ellagic acid, Leuteolin, Chebulinic acid, Corilagin.

Remarks: Haritaki is a safe and effective purgative mild laxative, stomachic. Haritaki churna is effective in constipation and elimination of toxins from the intestines.

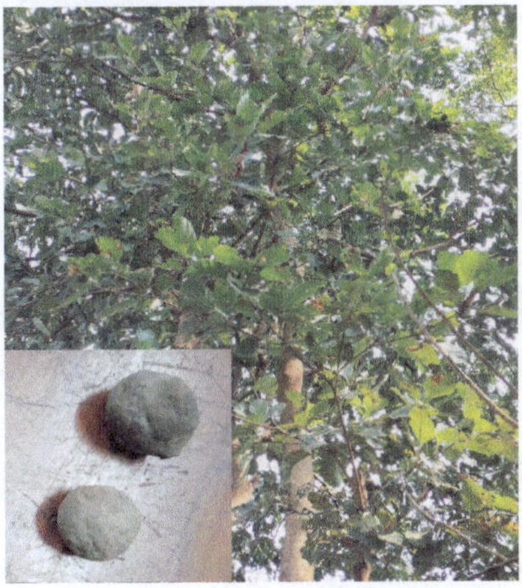

Scientific name: *Terminalia bellerica*

Common name: Bibhitaki, Baheda (Hindi)

Distribution: Bibhitaki is a huge deciduous tree that grows up to 30 meters tall and is found all over India. Madhya Pradesh, Uttar Pradesh, Punjab, and Maharashtra are the states in India where it is most prevalent.

Part used: Fruit rind

Bioactive principles: Chebulagic acid, Phyllemblin, Tannins, Elagic acid.

Remarks: It is a herb of triphala. It is laxative in nature and used in the purgation therapy.

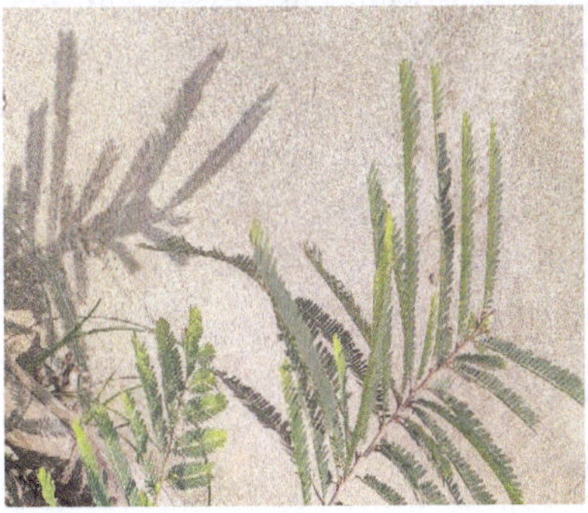

Scientific name: *Emblica officinalis*

Common name: Amla (Hindi)

Distribution: In India, amla is a fairly prevalent plant. The best subtropical regions for amla agriculture are Madhya Pradesh, Rajasthan, Tamil Nadu, and Uttar Pradesh.

Part used: Fruit

Bioactive principles: gallic acid, ellagic acid, chebulinic acid, corilagin

Remarks: It is an herb of triphala. It relieves constipated bowl when taken regularly.

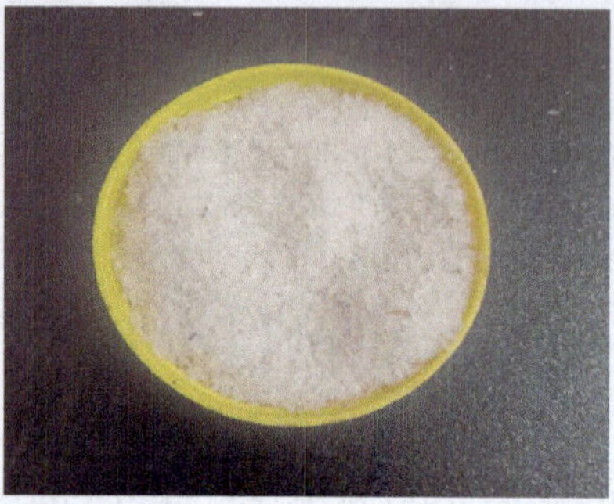

Scientific name: *Plantago ovata*

Common name: Ispaghula

Distribution: South Rajasthan, Punjab, and Gujarat are where the plant is most commonly grown.

Part used: Seeds and husk

Bioactive principles: husk contain mucilage.

Remarks: Psyllium is a laxative that forms bulk. Its primary function as dietary fiber is to alleviate the symptoms of moderate diarrhoea and constipation.

5. Dyspepsia or Indigestion

About the condition/Definition- It is discomfort in your upper abdomen.

Etiology- Eating a large or fatty meal is usually the cause of occasional indigestion.

Lifestyle choices such as overeating, eating too quickly, and consuming foods that are difficult for your body to digest; medical problems such as GERD, ulcers, hyperchlorhydria, and irritable bowel syndrome (IBS).

Symptoms- Some symptoms, like stomach pain and a feeling of fullness shortly after eating, are referred to as indigestion. Additional symptoms include gas, burping, and bloating. nausea, regurgitation, somehow Heartburn and acid reflux, your stomach growling or gurgling loudly.

Pathogenesis- There are multiple causes of indigestion. The most common cause is particular foods and drinks that can aggravate the lining of the stomach such as spicy foods, alcohol and caffeine. Stress and anxiety can also result in the increased production of gastric acids that cause indigestion. Physical causes such as obesity and pregnancy can also result in increased pressure in the stomach leading to indigestion. It's important to exclude medications such as non-steroidal anti-inflammatories as a potential cause.

General treatment- Avoid foods that cause indigestion

Over-the-counter (OTC) or prescription medicines like antacids (Sodium bicarbonate, Simethicone etc.), H2 blockers (Cimetidine, Famotidine etc.),

Proton pump inhibitors (Esomeprazole, Lansoprazole etc.), Prokinetics (Metoclopramide, Bethanechol etc.)

Herbal Treatment

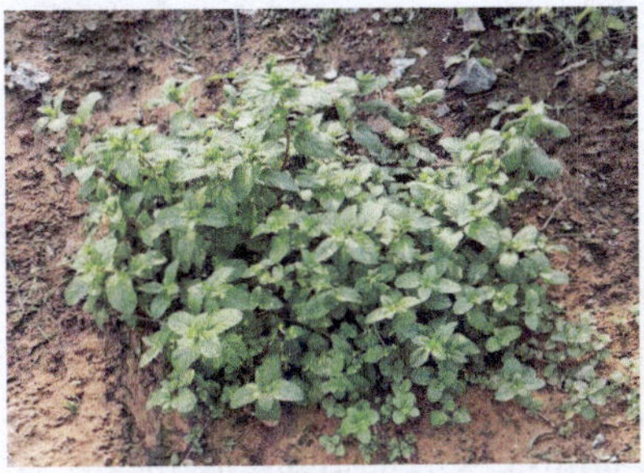

Scientific name: *Mentha piperita* L.

Common name: Pippermint/Mentha, Pudina

Distribution: It is said that mint began in the Mediterranean region and then expanded, both naturally and artificially, over the rest of the world. It is widely grown in Punjab and Uttar Pradesh, India.

Part used: Leaves

Bioactive principles: Menthol, Menthone.

Remarks: Mint leaves are renowned for being a delicious appetizer. Through the stimulation of digestive enzymes, it aids in the promotion of the digestive system. Because of its antibacterial and antiseptic qualities, mint oil can help with stomach infections and indigestion. Because it contains methanol, it has anti-spasmodic properties.

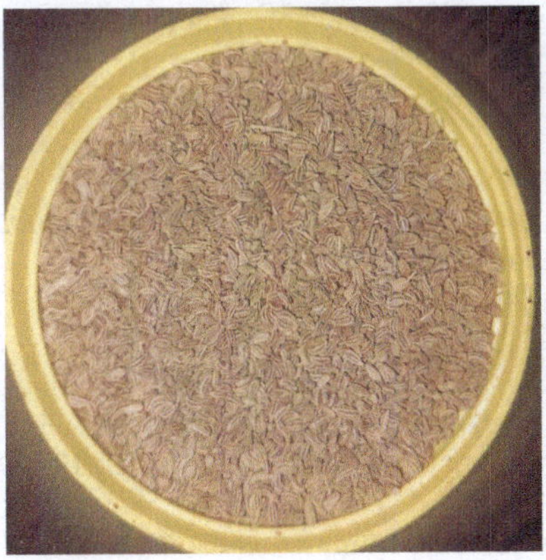

Scientific name: *Trachyspermum Ammi*

Common name: Ajwain

Distribution: It is an indigenous herb in Egypt. All across the world, this herb is commonly available. Rajasthan, West Bengal, Maharashtra, Gujarat, Punjab, Bihar, Uttar Pradesh, and Madhya Pradesh are among the Indian states where it is grown.

Part used: Seeds

Bioactive principles: carvacrol, thymol, p-cymene

Remarks: It helps with indigestion and stomach pain. Because of its protease action, it functions as a digestive tonic and is useful in treating issues with the stomach and small intestine.

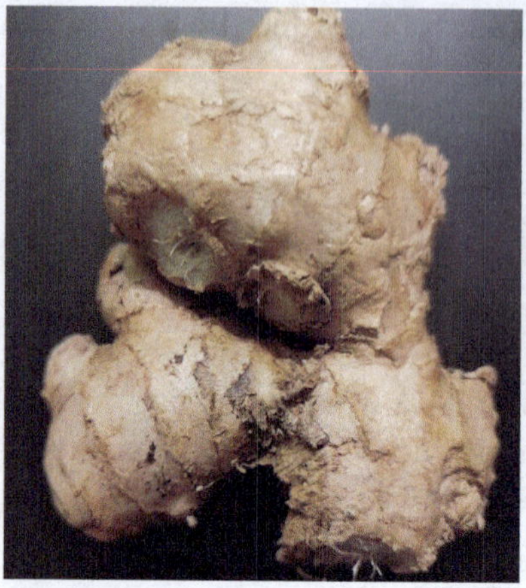

Scientific name: *Zingiber officinale*

Common name: Ginger, Adrakh

Distribution: Southern India, China

Part used: Rhizome

Bioactive principles: zingiberene, zingerone, gingerols

Remarks: Reduce gas and bloating by improving stomach emptying. Supplementing with ginger was associated with a decrease in heartburn, nausea, bloating, belching, and stomach pain.

Conclusion

Ancient cultures have long practiced herbal medicine, which focuses the use of plants to cure diseases and improve overall condition and well-being. Considering the fact that many herbs include strong active elements, certain medical products are made from these organic compounds, thus they should be used with the same precaution as pharmaceutical drugs.

References

Das BM, Barat SK. (1954). Astringency of some common Indian vegetable tanning materials. (Myrobalans), Osterr. Lederzig., Chern. Abstr., 48 (22): 47-51.

Gholkar MS, Mulik MB, Laddha KS. (2013). Fate of β-asarone in Ayurvedic sodhana process of vacha. J Ayurveda Integr Med.4(1):19-22.

Islam, M. N., Reyad-ul-Ferdous, M., Fahad, M. A. B., Hossain, M. R. and Mukti, M. (2014), In-vivo Antidiarrheal and In-vitro Antimicrobial Activities of the Leaf Extracts of Bauhinia acuminata, American Journal of Research Communication, pp. 158 -166.

Kamath JV, Rahul N, Kumar CKA, Lakshmi SM. (2014). Psidium guajava L: A review, International Journal of Green Pharmacy, pp. 9-11.

Panda SK, Nirvanashetty S, Parachur VA, et al. (2022). A randomized, double-blind, placebo-controlled, parallel-group, comparative clinical study to evaluate the efficacy and safety of OLNP-06 versus placebo in subjects with functional dyspepsia. J Diet Suppl. 19(2): 226-237.

Rita P., Animesh D.K. (2011). An Updated overview of Peppermint (Mentha Piperita L.), International Research Journal of Pharmacy. 2(8): 1-10.

Scartezzini P, Antognoni F, Raggi MA, Poli F, Sabbioni C. (2006). Vitamin C content and antioxidant activity of the fruit and of the Ayurvedic preparation of Emblica officinalis Gaertn, Journal of Ethnopharmacology, 104(1-2), 113-8.

Vimala G, Shoba FG. (2014). A Review on Antiulcer Activity of Few Indian Medicinal Plants. International Journal of Microbiology. 2014: 1-14.

Zhao L, Cao J, Shang JH, Liu YP, Khan A, et al. (2017). Airways antiallergic effect and pharmacokinetics of alkaloids from Alstonia scholaris. Phytomedicine, 27: 63-75.

11

Medicinal Plants Effective in Cardiovascular System Disorders in Animals

Matsyagandha K Patil

Department of Veterinary Pharmacology and Toxicology, College of Veterinary and Animal Sciences, Udgir-413517, Latur, Maharashtra
Maharashtra Animal and Fishery Sciences University, Nagpur, Maharashtra

Cardiovascular System Disorders in Domestic Animals

Cardiovascular system disorders in domestic animals include a range of conditions that affect the heart (pericardium, myocardium, endocardium), veins, arteries and lymphatic vessels. Infectious disorders like Heartworms (*Dirofilaria immitis*, vegetative endocarditis in pigs, equine viral arteritis). Patency of the foramen ovale, interventricular foramena, patent ductus arteriosus, persistence of the right aortic arch, coarctation of the aorta, transposition of the aorta, congenital aneurysm, pulmonic stenosis, subaortic stenosis, ectopia cardis, acardia, and diplocardia are examples of congenital and developmental disorders that can result in these conditions. Traumatic disorders like Traumatic reticulopericarditis and cardiac failure. Degenerative diseases like fatty and hyaline degeneration. Inflammatory disorders like pericarditis, myocarditis, endocarditis and phlebitis may also lead to cardiovascular system disorders. Some tumours associated with the cardiovascular system like rhabdomyosarcoma, fibroma and myxofibroma also cause cardiovascular system disorders.

Cardiovascular System Disorders Induced in Lab Animals

Laboratory animals are used to study cardiovascular system problems in order to test medications, comprehend disease mechanisms, and create remedies. The choice of model, method of induction, and animal species depends on the specific cardiovascular condition being studied. An outline of how cardiovascular diseases are created in lab animals can be seen below.

1. Hypertension

Pharmacological Models: Administration of drugs like angiotensin II, norepinephrine, or DOCA-salt (deoxycorticosterone acetate combined with high salt intake) to induce high blood pressure.

Renal Models: Surgical procedures like the two-kidney, one-clip (2K1C) or one-kidney, one-clip (1K1C) methods. These involve partially constricting the renal artery to simulate renovascular hypertension.

Dietary Models: Feeding animals high-salt diets to increase blood pressure.

Common Animals: Rats (e.g., Sprague Dawley, Wistar), mice.

2. Atherosclerosis

Dietary Models: High-fat, high-cholesterol diets induce plaque buildup in arteries.

Genetic Models: Use of genetically modified animals, such as ApoE-deficient or LDL receptor-deficient mice, which are prone to developing atherosclerosis.

Mechanical Injury: Inducing endothelial damage using balloon catheterization or wire injury to simulate plaque formation.

Common Animals: Mice, rabbits, pigs.

3. Myocardial Infarction (Heart Attack)

Surgical Models: Ligation (tying off) of the left anterior descending (LAD) coronary artery in rodents to mimic a heart attack.

Ischemia-Reperfusion (I/R) Models: Temporarily occluding the coronary artery, followed by reperfusion, simulating the restoration of blood flow after a heart attack.

Cryoinjury: Application of a freezing probe to the heart surface to cause localized tissue death.

Common Animals: Rats, mice, pigs.

4. Heart Failure

Post-Myocardial Infarction: Animals that survive induced myocardial infarction often develop heart failure.

Pressure Overload Models: Techniques like transverse aortic constriction (TAC) or pulmonary artery banding to increase pressure in the heart.

Volume Overload Models: Creating arteriovenous fistulas to increase blood volume and induce heart failure.

Common Animals: Rats, mice, dogs.

5. Arrhythmias

Pharmacological Models: Administration of drugs like isoproterenol or aconitine to induce abnormal heart rhythms.

Electrical Stimulation: Using pacemakers or direct current shocks to disrupt normal electrical activity.

Genetic Models: Mutant animals with specific ion channel defects (e.g., KCNQ1 or SCN5A mutations) to study inherited arrhythmias.

Common Animals: Rats, mice, rabbits.

6. Pulmonary Hypertension

Hypoxia-Induced Models: Exposing animals to low-oxygen environments to cause pulmonary hypertension.

Pharmacological Models: Use of monocrotaline, a toxic alkaloid, to induce damage to the pulmonary vasculature.

Surgical Models: Banding of the pulmonary artery to create pressure overload.

Common Animals: Rats, mice.

7. Heart Valve Disease

Endocarditis Models: Infusion of bacteria (e.g., Staphylococcus aureus) to induce infection of heart valves.

Calcification Models: Use of high-phosphate diets or specific mineralization promoters.

Common Animals: Rabbits, rats, mice.

8. Cardiomyopathy

Chemical Models: Administration of drugs like doxorubicin (Adriamycin) to induce toxic cardiomyopathy.

Genetic Models: Animals with mutations in sarcomeric proteins (e.g., troponins, myosin-binding proteins) to study hypertrophic or dilated cardiomyopathy.

Autoimmune Models: Inducing myocarditis using cardiac myosin immunization to model autoimmune-mediated cardiomyopathy.

Common Animals: Rats, mice, rabbits.

9. Thrombosis and Stroke

Chemical Models: Injection of thrombogenic agents like ferric chloride or collagen to induce blood clots.

Mechanical Models: Occlusion of arteries using embolic materials or ligation.

Genetic Models: Animals lacking anticoagulant proteins (e.g., antithrombin III).

Common Animals: Rats, mice, rabbits.

These models have contributed significantly to understanding cardiovascular disease and developing effective treatments, though the welfare of laboratory animals remains a priority in research.

Drugs Used to Treat Cardiovascular System Disorder

Many drugs used to treat cardiovascular system disorders. On the basis of mechanism of action of drugs, these are classified as Diuretic (Furosemide, Spironolactone, Hydrochlorothiazide), ACE Inhibitors (Enalapril, Benazepril), Angiotensin II Receptor Blockers (Telmisartan), Positive Inotropes (Pimobendan, Dobutamine, Digoxin), Beta-Blockers (Atenolol, Propranolol, Carvedilol), Calcium Channel Blockers (Amlodipine, Diltiazem), Antiarrhythmic Drugs (Lidocaine, Sotalol, Amiodarone, Mexiletine), Vasodilators (Nitroglycerin, Hydralazine, Sodium Nitroprusside), Anticoagulants and Antiplatelet Drugs (Aspirin, Clopidogrel, Heparin), Anti-Heartworm Drugs (Melarsomine, Ivermectin/Moxidectin), Hypertension-Specific Drugs (Amlodipine, ACE Inhibitors, Telmisartan), Antioxidants and Supplements (Omega-3 Fatty Acids, Taurine, L-Carnitine)

Cardioprotective Medicinal Plants

Numerous epidemiologic studies demonstrate that diets high in fruits and vegetables, or foods high in antioxidants, are linked to a lower incidence of cardiovascular diseases. The presence of phytonutrients such as carotenoids, cardiac glycosides, alkaloids, flavonoids, polyphenolic compounds, saponins, terpenoids [triterpenes], and fatty acids in many plants is thought to be the cause of their strong cardio-protective effects, according to traditional Indian medicine. Ayurveda has mentioned as different plants used to treat or prevent cardiovascular disorders ex: atherosclerosis, hypertension, myocardial infarction, arrhythmia, thrombosis, etc.

Cardiovascular Disorders

Atherosclerosis is caused by thickening of the artery walls due to deposition of fatty material and therefore affects the blood flow through the arterial blood vessels. It is also known as Arteriosclerotic Vascular Disease or ASVD. Low density lipoprotein promotes accumulation of macrophages that leads to a chronic inflammation of arterial walls and hardening of arteries.

Causes: Damage or injury to an artery's inner layer is the first step toward atherosclerosis. High blood pressure, high cholesterol, irritants like nicotine, and certain illnesses like diabetes can all contribute to the damage.

Pathophysiology: When endothelial damage occurs, the artery wall's chronic inflammatory reaction results in atherosclerosis. T-lymphocytes, monocyte-derived macrophages, changed lipoproteins, and the normal cellular component of the artery wall interact to cause the progression of lesions. The response-to-injury hypothesis is a statement of the modern perspective on atherosclerosis. The hypothesis involves the following steps: factor release, platelet adhesion, monocyte adhesion to the endothelium, buildup of lipoproteins, chronic endothelial damage, SMC proliferations, and the creation of extracellular matrix (ECM).

Medications: Anticoagulants (heparin, Coumadin), high density lipoproteins, blood pressure drugs (beta blockers, angiotensin-converting enzyme (ACE) inhibitors), calcium channel blockers, and antiplatelet drugs (aspirin).

Pulmonary Hypertension (PH): An increase in blood pressure within the pulmonary arteries, which transport blood from the heart to the lungs. The elevated pressure can hinder the ability of the right side of the heart to pump blood effectively, leading to further complications such as right-sided heart failure.

Causes : A variety of underlying conditions can lead to pulmonary hypertension in dogs. Some common causes include: Heartworm Disease, congenital heart defects, Left-sided heart disease and respiratory diseases can raise pulmonary vascular resistance.

Symptoms: Common signs include: exercise intolerance (dogs may exhibit reluctance to engage in physical activity), difficult breathing, cyanosis, fainting episodes.

Medications: Drugs like sildenafil (Viagra) and tadalafil (Cialis) are commonly prescribed as they help dilate pulmonary arteries, reducing pressure. Additionally, treating underlying conditions such as heartworm or congestive heart failure is crucial.

Cardiomyopathy: refers to various heart muscle diseases that affect both dogs and cats. This condition can lead to severe complications, including heart failure and arrhythmias, and may require prompt diagnosis and treatment.

Types of Cardiomyopathy : There are several types of cardiomyopathy observed in veterinary medicine, dilated cardiomyopathy (DCM), hypertrophic cardiomyopathy (HCM), and restrictive cardiomyopathy (RCM).

Breeds such as Doberman Pinschers, Great Danes, and Boxers are particularly predisposed to dilated cardiomyopathy. Hypertrophic cardiomyopathy is more common in cats, especially among breeds like the Maine Coon and Ragdoll.

Causes : vary widely. Genetic predispositions (DCM), Nutritional deficiencies, particularly in taurine and carnitine, are known to contribute to this condition, especially in certain breeds. Infectious agents, toxins, and secondary effects from other diseases can also contribute to the onset of cardiomyopathy in pets.

Symptoms: Common symptoms include lethargy, decreased appetite, coughing, difficulty breathing, and episodes of fainting or collapsing due to arrhythmias. In cats, rapid breathing and paralysis due to thromboembolism may indicate more severe complications of cardiomyopathy.

Medications: ACE inhibitors, diuretics, and positive inotropes like pimobendan, which enhance heart function.

Thrombosis and Stroke

The partial or total blockage of a blood artery by a thrombus is known as thrombosis, which can lead to ischemia or tissue damage. In animals, thrombosis can occur in both arterial and venous systems. Stroke, or cerebral vascular accident, refers to a sudden disruption of blood flow to the brain, effects in neurological deficits. Ischemic strokes, caused by thromboembolism, are more common than hemorrhagic strokes, which involve bleeding into the brain.

Causes: Underlying Diseases (hyperadrenocorticism, heart disease and immune-mediated disorders increase stroke risk), Age and Breed Predilections (Certain breeds, such as Cavalier King Charles Spaniels and Greyhounds, exhibit a higher incidence of strokes), Environmental Factors (stress and environmental changes can trigger thrombotic events, particularly in susceptible animals).

Clinical Signs: Neurological Symptoms (difficulty walking, head tilt, and personality changes)

Medications: Anticoagulants, thrombolytics , antiplatelet drugs.

Heart valve disease, often referred to as degenerative mitral valve disease (MVD) in dogs, predominantly impacts the mitral valve situated between the left atrium and left ventricle. This degenerative process results in the valve not closing effectively, allowing blood to flow backward into the heart. This leakage, known as regurgitation, can cause various heart-related problems, including heart murmurs and congestive heart failure (CHF).

Causes: commonly associated with aging and genetic predispositions in certain breeds. Factors contributing to the development of MVD include: Age (Older dogs are at great risk, particularly those over the age of 5 years), Breed (Specific breeds such as Cavalier King Charles Spaniels, Dachshunds, and Cocker Spaniels are more commonly affected), Sex (MVD is often reported to be more prevalent in male dogs compared to females).

Signs and Symptoms: Heart Murmurs: The earliest indicator of mitral valve disease, heard upon auscultation, Respiratory Issues: Signs such as coughing, rapid or labored breathing can indicate the development of CHF due to fluid build-up in the lungs, Exercise Intolerance: Affected dogs may tire quickly and exhibit reduced activity levels, Advanced Symptoms: As the disease progresses, dogs may develop severe conditions like ascites, an enlarged abdomen, or sudden fainting episodes.

Medications: Such as diuretics to reduce fluid retention, ACE inhibitors to lower blood pressure, and inotropes to improve heart muscle function.

Medicinal Plants

The plants are used to treat or prevent cardiovascular disorders and some of them are as follows.

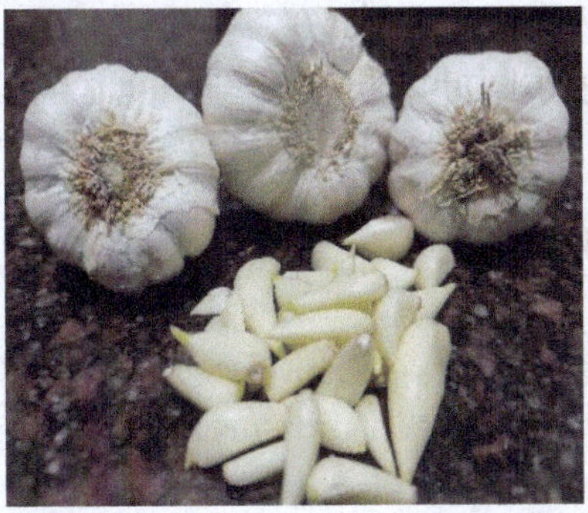

Scientific name: *Allium sativum*

Common name: Garlic

Distribution : Uttar Pradesh, Gujarat, and Punjab, Rajasthan

Part used : Entire garlic bulb

Bioactive principles: Allicin, Allin, Garlic sulfide, S-allyl-cysteine (SAC), diallyl sulfide, diallyl disulfide, and diallyl trisulfide, Ajoene.

Remarks : Garlic known for antioxidant, anti-inflammatory, vasodilatory, blood pressure lowering, reducing cholesterol, anticoagulant, reducing platelet aggregation qualities, and garlic is frequently used in traditional medicine for its ability to enhance heart health and is commonly used to lessen the symptoms of heart valve disease, to reduce the risk of myocardial infarction, helps to control atherosclerosis, to treat arrhythmias and pulmonary hypertension and helps to lower the risk of stroke and thrombosis.

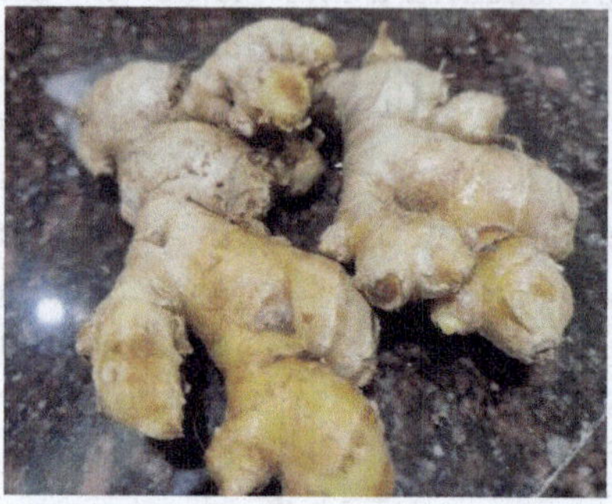

Scientific name: *Zingiber officinale Rosc*

Common name: Ginger

Distribution: Karnataka, Orissa, Assam, Meghalaya, Arunachal Pradesh, and Gujarat.

Part used: Root of the ginger plant

Bioactive principles: Gingerol, shogaol, zingerone, and paradol.

Remarks: Ginger is renowned for its cardioprotective, antioxidant, anti-inflammatory, vasodilatory, anticoagulant, antibacterial and digestive qualities, and helps to lower cholesterol, lower blood pressure, lower the risk of thrombosis and stroke and improves circulation - all of which can promotes heart health in general and possibly assist to manage heart valve disease, helps to control atherosclerosis, support in the treatment of arrhythmias, and helps to manage the symptoms of pulmonary hypertension and myocardial infarction.

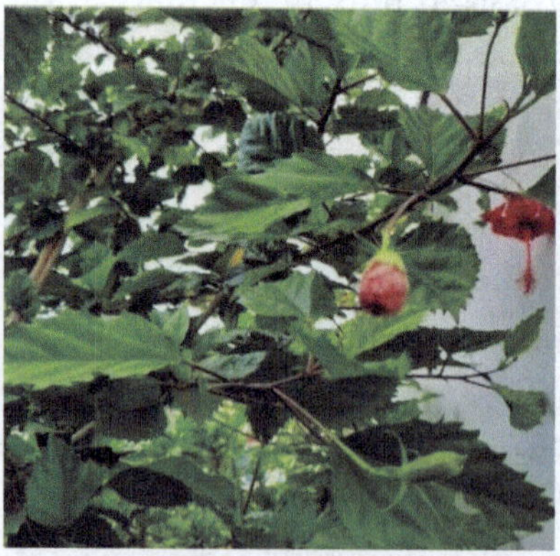

Scientific name: *Hibiscus rosasinesis*

Common name: *Hibiscus*

Distribution: Karnataka, Maharashtra, Kerla, Odisha

Parts used: flower pods, or calyces,

Bioactive principles: flavonoids (quercetin, hibiscetin, and gossypetin), anthocyanins (hibiscin), and organic acids (hydroxycitric and hibiscus)

Remarks: Hibiscus possesses anti-inflammatory, vasodilatory, cholesterol-lowering, and antioxidant qualities. By lowering blood pressure, enhancing circulation, and helping to control heart valve problems, it can promotes heart health.

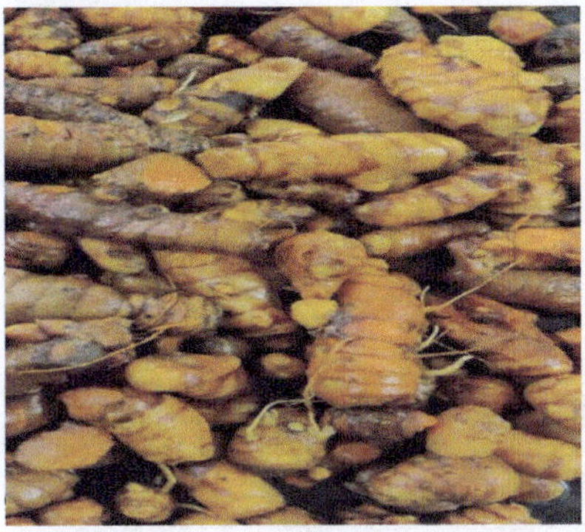

Scientific name: *Curcuma longa*

Common name: turmeric

Distribution : Andhra Pradesh, TamilNadu, Orissa, Karnataka, West Bengal, Gujarat, Meghalaya, Maharashtra.

Parts used: Rhizome

Bioactive principles: Curcumin, Curcuminoids, Zingiberene, Curcumenol, Curcumol, Eugenol, Tetrahydrocurcumin, Triethylcurcumin.

Remarks: Turmeric supports heart valve function and has anti-inflammatory, antioxidant, cardioprotective, lowering oxidative stress and vasodilatory qualities and frequently used to treat wounds, infections, arthritis, and heart diseases like cardiomyopathy, atherosclerosis, myocardial infarction, heart valve disease, pulmonary hypertension by lowering oxidative stress and vascular inflammation. It may strongly supports in preventing thrombosis and reducing stroke risk and promotes heart health.

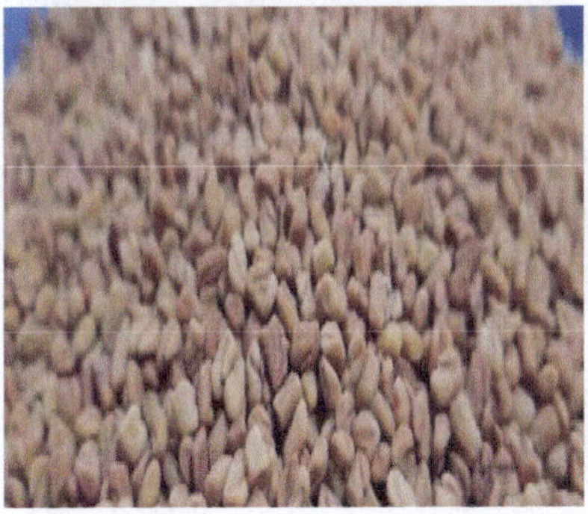

Scientific name : *Trigonella foenum-graecum*

Common name: Fenugreek seeds

Distribution: Maharashtra, Rajasthan, Gujarat, Madhya Pradesh, Uttar Pradesh, and Punjab

Parts used: Seed, Leaves

Bioactive principles: galactomannans, flavonoids, coumarins, saponins, alkaloids, and essential oils,

Remarks : Anti-inflammatory, vasodilatory, antioxidant, cardiotonic, diuretic, control blood sugar levels, improve digestion, anticoagulant, improves circulation and cholesterol-lowering qualities of fenugreek may helps to minimize the risk of atherosclerosis, myocardial infarction, pulmonary hypertension, cardiomyopathy, stroke and thrombosis and enhances cardiovascular health.

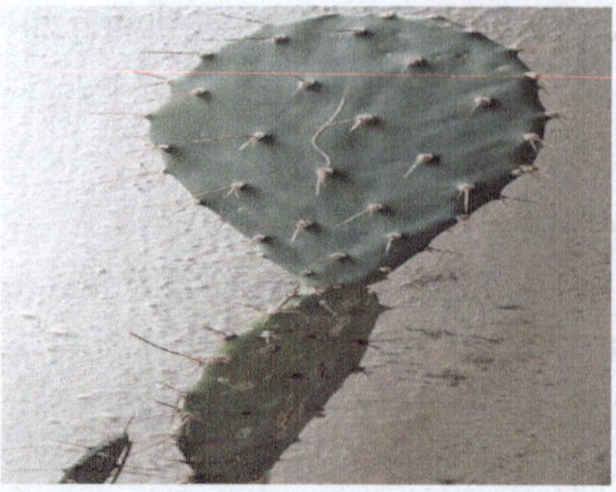

Scientific name: *Opuntia* spp.

Common name: Cactus

Distribution : Rajasthan, Gujarat, Haryana, Punjab

Part used: Fruits , pads

Bioactive principles: Flavonoids, Betalains, Triterpenoids, Polyphenols

Remarks: It is a promising option for promoting heart health because of its high antioxidant and fiber content. It has been used traditionally in some regions for managing or treating conditions like hypertension and high cholesterol

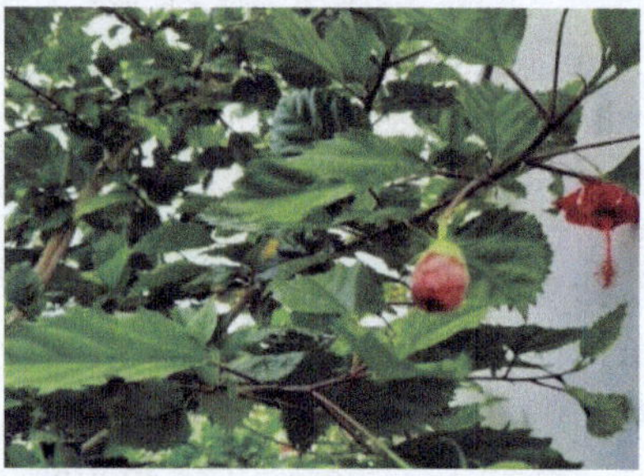

Scientific name: *Croton sparciflorus*

Common name: Ban Tulasi

Distribution: Andhra Pradesh, Karnataka, Kerala, Maharashtra, and Odisha

Parts used: Leaves, seed, stem whole plant

Bioactive principles: Saponins, Alkaloids, Phenols, Tannins, Flavoniods, Crotsparinine, Crotsparine

Remarks: It has antioxidant, anti-hypertensive, anti-inflammatory, lipid-lowering, blood sugar regulating and cardiac muscle protecting properties. Together, these characteristics may help shield the heart from a number of cardiovascular conditions like heart attack or reduced blood flow, arterial plaques, atherosclerosis, hypertension, and myocardial infarction.

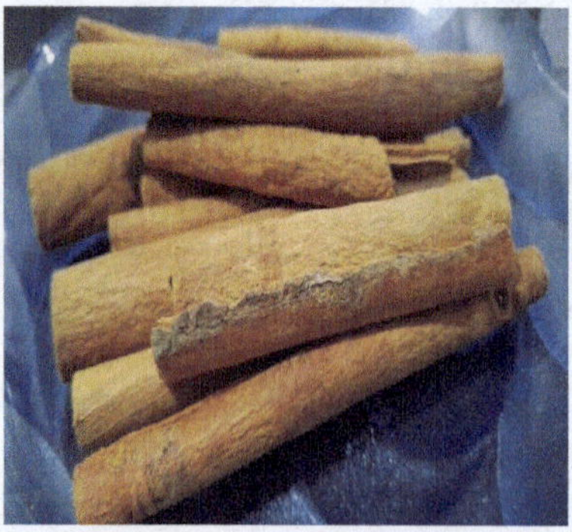

Scientific name: *Cinnamon tamala*

Common name: Cinnamon Indian bay, Indian cassia

Distribution: Himalaya

Parts used: Leaves, bark

Bioactive principles: Flavonoids, Polyphenols,

Alkaloids, Flavones and flavonols, Tannins, Saponins, Glycosides.

Remarks: Antibacterial, anti-inflammatory, anticoagulant, vasodilatory, cholesterol-lowering, and antioxidant qualities of cinnamon may help better digestion, heart health, increase blood flow, lessen oxidative stress, and blood sugar regulation which may helps to lower the risk of stroke and prevent thrombosis, heart valve damage, atherosclerosis, pulmonary hypertension, arrhythmias and maintain heart health by controlling blood sugar.

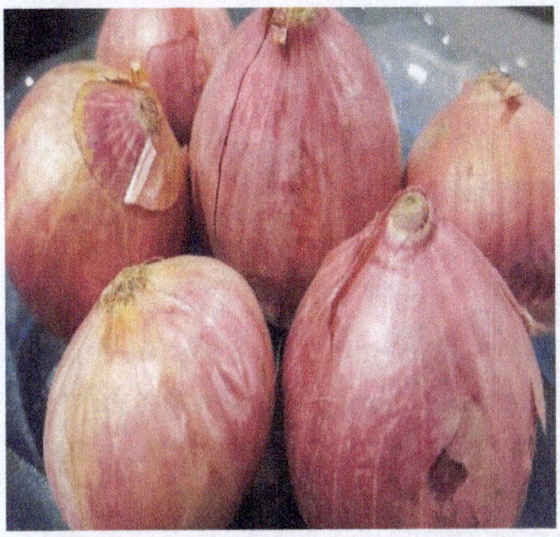

Scientific name : *Allium cepa*

Common name: Onion

Distribution: Maharashtra, Andhra Pradesh, Karnataka, and Tamil Nadu

Parts used: Bulb, leaf

Bioactive principles: Flavonoids (e.g., Quercetin), Alliin, Allicin, Thiosulfates,Fructooligosaccharides (FOS), Saponins

Remarks: The onion, or *Allium cepa*, is a great food and medicinal plant for heart health because of its many cardioprotective qualities. Onions can prevents and manage a number of cardiovascular problems because of their anti-inflammatory, antihypertensive, lipid-lowering, antithrombotic, antioxidant, and blood sugar-regulating properties.

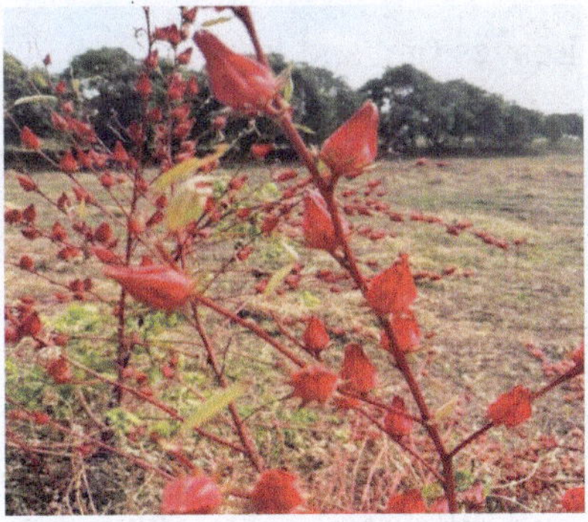

Scientific name: *Hibiscus sabdariffa*

Common name: Laal Ambadi, Patwa, or Tambdi-ambadi.

Distribution: Karnataka, Maharashtra, Kerla, Odisha

Parts used: Flower pods, or calyces

Bioactive principles: Anthocyanins, flavonoids, Glycosides, Hibiscin, Organicacids, Saponins, Steroids, Tannins.

Remarks: It possess anti-inflammatory, blood pressure-lowering, vasodilatory and antioxidant qualities and helps to manage pulmonary hypertension and lessen the risk of thrombosis and stroke by enhancing blood circulation and lowering oxidative stress.

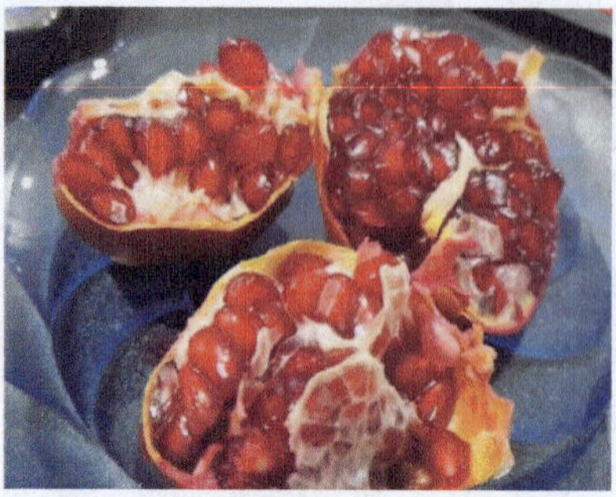

Scientific name: *Punica granatum*

Common name: Pomegranate

Distribution in India: Grown mainly in Maharashtra, Gujarat, Andhra Pradesh, and Rajasthan.

Part used: Fruit (Seeds and juice)

Bioactive principles: Punicalagins, Anthocyanins, Ellagic acid

Remarks: It possess anticoagulant, anti-inflammatory, vasoprotective and antioxidant properties, which are good for the heart, lowers cholesterol, lowering blood pressure, enhancing heart function, lowering inflammation and oxidative stress and enhance circulation. Pomegranate may help in preventing and treating atherosclerosis, managing heart valve disease, lower the risk of arrhythmias, lessen the risk of stroke and thrombosis, and supports in the treatment of pulmonary hypertension.

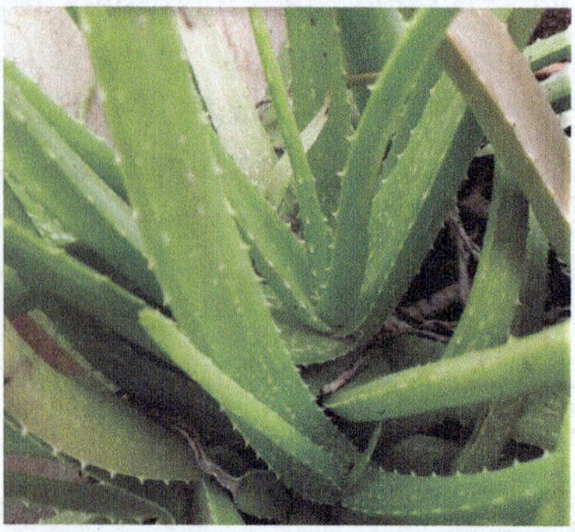

Scientific name: *Aloe vera*

Common name: *Aloe Vera*

Distribution: Grown in arid and semi-arid regions, especially in Rajasthan, Gujarat, and Haryana.

Part used: Leaves (gel and latex)

Bioactive principles: Aloin, Acemannan, Anthraquinones

Remarks: It has cooling, anti-inflammatory, restortative, anticoagulant, vasodilatory and antioxidant qualities. By lowering cholesterol and oxidative stress, enhancing circulation, and providing overall cardiovascular protection—all of which might be beneficial for heart valve disease, helps to manage atherosclerosis, also lowers oxidative stress and inflammation in pulmonary hypertension and lowers the risk of stroke and thrombosis — It may helps to improve cardiovascular health. In addition, it is well-known for its ability to cure skin, and used to promote digestive health, reduce inflammation, and treat burns and wounds naturally.

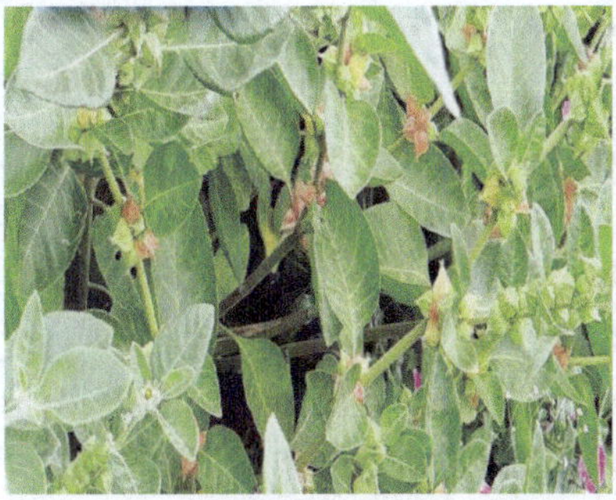

Scientific name: *Withania somnifera*

Common name: Ashwagandha

Distribution in India: Grown primarily in dry regions of India, including Rajasthan, Madhya Pradesh, and Uttar Pradesh.

Part used: Root

Bioactive principles: Withanolides, Alkaloids

Remarks: Ashwagandha well-known for its cardioprotective, adaptogenic, antioxidant, cardiotonic, diuretic, vasodilatory and anti-inflammatory qualities, which lowers stress, boosts endurance, lowers inflammation, improves cognitive function, strengthens the heart, lowers blood pressure and improves general wellbeing. It could helps to treat conditions like pulmonary hypertension, myocardial infarction, cardiomyopathy, heart valve disease and lowers the risk of stroke.

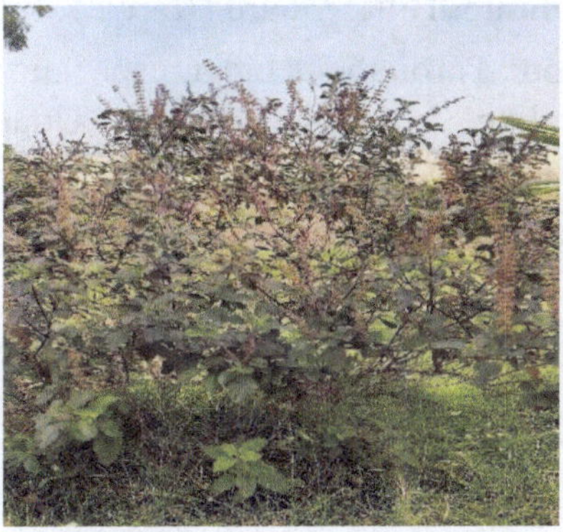

Scientific name*:* *Ocimum sanctum*

Common name: Tulsi (Holy Basil)

Distribution in India: Grown throughout India, especially in home gardens and rural areas.

Part used: Leaves

Bioactive principles: Eugenol, Ursolic acid, Rosmarinic acid

Remarks: The adaptogenic, anti-inflammatory, vasodilatory, cardiotonic, diuretic, antioxidant and antibacterial qualities of tulsi are well-known. It can promotes heart health by maintaining heart functions and lowers oxidative stress, lowers blood pressure, increase immunity and lessen stress, all of which may help with diseases like heart valve disease, regulate arrhythmias, pulmonary hypertension, myocardial infarction, lowers the risk of stroke and thrombosis.

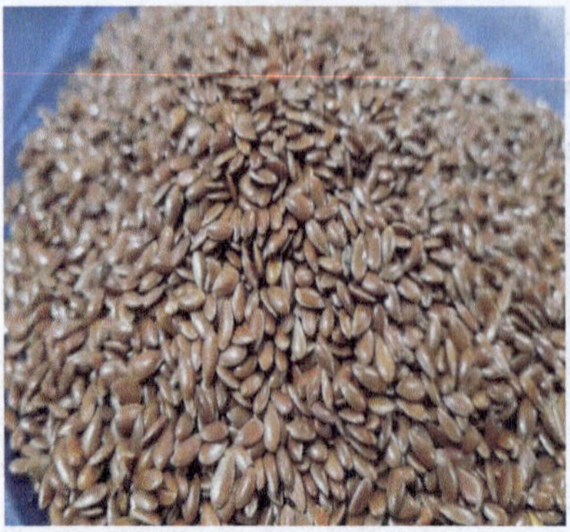

Scientific name: *Linum usitatissimum*

Common name: Flax seeds

Distribution in India: Grown in cooler regions of India, such as Rajasthan, Madhya Pradesh, and Punjab.

Part used: Seeds

Bioactive principles: Alpha-linolenic acid (ALA), Lignans, Fiber

Remarks: Flax seeds are rich in omega-3 fatty acids, fiber, and antioxidants. It improves digestion, lower cholesterol, balancing blood sugar levels, lower inflammation and promote heart health therefore used to treat atherosclerosis and myocardial infarction.

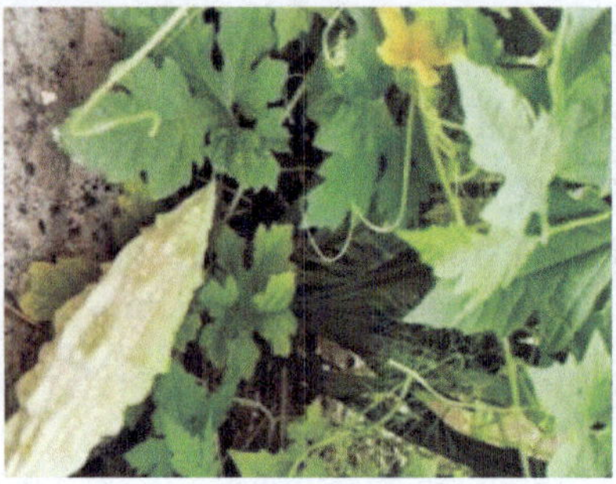

Scientific name: *Momordica charantia*

Common name: Bitter Gourd (Karela)

Distribution: Throughout India, especially in states like Madhya Pradesh, Uttar Pradesh, Tamil Nadu, and Andhra Pradesh.

Part used: Fruit

Bioactive principles: Charantin, Momordicin, Polypeptide-p

Remarks: Bitter gourds (*Momordica charantia*) are a promising natural remedy for heart health because of their anti-inflammatory, lipid-lowering, blood sugar-regulating, antioxidant, and antihypertensive qualities. It prevents development of a blood clot and decrease the risk of stroke and heart attack, promoting healthy blood vessels and regulating blood pressure, maintaining healthy arteries prevents atherosclerosis, and reduces chronic inflammation associated with CVDs.

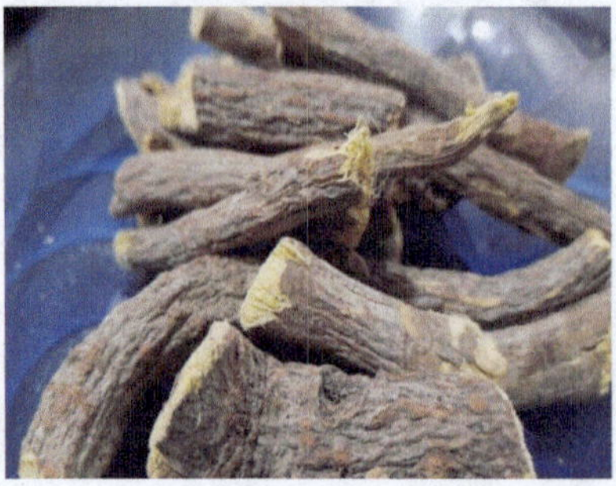

Scientific name: *Glycyrrhiza glabra*

Common name: Licorice

Distribution in India: Grown in regions like Jammu & Kashmir, Uttar Pradesh, and Himachal Pradesh.

Part used: Root

Bioactive principles: Glycyrrhizin, Flavonoids, Saponins

Remarks: Licorice contains immune-stimulating, cardioprootective, cardiotonic, diuretic, vasodilatory, immunomodulatory, anti-inflammatory, calming and antioxidant qualities. By lowering inflammation and enhancing circulation, it may promote and strengthen heart health, and lessen the signs of heart-related conditions. But its overuse can harm heart health and increase the risk of arrhythmias because it alters potassium levels.

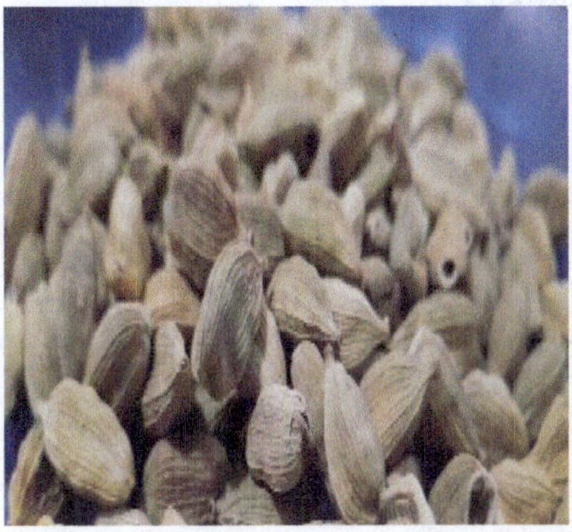

Scientific name: *Elettaria cardamomum*

Common name: Cardamom

Distribution in India: Primarily grown in Kerala, Karnataka, and Tamil Nadu.

Part used: Seeds (from the fruit)

Bioactive principles: 1,8-cineole, terpinyl acetate, alpha-terpineol, flavonoids

Remarks: With its anti-inflammatory, antihypertensive, lipid-lowering, blood sugar-regulating, antioxidant, and other cardioprotective properties, cardamom is a potent spice that can help prevent and treat cardiovascular illnesses.

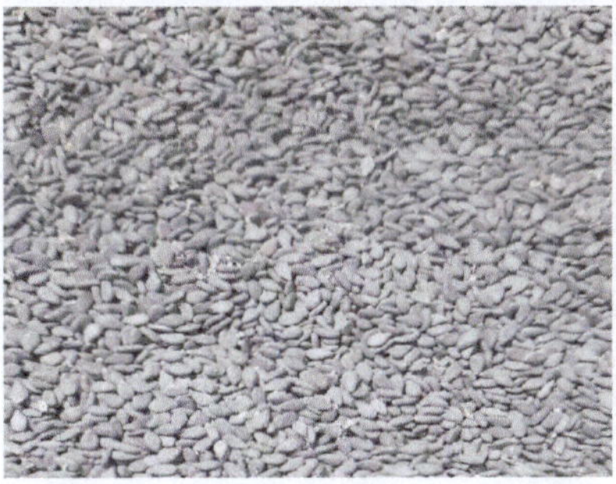

Scientific name: *Nigella sativa*

Common name: Black cumin, Nigella

Distribution: South and Southwest Asia, widely cultivated in the Middle East, Mediterranean, and India.

Part used: Seeds

Bioactive principles: Thymoquinone, carvacrol, nigellidine, fatty acids

Remarks: Because of its anti-inflammatory, antihypertensive, lipid-lowering, antidiabetic, antioxidant, anti-thrombotic and anticoagulant qualities, black cumin may helps to lower the blood pressure, lower the risk of stroke and thrombosis, improves endothelial functions while promoting cardiovascular health in general.

References

Anjaria, J. (2002) Ethanovet Heritage Indian Ethnoveterinary Medicine An Overview. Pathik Enterprise, Ahmedabad.

Chavan RS. (2006) Veterinary Pathology. 1st ed. CBS Publishers & Distributors, New Delhi.

Gupta, S. K. (2016) Drug Screening Methods. Jaypee Brothers Medical Publishers Pvt. Ltd., New Delhi.

Koshma M, Reddy VJ, Aditya TN, Basha SJ, Rani YS, Swaroopa P. Cardioprotective activity of medicinal plants: a review. Int. Res. J. Pharm. 2018;8:4-11.

Parmar, NS, and Prakash, S. (2006) Screening Methods in Pharmacology. Narosa Publishing House Pvt. Ltd., New Delhi.

Prasad VV and Koley KM (2006) Veterinary Pharmacology and Toxicology. 1st ed. Jaypee Brothers Medical Publishers, New Delhi.

Roy, B. K. (2023) Veterinary pharmacology and toxicology (7th ed.) Kalyani Publishers, New Delhi – 110002.

Tilak-Jain JA, Devasagayam TP. Cardioprotective and other beneficial effects of some Indian medicinal plants. Journal of Clinical Biochemistry and Nutrition. 2006;38(1):9-18.

Zaragoza C, Gomez-Guerrero C, Martin-Ventura JL, Blanco-Colio L, Lavin B, Mallavia B, Tarin C, Mas S, Ortiz A, Egido J. Animal models of cardiovascular diseases. BioMed Research International. 2011;2011(1):497841.

12

Medicinal Plants Effective in Respiratory Disorders in Animals

R. D. Singh[1], Santwana Palai[2], Sarita Devi[3], and Abhishek Gupta[4]

[1]*Department of Veterinary Pharmacology & Toxicology, College of Veterinary Science & Animal Husbandry, Kamdhenu University, Sardarkrushinagar - 385506, Gujarat*
[2]*Department of Veterinary Pharmacology & Toxicology, College of Veterinary Science & Animal Husbandry, OUAT, Bhubaneswar-751003, Odisha*
[3]*Department of Veterinary Medicine, College of Veterinary Science & Animal Husbandry, Kamdhenu University, Sardarkrushinagar - 385506, Gujarat*
[4]*Department of Veterinary Pharmacology and Toxicology, College of Veterinary Science & Animal Husbandry, Kamdhenu University, Sardarkrushinagar - 385506, Gujarat*

Respiratory tract disorders in domestic animals

The respiratory system is vital for efficient oxygen exchange, metabolic function, and overall health. Respiratory tract disorders in livestock species are among the most significant health challenges, leading to economic losses in terms of reduced productivity, treatment costs, and mortality. These disorders can affect the upper respiratory tract (URT), lower respiratory tract (LRT), or both. Overview of common respiratory diseases in livestock, their aetiology, clinical manifestations, pathophysiology, diagnostic approaches, and management strategies are summarized as follows: -

1. Bovine Respiratory Disease Complex (BRDC)

- ***Species affected:*** Cattle
- ***Etiology:*** Multifactorial; involves viruses (Bovine herpesvirus-1, Bovine respiratory syncytial virus, Parainfluenza-3, Bovine viral diarrhea virus), bacteria (*Mannheimia haemolytica*, *Pasteurella multocida*, *Mycoplasma bovis*), and environmental stressors.

- ***Pathophysiology:*** Stress or viral infections compromise mucociliary clearance, allowing bacterial colonization and secondary infections.
- ***Clinical signs:*** Pyrexia, nasal discharge, coughing, dyspnoea, anorexia, and weight loss.
- ***Diagnosis:*** Nasopharyngeal swabs for PCR, serology, bacterial culture, and thoracic ultrasonography.
- ***Management:*** Antibiotics, supportive care, vaccination, and minimizing stress through proper husbandry.

2. Contagious Caprine Pleuropneumonia (CCPP)

- ***Species affected***: Goats
- ***Etiology:*** *Mycoplasma capricolum* subsp. *Capripneumoniae*
- ***Pathophysiology:*** Severe fibrinous pleuropneumonia with serofibrinous exudation and pleural adhesion.
- ***Clinical signs:*** Fever, cough, dyspnoea, nasal discharge, and sudden death in severe cases.
- ***Diagnosis:*** PCR, serological assays (ELISA), and necropsy findings (fibrinous pleuritis).
- ***Management:*** Tylosin, oxytetracycline, or fluoroquinolones, along with vaccination programs.

3. Enzootic Pneumonia in Pigs

- ***Species affected:*** Swine
- ***Etiology:*** *Mycoplasma hyopneumoniae*, often in combination with secondary pathogens like *Pasteurella multocida*.
- ***Pathophysiology:*** Chronic inflammation of the bronchial and peribronchial tissues, impairing gas exchange.
- ***Clinical signs:*** Chronic, non-productive cough, growth retardation, and reduced feed efficiency.
- ***Diagnosis:*** Clinical signs, serology, PCR, and post-mortem lung lesions (consolidation of the cranial lobes).
- ***Management:*** Antibiotics (*e.g.*, macrolides), biosecurity, and vaccination.

4. Infectious Bovine Rhinotracheitis (IBR)

- ***Species affected:*** Cattle
- ***Etiology:*** Bovine herpesvirus-1 (BHV-1).
- ***Pathophysiology:*** Infection of the upper respiratory tract leading to necrosis of the mucosa and secondary bacterial infections.
- ***Clinical signs:*** Fever, hyperaemia of nasal mucosa, conjunctivitis, nasal discharge, and abortion in pregnant cows.
- ***Diagnosis:*** Virus isolation, PCR, ELISA, and immunofluorescence.
- ***Management:*** Vaccination (modified-live or inactivated), biosecurity measures, and symptomatic treatment.

5. Equine Influenza

- ***Species affected:*** Horses
- ***Etiology:*** Influenza A virus (subtypes H_3N_8 and H_7N_7).
- ***Pathophysiology:*** Replication in the respiratory epithelium, leading to inflammation and impaired mucociliary clearance.
- ***Clinical signs:*** Fever, dry cough, nasal discharge, anorexia, and muscle stiffness.
- ***Diagnosis:*** Virus isolation, PCR, and serology (hemagglutination inhibition test).
- ***Management:*** Antiviral agents, supportive therapy, and vaccination.

6. Ovine Progressive Pneumonia (OPP)

- ***Species affected:*** Sheep
- ***Etiology:*** Maedi-Visna virus, a lentivirus.
- ***Pathophysiology:*** Chronic interstitial pneumonia and progressive fibrosis of lung parenchyma.
- ***Clinical signs:*** Chronic cough, weight loss, dyspnea, and reduced milk production.
- ***Diagnosis:*** ELISA, PCR, and post-mortem examination of lungs.
- ***Management:*** There is no cure; control measures include culling infected animals and maintaining closed flocks.

7. Peste des Petits Ruminants (PPR)

- ***Species affected:*** Sheep and goats (mainly).
- ***Etiology:*** Peste des Petits Ruminants virus (PPRV), a Morbillivirus in the Paramyxoviridae family.
- ***Pathophysiology***: PPRV primarily infects epithelial cells of the respiratory and gastrointestinal tracts. It causes immunosuppression by targeting lymphoid tissues, leading to secondary bacterial infections.
- ***Clinical Signs:*** High fever, nasal/ocular discharge, coughing, Oral erosions, diarrhea, dehydration. High morbidity (100%) and mortality (50–90%).
- ***Diagnosis:*** Clinical signs, RT-PCR, ELISA, virus isolation.
- ***Management:*** supportive care like rehydration, antipyretics, antibiotics for secondary infections, Vaccination, quarantine, and movement restrictions.

8. Pneumonic Pasteurellosis/ Shipping fever

- ***Species affected:*** Multiple species, including sheep, goats, and cattle.
- ***Etiology:*** *Mannheimia haemolytica*
- ***Pathophysiology:*** Opportunistic invasion leading to fibrinous pneumonia
- ***Clinical signs:*** Fever, dyspnoea, nasal discharge, and sudden death.
- ***Diagnosis:*** Bacterial culture, PCR, and necropsy findings.
- ***Management:*** Early antibiotic treatment (e.g., ceftiofur, florfenicol) and vaccination.

9.Haemorrhagic *Septicaemia*

- ***Species affected:*** Cattle and buffalo.
- ***Etiology:*** *Pasteurella multocida* serotypes B and E.
- ***Pathophysiology:*** Acute septicaemia with lung congestion, oedema, and haemorrhage.
- ***Clinical signs:*** Fever, respiratory distress, swelling in the throat region, and sudden death.
- ***Diagnosis:*** Bacterial culture, PCR, and post-mortem findings.

- ***Management:*** Early antibiotic therapy, vaccination, and environmental hygiene.

10. Tuberculosis

- ***Species affected*:** Cattle, sheep, goats, and pigs.
- ***Etiology*:** *Mycobacterium bovis* (cattle) and *Mycobacterium avium* (pigs).
- ***Pathophysiology*:** Granuloma formation in lungs, lymph nodes, and other tissues.
- ***Clinical signs:*** Chronic cough, emaciation, and reduced productivity.
- ***Diagnosis:*** Tuberculin skin test, gamma-interferon assay, and culture of biopsy samples.
- ***Management:*** Test-and-slaughter programs and biosecurity measures.

11. Respiratory Syncytial Virus Infection (RSV)

- ***Species affected:*** Cattle, sheep, and goats.
- ***Etiology:*** Bovine respiratory syncytial virus (BRSV).
- ***Pathophysiology:*** Virus replicates in respiratory epithelium, causing necrosis, interstitial pneumonia, and emphysema.
- ***Clinical signs:*** Fever, coughing, nasal discharge, respiratory distress, and wheezing.
- ***Diagnosis:*** PCR, virus isolation, and paired serology.
- ***Management:*** Supportive therapy, anti-inflammatory drugs, and vaccination.

12. Rhodococcosis

- ***Species affected:*** Horses (primarily foals).
- ***Etiology:*** *Rhodococcus equi.*
- ***Pathophysiology:*** Chronic pyogranulomatous bronchopneumonia due to intracellular bacterial survival within macrophages.
- ***Clinical signs:*** Cough, nasal discharge, fever, weight loss, and exercise intolerance.
- ***Diagnosis:*** Thoracic radiography, tracheal wash culture, and PCR.

- ***Management:*** Combination therapy with rifampin and macrolides, alongside supportive care.

13. Aspergillosis

- ***Species affected:*** Poultry, cattle, and horses.
- ***Etiology:*** *Aspergillus fumigatus* and other *Aspergillus* species.
- ***Pathophysiology:*** Inhalation of fungal spores causes granulomatous inflammation, leading to necrosis in the lungs and air sacs.
- ***Clinical signs:*** Dyspnea, gasping, nasal discharge, reduced egg production (poultry), and chronic cough (horses).
- ***Diagnosis:*** Fungal culture, histopathology, and PCR.
- ***Management:*** Antifungals (e.g., itraconazole), improved ventilation, and hygiene.

14. Strangles

- ***Species affected:*** Horses.
- ***Etiology:*** *Streptococcus equi* subsp. *equi*.
- ***Pathophysiology:*** Bacterial infection causes abscess formation in lymph nodes, which may compress the trachea, leading to respiratory distress.
- ***Clinical signs:*** Fever, nasal discharge, swollen lymph nodes, and dyspnoea.
- ***Diagnosis:*** Culture, PCR, and serology.
- ***Management:*** Antibiotics, drainage of abscesses, and vaccination.

15. Guttural Pouch Mycosis

- ***Species affected:*** Horses.
- ***Etiology:*** *Aspergillus* spp.
- ***Pathophysiology:*** Fungal invasion of the guttural pouch can cause necrotizing inflammation, vascular erosion, and haemorrhage.
- ***Clinical signs:*** Epistaxis, dysphagia, nasal discharge, and head shaking.
- ***Diagnosis:*** Endoscopy, fungal culture, and imaging.
- ***Management:*** Antifungals, surgical intervention, and supportive care.

16. Parasitic Bronchitis (Husk)

- ***Species affected:*** Cattle and sheep.
- ***Etiology*:** *Dictyocaulus viviparus* (cattle) and *Dictyocaulus filaria* (sheep and goats).
- ***Pathophysiology:*** Larval migration and adult worms in the bronchi cause inflammation, leading to bronchitis and emphysema.
- ***Clinical signs:*** Coughing, dyspnea, nasal discharge, and poor weight gain.
- ***Diagnosis:*** Baermann technique, fecal larval culture, and clinical signs.
- ***Management:*** Anthelmintics (e.g., ivermectin), grazing management, and vaccination (for *D. viviparus* in endemic areas).

17. Fungal Rhinitis

- ***Species affected:*** Dogs, horses, and cattle.
- ***Etiology:*** *Cryptococcus* spp. and *Aspergillus* spp.
- ***Pathophysiology:*** Localized fungal infection of nasal passages and sinuses causing chronic inflammation.
- ***Clinical signs:*** Nasal discharge, sneezing, and facial swelling.
- ***Diagnosis:*** Fungal culture, cytology, and imaging.
- ***Management:*** Long-term antifungal therapy (*e.g.*, amphotericin B, itraconazole).

18. Allergic Rhinitis

- ***Species affected:*** Cattle, sheep, goats, and horses.
- ***Etiology:*** Hypersensitivity reaction to environmental allergens such as pollen, fungal spores, or dust.
- ***Pathophysiology:*** Inhalation of allergens triggers an immune response characterized by mast cell degranulation, histamine release, and inflammation of nasal mucosa.
- ***Clinical signs:*** Sneezing, nasal discharge (clear or mucoid), head shaking, pruritus around the nose, and reduced feed intake due to discomfort.

- ***Diagnosis:*** Clinical signs, exclusion of infectious causes, and intradermal allergy testing.
- ***Management:*** Antihistamines, corticosteroids, and environmental control (*e.g.*, reducing exposure to allergens).

19. Chronic Obstructive Pulmonary Disease (COPD) / Recurrent Airway Obstruction (RAO)

- ***Species affected:*** Horses (commonly), occasionally cattle.
- ***Etiology:*** Chronic exposure to airborne irritants such as dust, mold, and endotoxins in poorly ventilated environments.
- ***Pathophysiology:*** Hypersensitivity reaction in the lower respiratory tract leads to bronchoconstriction, mucus hypersecretion, and airway inflammation, resulting in impaired gas exchange.
- ***Clinical signs:*** Chronic cough, dyspnoea (especially during expiration), nasal discharge, wheezing, and a characteristic "heave line" due to abdominal muscle hypertrophy from laboured breathing.
- ***Diagnosis:*** Clinical signs, endoscopy, bronchoalveolar lavage (cytology showing neutrophilia), and pulmonary function testing.
- ***Management:*** Improved ventilation, soaking hay to reduce dust, or feeding haylage, dietary modifications, use of bronchodilators (*e.g.*, clenbuterol, albuterol), corticosteroids (*e.g.*, dexamethasone) and mucolytics.

General Treatment drugs in Respiratory System Disorders

Respiratory diseases in livestock are complex and require a multidisciplinary approach for effective management. The management of respiratory conditions in animals requires a tailored approach, often employing a combination of pharmacological agents to address the underlying pathology and alleviate symptoms. Among these, bronchodilators and anti-inflammatory drugs play a pivotal role in managing airway diseases characterized by obstruction and inflammation.

Bronchodilators relax the smooth muscles of the airway, improving airflow and reducing respiratory distress. Bronchodilators enhances the respiratory functions as well as serve as potent peripheral antitussive agents due to their ability to alleviate the stimulation of irritant receptors in the bronchial walls. This stimulation often arises from the mechanical distortion caused by bronchoconstriction, a common feature in many respiratory conditions. By addressing the underlying bronchoconstriction, bronchodilators reduce the reflexive cough response associated with irritant receptor activation. The mechanism behind this antitussive effect lies in the ability of bronchodilators to relax the smooth muscle of the airways. Beta-adrenergic agonists, methylxanthines, and anticholinergics are common classes of bronchodilators that act through distinct pathways to achieve this relaxation. By reducing bronchial wall tension and restoring normal airway patency, these drugs minimize the mechanical triggers that activate cough reflex pathways. In conditions such as asthma, chronic obstructive pulmonary disease (COPD), or allergic bronchitis, where bronchoconstriction is a primary component, bronchodilators not only improve airflow but also mitigate cough severity.

Anti-inflammatory drugs, including corticosteroids and non-steroidal anti-inflammatory drugs (NSAIDs), are essential in mitigating the inflammation that frequently exacerbates respiratory conditions.

Another critical aspect of respiratory pharmacology involves drugs that modify respiratory secretions. Expectorants, also known as mucokinetic drugs, enhance the clearance of respiratory secretions by improving ciliary movement or altering mucus viscosity. These agents stimulate the production of thinner mucus, facilitating its expulsion and playing a supportive role in managing coughs associated with thick or sticky secretions. For example, guaifenesin increases mucus fluidity, aiding expectoration in conditions like chronic bronchitis or pneumonia. Mucokinetics are particularly valuable in addressing the accumulation of inspissated mucus in chronic bronchial diseases, where it can obstruct airways and impair respiratory efficiency. Improving ciliary activity is one mechanism for enhancing mucus clearance. Beta-receptor agonists and methylxanthines stimulate ciliary motion, ensuring more efficient mucus transport, which is especially important when ciliary function is impaired. Another approach is reducing mucus viscosity to improve mobility. Hydration with sterile water or saline, increasing pH with agents like sodium bicarbonate, or enhancing ionic strength with saline solutions can all thin bronchial secretions, easing their expulsion and alleviating respiratory discomfort.

Mucolytics are drugs that decrease the viscosity of mucus in the respiratory tract, making it easier to expel through expectoration or mucokinesis. Mucolytic agents target the biochemical structure of mucus. Acetylcysteine, for instance, breaks disulfide bonds in thick mucus proteins, reducing its thickness and facilitating its clearance from the respiratory tract or promoting clearance.

Similarly, iodine-based compounds disrupt mucus structure, enhancing its fluidity and improving overall respiratory function.

Antitussive drugs (cough suppressants) are a vital component of respiratory therapy, specifically designed to suppress the cough reflex in cases where coughing is excessive, non-productive, or causing distress to the animal. Unlike productive coughs, which help clear mucus and foreign material from the airways, non-productive coughs offer no physiological benefit and can worsen airway irritation, leading to further inflammation and discomfort. Typically, dry coughs are addressed using antitussive agents, which suppress the cough reflex at the cough center. In contrast, productive coughs, characterized by the production of substantial amounts of phlegm, are managed by facilitating the expulsion of thickened mucus. Management strategies for such cases include the use of expectorants, mucolytics, and plain water nebulization.

Commonly used antitussives in veterinary medicine include codeine, a centrally acting opioid, and butorphanol, a mixed opioid agonist-antagonist. Both act on the cough center in the brain to reduce the frequency and intensity of coughing. The choice of antitussive depends on the underlying cause and severity of the cough. Codeine, known for its strong cough-suppressing properties, is particularly effective in managing severe, chronic coughs associated with conditions like tracheitis or bronchitis. Butorphanol, on the other hand, offers a balanced approach by providing antitussive effects alongside mild analgesia, making it suitable for cases where coughing is accompanied by pain or irritation. The careful use of these drugs can significantly enhance an animal's comfort and quality of life during recovery from respiratory illnesses. However, it is essential to recognize that antitussives should be used judiciously and as part of a broader treatment plan. Suppressing a productive cough without addressing the underlying cause, such as infection or obstruction, can lead to mucus retention and secondary complications like pneumonia. In veterinary practice, these drugs are often combined with other therapies, such as antibiotics, mucolytics, or anti-inflammatory agents, to provide comprehensive respiratory care. Proper diagnosis and a clear understanding of the cough's origin are crucial to ensuring that the use of antitussive medications is both safe and effective.

Decongestants reduce nasal and upper airway congestion by shrinking swollen mucosal tissues through vasoconstriction. These agents are commonly used in conditions involving rhinitis or sinusitis, where nasal blockages impair breathing and overall comfort. An example of a nasal decongestant commonly used in veterinary medicine is phenylephrine. This drug is a selective alpha-adrenergic agonist that works by causing vasoconstriction of the nasal mucosa, reducing swelling and congestion. It is often used in conditions such as rhinitis or sinusitis to alleviate nasal obstruction and improve airflow. Other decongestants, like oxymetazoline or pseudoephedrine, may also be employed in specific cases, though their use in animals requires careful dosing and monitoring to avoid potential side effects, such as hypertension or rebound congestion.

Aerosol therapy, including nebulization and metered-dose inhalers, has gained importance as an adjunctive approach in respiratory treatment. Aerosolized medications allow for direct delivery to the respiratory tract, ensuring higher local drug concentrations with minimal systemic effects. However, the success of aerosol therapy depends on several factors, including the animal's tolerance, the particle size of the aerosolized drug, and the environmental conditions during administration. Proper techniques and equipment maintenance are essential to maximize the efficacy of this approach.

Analeptics (respiratory stimulants) are drugs that stimulate respiratory activity, primarily used to counteract respiratory depression caused by anesthesia overdose or toxicity from other central nervous system (CNS) depressants. These agents work by enhancing the responsiveness of the respiratory centers in the brain to carbon dioxide levels, thereby restoring normal breathing. Common examples include doxapram, nikethamide, methylxanthines, and bemegride.

Infectious diseases are a significant subset of respiratory disorders in veterinary medicine, with bacterial pneumonia, viral infections, and mycoplasma-associated diseases being frequently encountered. Antibiotics remain the cornerstone of treatment for bacterial respiratory infections, with the choice of antibiotic guided by microbial sensitivity testing and the pharmacokinetic properties of the drug in the respiratory system. For optimal outcomes, veterinarians must combine these pharmacological strategies with supportive care, including hydration, nutritional support, and environmental management, ensuring a comprehensive approach to respiratory health.

Herbal Treatment in Respiratory System Disorders

Herbal medicines have been used for centuries to treat respiratory tract disorders in domestic animals and are now gaining renewed interest due to their safety, efficacy, and minimal risk of residues in animal products. Respiratory diseases such as bronchitis, pneumonia, asthma, and cough often challenge the livestock industry due to their impact on productivity and animal welfare. Herbal treatments, derived from plants with bioactive compounds, are increasingly recognized for their antimicrobial, anti-inflammatory, and immunomodulatory effects. These natural remedies offer an alternative or adjunctive approach to conventional pharmaceuticals, addressing concerns such as antimicrobial resistance and adverse drug reactions.

Several herbal plants are commonly employed in the treatment of respiratory diseases including pneumonia in animals. *Adhatoda vasica* (vasaka) is one of the most effective herbs used for its potent expectorant and bronchodilator properties. It contains alkaloids like vasicine, which help to clear mucus and ease breathing in cases of chronic bronchitis and asthma in large as well as small ruminants. Similarly, *Glycyrrhiza glabra* (licorice) is widely used for its soothing, demulcent, and anti-inflammatory effects on the respiratory tract, making it valuable for animals suffering from dry or irritating coughs. Methylxanthines, such as theobromine and theophylline, are naturally occurring compounds with significant bronchodilator properties. Found in plants like *Camellia sinensis* (green tea), these compounds are effective in relaxing bronchial smooth muscles, thereby improving airflow and relieving symptoms of obstructive airway diseases

Ocimum sanctum (holy basil) is a versatile herb with adaptogenic and immunomodulatory properties. It is used to manage respiratory stress and allergic rhinitis in animals exposed to environmental stressors like dust or smoke. *Terminalia bellerica* is valuable herb known for its bronchodilator and antimicrobial activity, useful in treating chronic coughs and respiratory infections. The resin from *Boswellia serrata* (Indian frankincense) is used for its anti-inflammatory properties in managing conditions like equine asthma and other chronic respiratory disorders.

Zingiber officinale (ginger) and *Curcuma longa* (turmeric) are also widely employed for their antimicrobial and anti-inflammatory properties, offering relief in cases of bacterial or viral respiratory infections. Turmeric, with its active component curcumin, helps reduce inflammation in chronic respiratory conditions, while ginger aids in enhancing mucus clearance and reducing airway inflammation. Another notable herb is *Allium sativum* (garlic), which has antimicrobial and mucolytic properties, beneficial for respiratory infections in animals.

Essential oils derived from aromatic plants offer natural, effective treatments for respiratory diseases in domestic animals and livestock. Oils like *Eucalyptus globulus* (eucalyptus), *Mentha piperita* (peppermint), and *Thymus vulgaris* (thyme) possess antimicrobial, anti-inflammatory, and bronchodilator properties that help alleviate symptoms of conditions like bronchitis, asthma, pneumonia, and nasal congestion. As inhalants they are used to relieve nasal congestion and improve respiration, especially in conditions such as nasal discharge and upper respiratory tract infections These oils are commonly used in inhalation therapies, diffused in the environment, or applied topically when diluted with carrier oils to clear airways, reduce inflammation, and improve breathing in animals such as cattle, goats, and horses. Other essential oils like *Lavandula angustifolia* (lavender) and *Melaleuca alternifolia* (tea tree) are beneficial for stress-related respiratory issues and microbial infections. They also support the immune system in fighting respiratory pathogens. When used appropriately, essential oils can complement traditional therapies and support the respiratory health of animals.

Herbal medicines offer effective natural alternatives for managing parasitic respiratory disorders in livestock and domestic animals. Plants like *Artemisia absinthium* (wormwood), *Nigella sativa* (black cumin), and *Allium sativum* (garlic) are known for their anthelmintic and antimicrobial properties. Wormwood helps expel lungworms from the respiratory tract, while black cumin boosts the immune system and alleviates respiratory symptoms caused by parasitic infestations. Garlic helps expel respiratory parasites and supports lung health, making it effective against lungworms and other nematodes. Other herbs like *Tanacetum vulgare* (tansy) and *Cinnamomum verum* (cinnamon) also target parasitic respiratory diseases, with compounds that have strong anti-parasitic effects. These herbs can be administered through oral supplements or in herbal formulations.

Various plant-derived compounds, including alkaloids, flavonoids, glycosides, lignans, polyphenols, and saponins, have been widely studied for their therapeutic potential against respiratory diseases and inflammation. These compounds exhibit a variety of bioactive properties, such as anti-inflammatory, antioxidant, and antimicrobial effects, making them valuable in managing respiratory conditions. Notable compounds like glycyrrhizin, mangiferin, piperine, zingerone, and forsythiaside-A have shown promising results in animal studies, demonstrating efficacy in reducing inflammation, alleviating respiratory symptoms, and improving overall lung function. The increasing evidence highlights the potential of these plant-based substances as natural alternatives or adjuncts to conventional treatments for respiratory disorders in animals.

The scope of herbal treatments is vast and promising. These remedies not only treat symptoms but also enhance the overall immune response of animals, reducing susceptibility to recurrent infections. With increasing consumer demand for organic and residue-free animal products, the use of herbal medicines aligns well with sustainable and eco-friendly livestock practices. Future research should focus on standardizing herbal extracts, validating their efficacy through clinical trials, and ensuring quality control. By integrating traditional knowledge with modern veterinary medicine, herbal treatments can provide holistic and effective solutions for managing respiratory diseases in domestic animals.

Medicinal plants used in Respiratory System Disorders

Medicinal plants used in respiratory system disorders can be sub-grouped in four major clusters as follow: -

1. Plants (active principles) with bronchodilator properties

- *Camellia sinensis* (Theobromine and Theophylline)
- *Coleus barbatus (C. forskohlii)* (Forskolin)
- *Datura stramonium* (Atropine and Scopolamine)
- *Ephedra sinica* (Ephedrine)
- *Lobelia inflata* (Lobeline)

2. Plants with Expectorant & Mucolytic Properties

- Expectorant botanicals may be divided into 'Stimulating' and 'Relaxing' expectorants. Stimulating expectorants induce coughing, tend to loosen mucus and are indicated for patients with productive coughs whereas relaxing expectorants are mainly antispasmodic in nature, indicated for patients with spasmodic or nonproductive coughs.
- Examples of stimulating expectorant plants (common name) are:
- *Aralia californica* (Elk's Clover)
- *Asclepias tuberosa* (Butterfly weed)
- *Aspidosperma quebracho* (Kebrako)
- *Bellis perennis* (Common daisy)
- *Cephaelis ipecacuanha* (Ipecac)
- *Glycyrrhiza glabra* (Licorice)
- *Hedera helix* (Common Ivy)

- *Lobelia inflata* (Indian tobacco)
- *Polygala senega* (Seneca snakeroot)
- *Primula veris* (Cowslip Primrose)
- *Sanguinaria canadensis* (Bloodroot)
- *Trifolium pratense* (Red Clover)
- *Urginea maritima* (Red squill)
- Example of relaxing expectorants are:
- *Angelica archangelica* (Wild celery)
- *Drosera rotundifolia* (Roundleaf sundew)
- *Grindelia spp.* (Gumweed)
- *Hyssopus officinalis* (Hyssop)
- *Pimpinella anisum* (Aniseed, Anise)
- *Prunus serotina* (Wild Cherry)
- *Verbascum thapsus* (Common mullein)

3. Plants with Anti-tussive (cough-suppressant) Properties

- *Allium sativum* (Garlic)
- *Caephalis ipecacuanha* (Ipecac)
- *Calotropis gigantea* (Giant milkweed)
- *Cuminum cyminum* (Cumin)
- *Justicia adathoda or Adhatoda vasica* (Malabar nut, Adusa)
- *Leonotis nepetifolia* (Lion's ear plant)
- *Papaver somniferum* (Opium poppy) (Codeine & Noscapine)
- *Prunus serotina* bark (Wild or black cherry) (Amygdalin)
- *Solanum virginianum* (Yellow-fruit nightshade, Kantakari)
- *Tussilago farfara* (Coltsfoot)
- *Vincetoxicum indicum* (Indian Ipecac)

4. Plants with Herbal Demulcents Property on Respiratory Tract

- *Agropyrum (Elymus) repens* (Couch grass)
- *Avena sativa* (Oatmeal)
- *Glycyrrhiza glabra* (liquorice)
- *Linum usitatissimum* (Flaxseed, Linseed)
- *Malva sylvestris* (Common Mallow)
- *Pulmonaria officinalis* (Lungwort)
- *Symphytum officinale* (Comfrey)
- *Zea mays* (Corn silk)

5. Plants Active Against Respiratory Pathogens

Sr. No.	Botanical Name of the Plant (common name)	Active compounds	Pathogens targeted
1.	*Ocimum sanctum* (Tulsi or Holy Basil)	Eugenol, ursolic acid, and rosmarinic acid	*Staphylococcus spp.*, *Escherichia coli*, and certain respiratory viruses
2.	*Adhatoda vasica* (Malabar Nut)	Vasicine and vasicinone	*Mycoplasma spp.*, *Pasteurella multocida*
3.	*Allium sativum* (Garlic)	Allicin and sulfur-containing compounds	*Bordetella bronchiseptica, Mycoplasma spp. and fungus*
4.	*Zingiber officinale* (Ginger)	Gingerol, shogaol	*E. coli, Pseudomonas aeruginosa, Staphylococcus aureus*
5.	*Curcuma longa* (Turmeric)	Curcumin	*Pasteurella multocida, Streptococcus spp.*
6.	*Eucalyptus globulus* (Eucalyptus)	Eucalyptol, terpenes	*Staphylococcus spp., Pseudomonas spp.*
7.	*Azadirachta indica* (Neem)	Azadirachtin, nimbin	*Mycoplasma spp., E. coli*
8.	*Mentha piperita* (Peppermint)	Menthol	*Streptococcus pneumoniae, E. coli*
9.	*Nigella sativa* (Black cumin seed)	Thymoquinone	*Pasteurella spp., Mycoplasma spp*
10.	*Terminalia chebula* (Haritaki)	Chebulagic acid, gallic acid	*Staphylococcus aureus, Bacillus subtilis.*
11.	*Thymus vulgaris* (Thyme)	Thymol, carvacrol	*Pseudomonas spp., Mycoplasma spp.*
12.	Andrographis paniculata (Kalmegh)	Andrographolide	*Mycoplasma spp., Pasteurella spp.*
13.	*Aloe vera*	Aloin, acemannan	*E. coli, Pseudomonas spp.*

14.	*Glycyrrhiza glabra* (Licorice)	Glycyrrhizin, liquiritin	*Mycoplasma spp., Staphylococcus aureus,* certain viruses
15.	*Tylophora indica* (Indian Ipecacuanha)	Tylophorine, tylophorinidine	*Mycoplasma* spp., *Pasteurella multocida, Staphylococcus aureus*
16.	*Inula helenium* (Elecampane or Horseheal)	Sesquiterpene lactones (alantolactone, isoalantolactone)	*Staphylococcus aureus, E. coli, Acinetobacter baumanni*

Medicinal Plants Effective To Treat Respiratory Tract Disorders

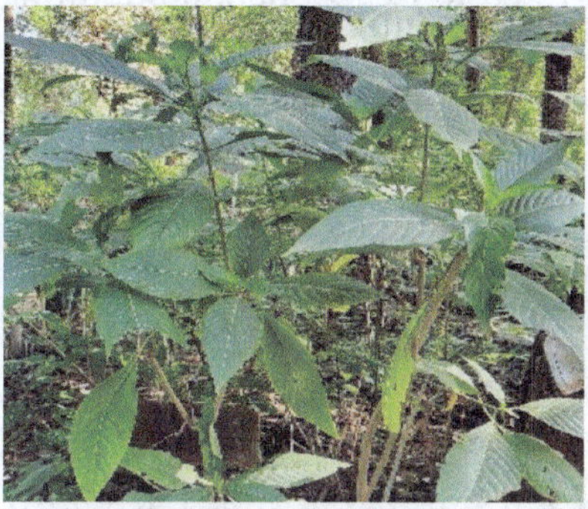

Scientific name: *Adhatoda vasica*

Common name: Malabar nut, Vasaka

Distribution: Tropical regions of Southeast Asia including India

Part used: Leaves, flower and bark

Bioactive principles: Vasicine, vasicinone, quinazoline alkaloids

Remarks: Used to treat asthma and chronic bronchitis

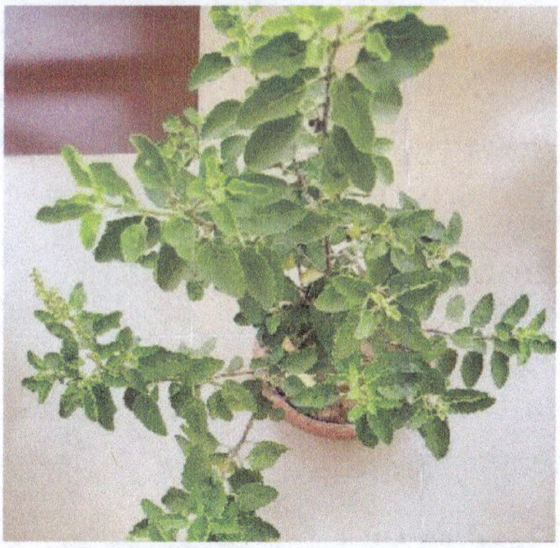

Scientific name: *Ocimum sanctum*

Common name: Holy basil, Tulsi

Distribution: Widely distributed across India and Southeast Asia

Part used: Leaves, seeds

Bioactive principles: Eugenol, camphene, cineole, flavonoids

Remarks: Anti-inflammatory, antimicrobial / antiviral effects, alleviates congestion

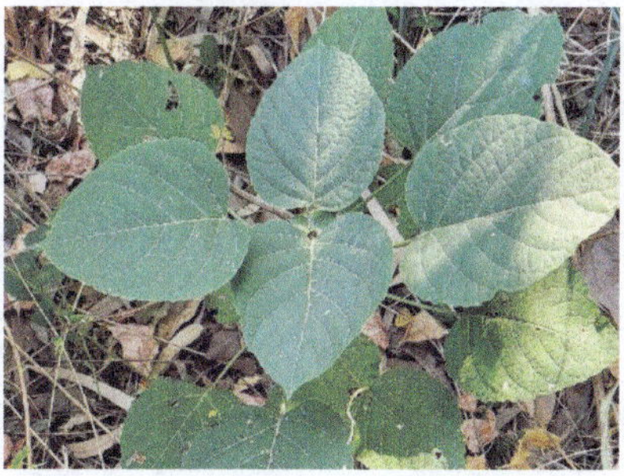

Scientific name: *Tylophora indica (Vincetoxicum indicum, Cynanchum indicum)*

Common name: Arkaparni, Indian-Ipecacuanha, Anantmool

Distribution: Asia, Africa, Australia

Part used: Roots and Leaves

Bioactive principles: Tylophorine, tylophorinidine (alkaloids)

Remarks: Used to treat asthma and certain allergies.

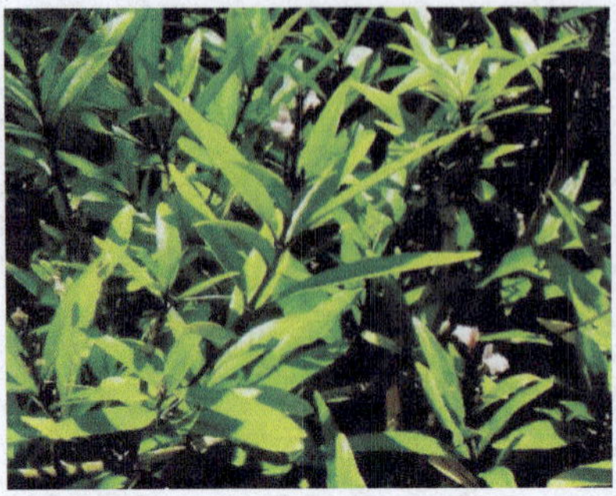

Scientific name: *Justicia gendarussa*

Common name: Willow-leaved Justicia

Distribution: Indian subcontinent

Part used: Leaves

Bioactive principles: Gendarussin (saponin)

Remarks: Used to treat cough, cold, throat and pulmonary infections and allergic bronchial asthma.

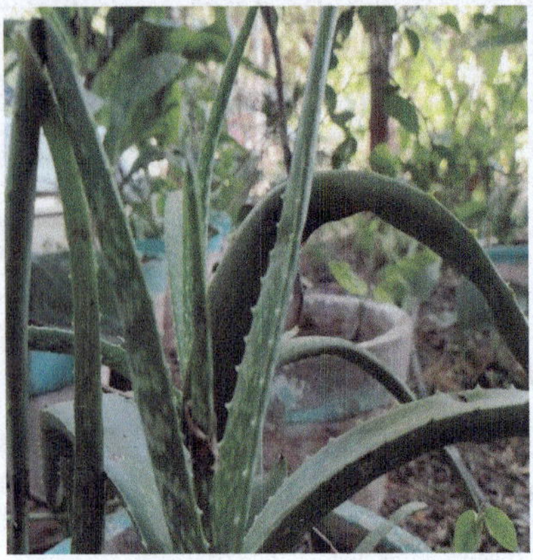

Scientific name: *Aloe vera*

Common name: Aloe, Ghritkumari

Distribution: Tropical and subtropical regions worldwide

Part used: Leaves (gel and latex)

Bioactive principles: Aloin, barbaloin, anthraquinones, polysaccharides

Remarks: Exhibits anti-inflammatory and soothing properties; helps alleviate irritation in the respiratory tract.

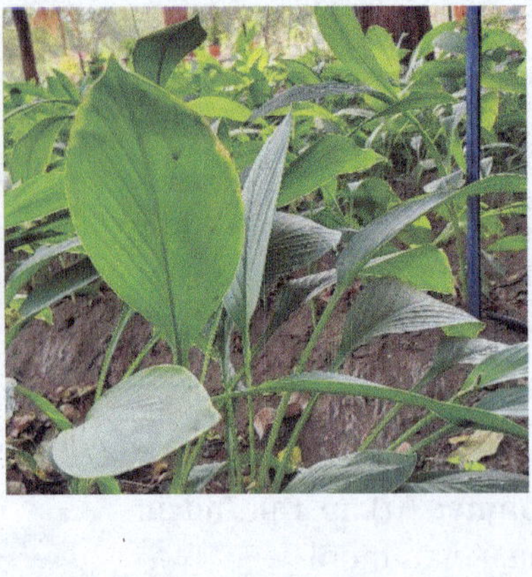

Scientific name: *Curcuma Longa*

Common name: Turmeric, Haldi

Distribution: High rainfall areas of Asia and Southeast Asia

Part used: Rhizomes

Bioactive principles: Curcumin

Remarks: Possess anti-inflammatory, antimicrobial and antioxidant properties

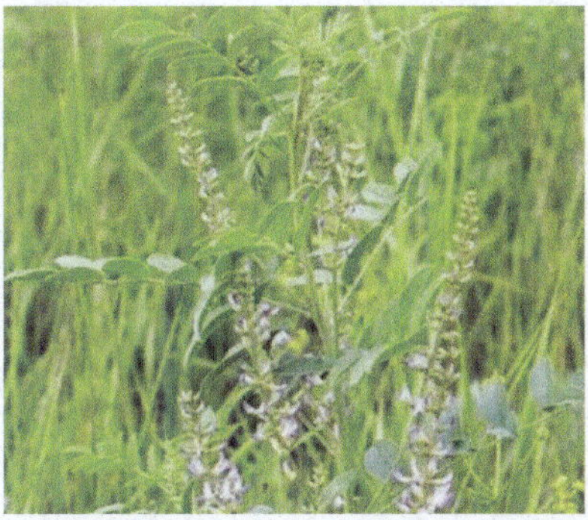

Scientific name: *Glycyrrhiza glabra*

Common name: Licorice, Mulethi

Distribution: Mediterranean region and Central and south-western Asia

Part used: Roots

Bioactive principles: Glycyrrhizin

Remarks: Immunity booster, anti-tussive, anti-inflammatory, anti-viral, expectorant

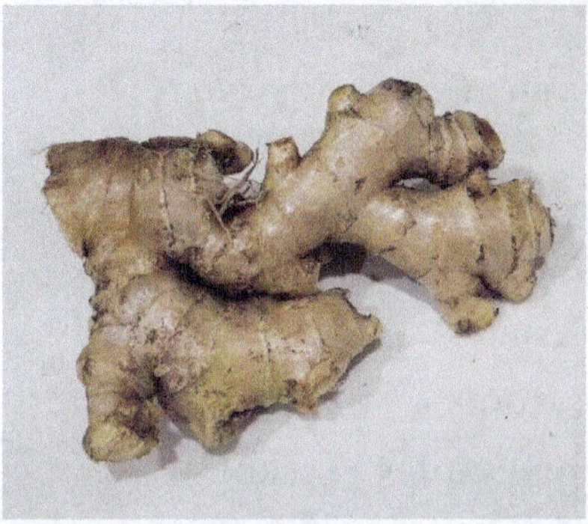

Scientific name: *Zingiber officinale*

Common name: Ginger

Distribution: South and south-east Asia

Part used: Rhizomes

Bioactive principles: Gingerol, shogaol, zingerone

Remarks: Anti-tussive, anti-inflammatory, anti-microbial properties and bronchodilator

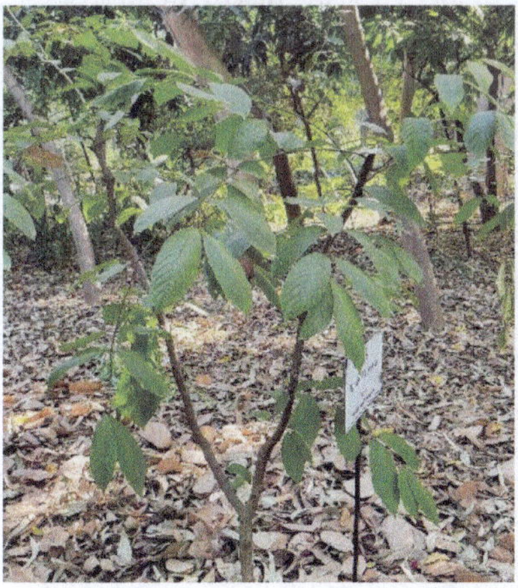

Scientific name: *Terminalia chebula*

Common name: Haritaki, Harad

Distribution: Indian subcontinent, China

Part used: Fruits and Bark

Bioactive principles: Chebulagic acid, chebulinic acid, ellagic acid and gallic acid (Tannins)

Remarks: Antitussive, antimicrobial property

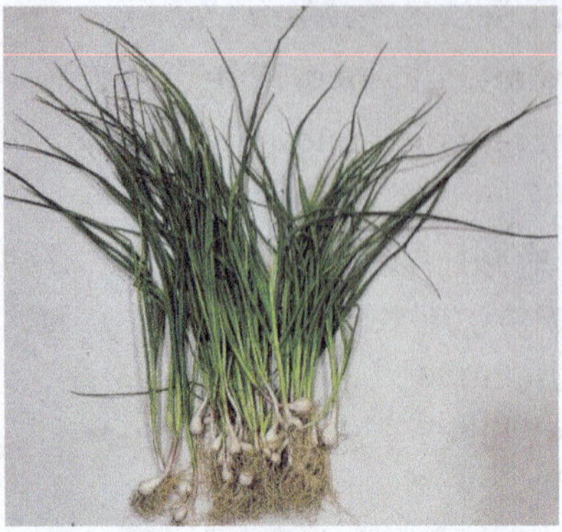

Scientific name: *Allium sativum*

Common name: Garlic

Distribution: Cultivated worldwide, with origins in Central Asia

Part used: Bulbs, cloves

Bioactive principles: Allicin

Remarks: Natural expectorant, antimicrobial, antifungal

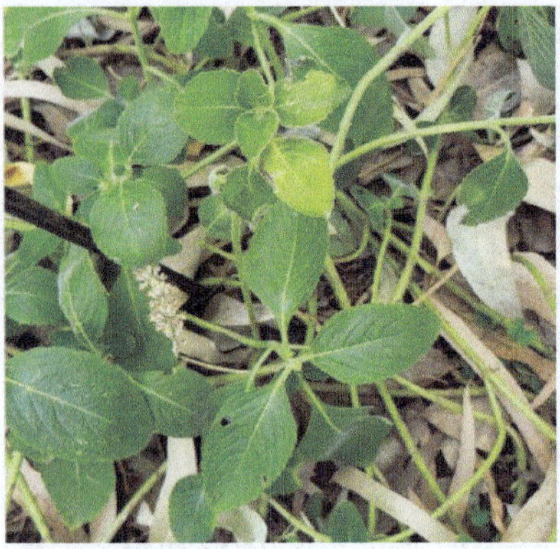

Scientific name: *Coleus forskolii (C. barbatus)*

Common name: Woolly plectranthus

Distribution: India, Nepal, and parts of Southeast Asia

Part used: Roots

Bioactive principles Forskolin (diterpene)

Remarks: Potent bronchodilator, act by stimulating adenylate cyclase activity

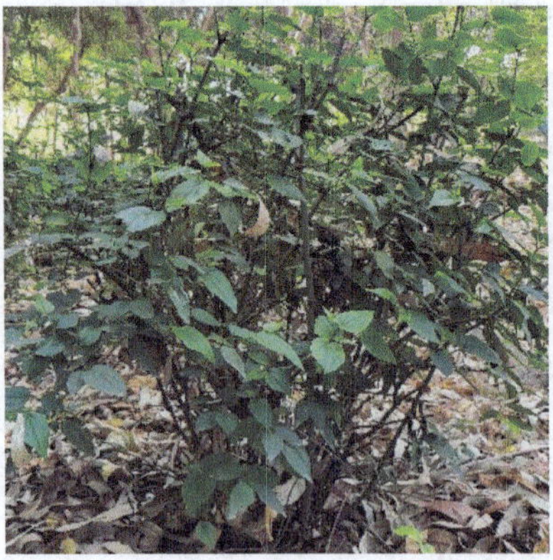

Scientific name: *Scindapsus officinalis*

Common name: Gaja pippali, Betel vine

Distribution: Indian subcontinent, China

Part used: Ripened fruit (powder)

Bioactive principles: Scindapsins, piperine, flavonoids

Remarks: Used to treat cough with phlegm, sinusitis, throat disorder, asthma, chronic respiratory disorders

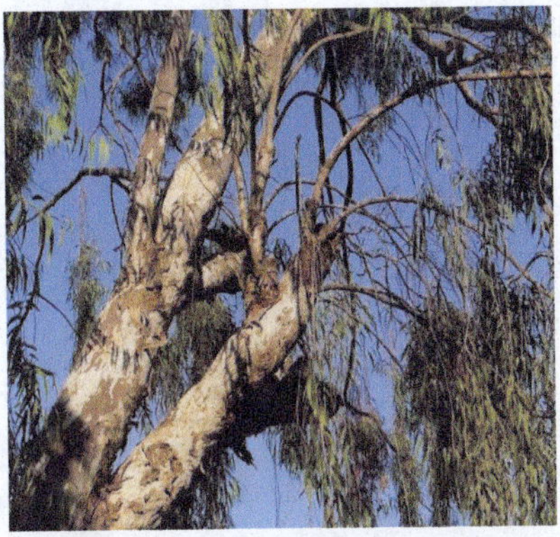

Scientific name: *Eucalyptus globulus*

Common name: Blue gum eucalyptus

Distribution: Native to south-eastern Australia, cultivated worldwide

Part used: Leaves

Bioactive principles: Eucalyptol (1,8-cineol), Terpinen-4-ol

Remarks: Essential oil used to treat nasal congestion, sinusitis, bronchitis, asthma

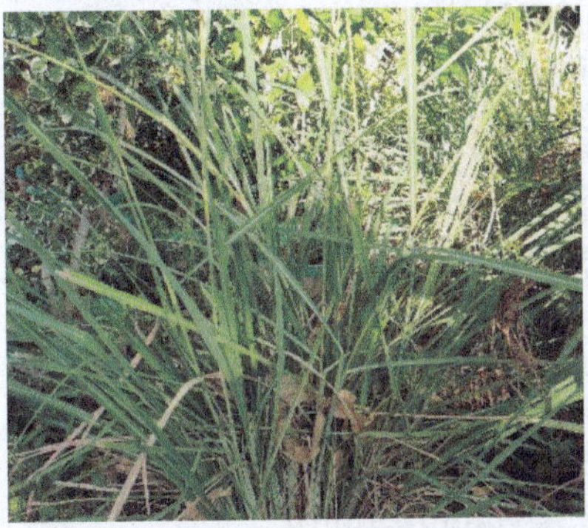

Scientific name: *Cymbopogon citratus*

Common name: Lemongrass

Distribution: Tropical and subtropical regions worldwide

Part used: Leaves

Bioactive principles: Citral, geraniol, flavonoids, Vitamin C

Remarks: Anti-spasmodic, antioxidant, helps reducing mucus production

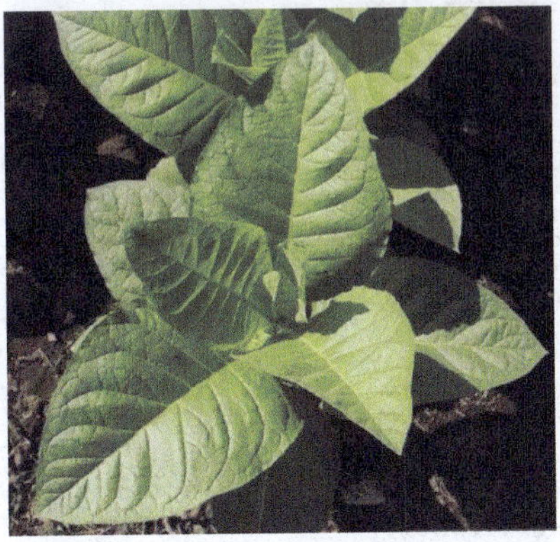

Scientific name: *Lobelia inflata*

Common name: Indian Tobacco

Distribution: Temperate regions worldwide

Part used: Leaves, seeds

Bioactive principles: Lobeline

Remarks: Effective bronchodilator, relaxant, antispasmodic, respiratory stimulant

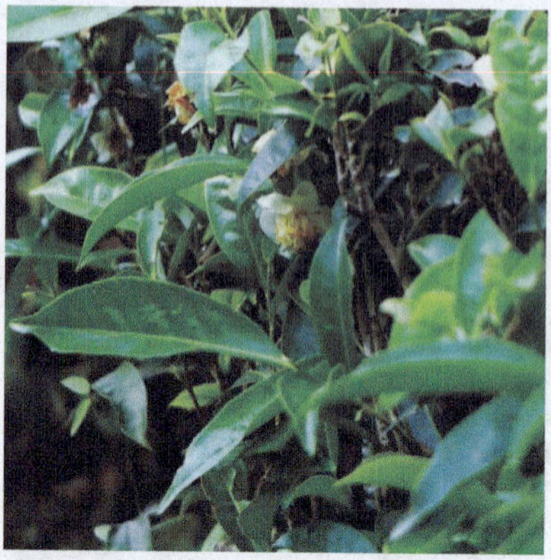

Scientific name: *Camellia sinensis*

Common name: Tea Plant

Distribution:

Part used: Leaves

Bioactive principles: Methylxanthines, catechins

Remarks: Mild bronchodilator, and antioxidant properties

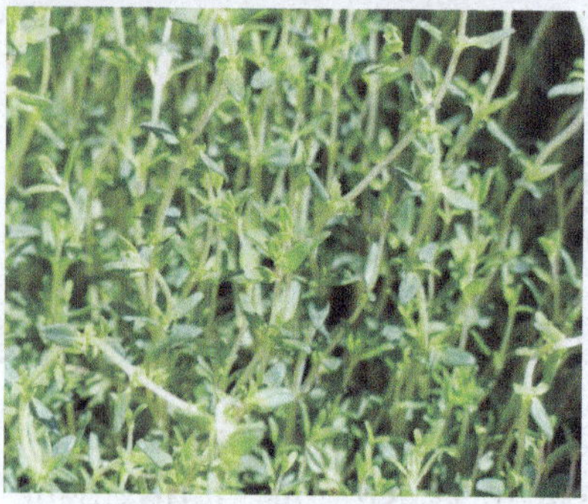

Scientific name: *Thymus vulgaris*

Common name: Thyme

Distribution: Native to the Mediterranean region; cultivated worldwide

Part used: Leaves and flowers

Bioactive principles: Thymol, carvacrol

Remarks: Bronchodilator and antimicrobial agent

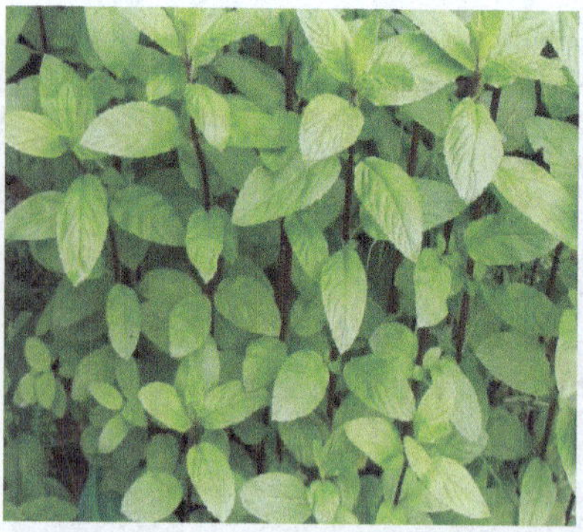

Scientific name: *Mentha piperita*

Common name: Peppermint

Distribution: Europe, North America, and Asia, cultivated worldwide

Part used: Leaves

Bioactive principles: Menthol, limonene

Remarks: Bronchodilator and decongestant effects

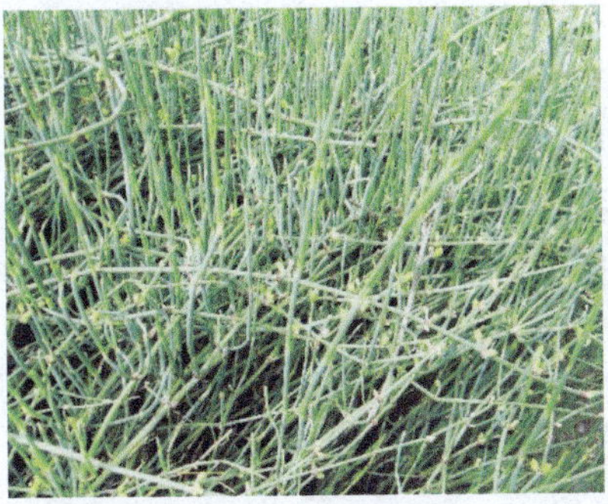

Scientific name: *Ephedra sinica*
Common name: Ma huang, Yellow horse
Distribution: Native to China, India, and Central Asia
Part used: Stems
Bioactive principles: Ephedrine, pseudoephedrine
Remarks: Effective bronchodilator

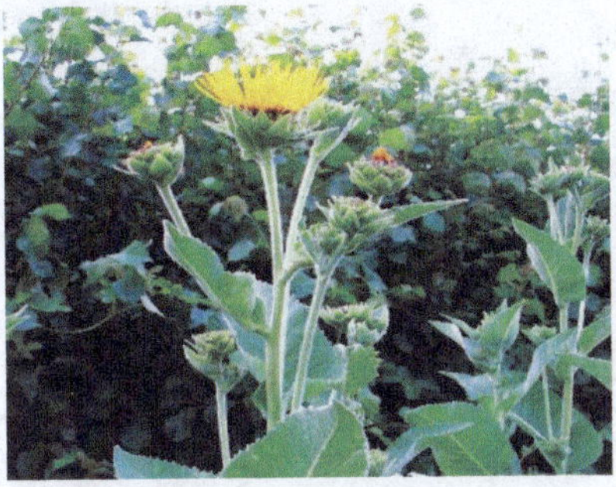

Scientific name: *Inula helenium*
Common name: Elecampane, horseheal
Distribution: Native to Europe & Asia
Part used: Dried Roots/ Rhizome
Bioactive principles: Alantolactone, isoalantolactone, inulin
Remarks: Anti-inflammatory/ antibacterial

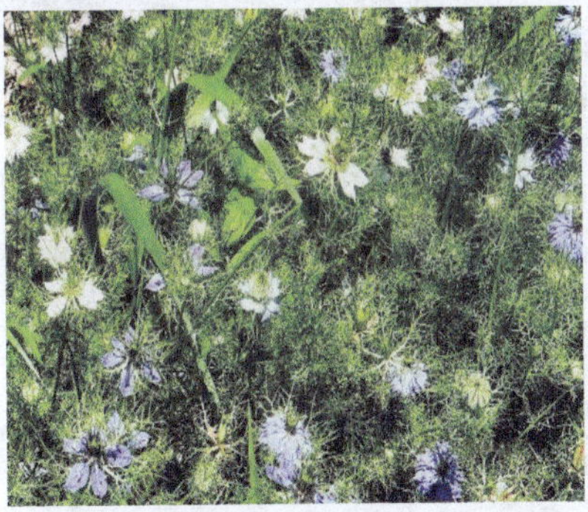

Scientific name: *Nigella sativa*
Common name: Black Cumin
Distribution: South Asia, the Middle East, and North Africa
Part used: Seeds
Bioactive principles: Thymoquinone, nigellone, alkaloids
Remarks: Anti-inflammatory and bronchodilator properties

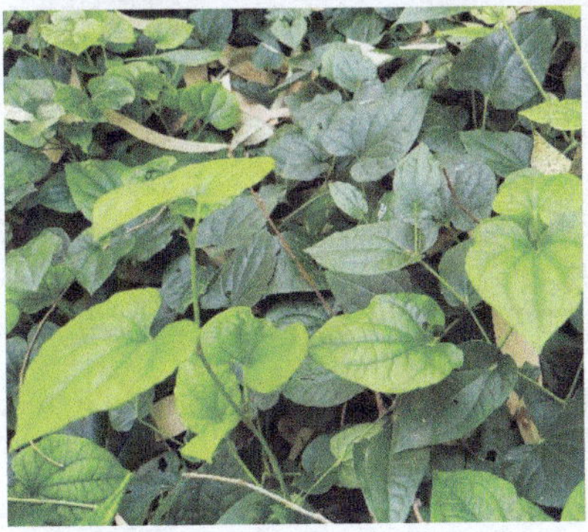

Scientific name: *Piper longum*
Common name: Long Pepper, Pipli
Distribution: Native to Southeast Asia and India
Part used: Fruits, roots
Bioactive principles: Piperine, Piperlonguminine
Remarks: Expectorant, decongestant, expel excessive mucus from the lungs

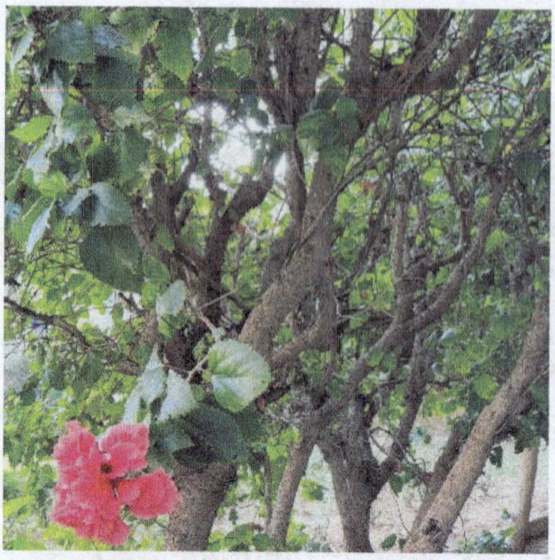

Scientific name: *Hibiscus rosa-sinensis*

Common name: Hibiscus, China rose

Distribution: Tropical and subtropical regions worldwide

Part used: Flower and Leaves

Bioactive principles:

Remarks: Anti-tussive properties, mucilage provides soothing effects

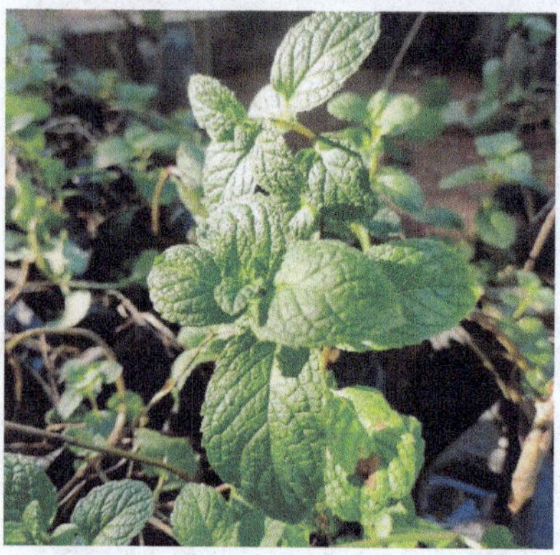

Scientific name: *Mentha arvensis*

Common name: Field Mint, Pudina

Distribution: Temperate and tropical regions of Asia

Part used: Leaves

Bioactive principles: Menthol, menthone, carvone

Remarks: Bronchodilator, decongestant, soothing effect

References

Ackermann MR, Brogden KA. Response of the ruminant respiratory tract to Mannheimia haemolytica. Microbes Infect. 2000;2(9):1079-88.

Aggarwal BB, Sundaram C, Malani N, Ichikawa H. Curcumin: the Indian solid gold. Adv Exp Med Biol. 2007; 595:1-75.

Ahmad A, Husain A, Mujeeb M, Khan SA, Najmi AK, Siddique NA, et al. A review on therapeutic potential of Nigella sativa: A miracle herb. Asian Pac J Trop Biomed. 2013;3(5):337-352.

Asl MN, Hosseinzadeh H. Review of pharmacological effects of Glycyrrhiza sp. and its bioactive compounds. Phytother Res. 2008;22(6):709-724.

Banyard AC, Parida S, Batten C, Oura C, Kwiatek O, Libeau G. Global distribution of peste des petits ruminants virus and prospects for improved diagnosis and control. J Gen Virol. 2010;91(12):2885-2897.

Benkirane A, De Alwis MC. Hemorrhagic septicemia: Its significance, prevention and control. Vet Med Sci. 2002;55(6):341-346.

Blackall PJ. Infectious coryza: Overview of the disease and new diagnostic options. Clin Microbiol Rev. 1999;12(4):627-632.

Cermelli C, Fabio A, Fabio G, Quaglio P. Effect of eucalyptus essential oil on respiratory bacteria and viruses. Curr Microbiol. 2008;56(1):89-92.

Ellis JA. Bovine respiratory syncytial virus: Immune responses and vaccination. Anim Health Res Rev. 2017;18(1):6-15.

Ghotge NS, Ramdas SR, editors. Plants used in animal care. ANTHRA publication; 2008.

Gyles CL, Prescott JF, Songer JG, Thoen CO. Pathogenesis of Bacterial Infections in Animals. 4th ed. Wiley-Blackwell; 2010. p. 144-150.

Khare CP. Indian Medicinal Plants: An Illustrated Dictionary. Springer; 2007. p. 676.

Kumar A, Kaur P, Sharma A, Reddy AV. Pharmacological review on Terminalia chebula. Int J Res Ayurveda Pharm. 2013;4(3):392-396.

Kumar RA, Sridevi K, Vijaya C, Nanduri S, Rajagopal S. Anticancer and immunostimulatory compounds from Andrographis paniculata. J Ethnopharmacol. 2004;92(2-3):291-295.

Lawson LD, Bauer R. Garlic: composition, medicinal history, and therapeutic use. In: Koch HP, Lawson LD, editors. Garlic: The science and therapeutic application of Allium sativum L. and related species. 2nd ed. Williams & Wilkins; 1996. p. 1-24.

McKay DL, Blumberg JB. A review of the bioactivity and potential health benefits of peppermint tea (Mentha piperita L.). Phytother Res. 2006;20(8):619-633.

Newton JR, Verheyen K, Talbot NC, Timoney JF. Strangles: Epidemiology, treatment and control. Equine Vet J. 1997;29(5):373-382.

Nicholas R, Churchward C. Contagious caprine pleuropneumonia: An update on the disease and its treatment. Vet J. 2012;193(2):146-53.

OIE. Bovine Tuberculosis. [Internet]. 2023. Available from: https://www.woah.org

Prescott JF. Rhodococcus equi: An animal and human pathogen. Clin Microbiol Rev. 1991;4(1):20-34.

Radostits OM, Gay CC, Hinchcliff KW, Constable PD. Veterinary Medicine: A Textbook of the Diseases of Cattle, Horses, Sheep, Pigs and Goats. 10th ed. Elsevier Health Sciences; 2007.

Satyavani K, Gurumurthy P, Kannan N. Ethnomedicinal plants used for the treatment of respiratory disorders among the tribals of Western Ghats, India. Int J Pharm Sci Res. 2012;3(9):2992-2997.

Soković M, Glamočlija J, Marin PD, Brkić D, van Griensven LJ. Antibacterial effects of the essential oils of commonly consumed medicinal herbs using an in vitro model. Molecules. 2010;15(11):7532-7546.

Surjushe A, Vasani R, Saple DG. Aloe vera: a short review. Indian J Dermatol. 2008;53(4):163-166.

Taylor MA, Coop RL, Wall RL. Veterinary Parasitology. 4th ed. Wiley-Blackwell; 2015..

Ved DK, Tagadur S, Sureshchandra V, Barve V, Srinivas V, Sangeetha S, Ravikumar K, Kartikeyan R, Kulkarni V, Kumar AS, Venugopal SN, Somashekhar BS, Sumanth MV, Begum N, Rani S, Surekha KV, Desale N. 2016. FRLHT's ENVIS Centre on Medicinal Plants, Bengaluru. Available from: http://envis.frlht.org/plant_details.php?disp_id=1187.

Whittemore JC, Lappin MR. Diagnosis, treatment, and prognosis of Cryptococcus infections in cats and dogs. Vet Med. 2013;108(2):87-96.

Williams J, Robinson NE, editors. Current Therapy in Equine Medicine. 6th ed. Saunders; 2008.

Wynn SG, Fougère B. Veterinary herbal medicine. Elsevier Health Sciences; 2006.

Yarnell E, Abascal K, Rountree R. Clinical botanical medicine. Mary Ann Liebert, Inc., publishers; 2009.

Yarnell E. Nature's Cures: What You Should Know. Healing Mountain Publishing; 2006.

Yarnell E. Nature's Miracle Medicines Amazing Remedies. Healing Mountain Publishing; 2007.

13

Medicinal Plants Effective in Kidney Disorders in Animals

V. N. Sarvaiya, K.A. Sadariya, and S.K. Bhavsar

Department of Veterinary Pharmacology and Toxicology, College of Veterinary Science and A.H., Kamdhenu University, Anand-388001, Gujarat

The kidney plays a role in controlling the volume of different bodily fluids, fluid osmolality, acid-base balance, toxin elimination, and different electrolyte concentrations. The glomerulus filters one-fifth of the volume of blood that enters the kidneys. Among the compounds that are reabsorbed include amino acids, salt, bicarbonate, glucose, and solute-free water. Among the chemicals that are released are ammonium, potassium, hydrogen, and uric acid. The kidneys maintain homeostasis, eliminate metabolic waste products like uric acid, urea, creatinine and ammonia, regulate extracellular fluid volume, blood pressure (via the rennin-angiotensin system) and controlling systemic pH (via regulation of H^+ and HCO^{3-} concentration).

Among various kidney diseases, especially chronic kidney disease (CKD) is a slow loss of kidney function in which, kidney dysfunction is present for more than three months. There are six progressive stages of CKD *i.e.* stages 1, 2, 3a, 3b, 4 and 5. The stages are based on the results of glomerular filtration rate (GFR) test (1). In stage 1 there is mild kidney damage, while in stage 5 kidneys lost their working capacity. Chronic kidney disease (CKD) is a worldwide health issue that is becoming more prevalent in both developed and developing nations. It typically affects adults. .

Models for Chronic Kidney Disease

To investigate the origins and management of chronic kidney disease (CKD), numerous animal models have been created. These models are developed to study patho-physiology of CKD and to observe the effects of allopathic or herbal drugs on disease model.

1. Adenine-induced (0.25%(w/w) for 35 days) chronic renal disease had similar biochemical findings to that of human chronic kidney disease (2). Pathological alterations in the proximal tubules, distal tubules and glomerular abnormalities were confirmed by histological findings.
2. Intraperitoneal injection of gentamicin (100 mg/kg) for 8 days produced nephrotoxicity in wistar rats (3).
3. Another method was to develop 5/6 nephrectomized animal model. Rats with 5/6 nephrectomies are employed as a model for renal failure in order to assess *the* renoprotective properties of compounds (4).
4. Single intraperitoneal injection of cisplatin (5 mg/kg b.w.) produced nephrotoxicity in Wistar rats (5). Abamectin for 28 days at a dose of 2 mg/kg body weight was also used to produce CKD in rats (6).

Treatment for Chronic Kidney Disease

To treat the complications of CKD, generally medications for controlling high blood pressure; relieving pain and inflammation are given; low protein diets are recommended, but again dialysis is the only option to take care of the patient in end stage kidney disease. The potential to prevent or halt the progression of a disease and lower healthcare expenses are two factors that contribute to interest in the health-promoting qualities of herbal medicines. Worldwide, hospital stays and CKD treatment place a huge financial strain on the healthcare system, and this cost is only going to grow.

Herbal Treatment for Chronic Kidney Disease

Over several decades, people with chronic kidney disease have been treated with complementary and alternative therapies, with varying degrees of improvement in their condition. These treatments are probably used in conjunction with traditional medications in Western nations, but alternative medications are only used for individuals with chronic kidney disease in China and other Asian and African nations.

There are several medicinal plants effective in chronic kidney disorders. Various plant parts, including the leaves, fruits, barks, roots and even the seeds are utilised in the preparation of medicines.

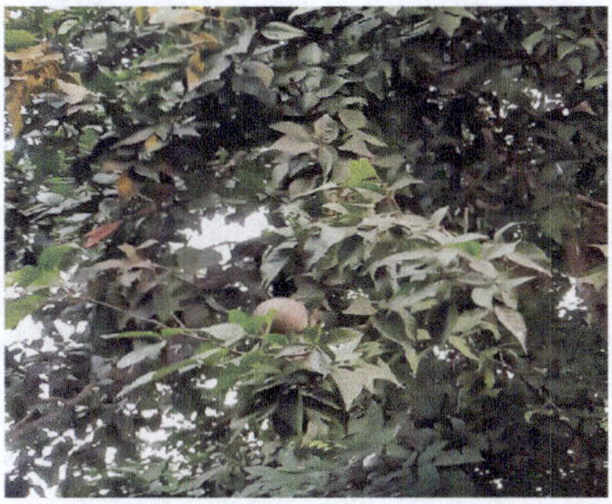

Scientific name: *Aegle marmelos*

Common name: Bael, Bel, Belgiri

Distribution: Indian Subcontinent

Parts used: Root, bark, leaf, flower and fruit

Bioactive principles: Marmeline, Agelin, Aegelenine, Dictamine, Fragrine

Remark: It protects renal cells through its anti-inflammatory and antioxidant effects, decreasing inflammation and oxidative stress in kidney tissues

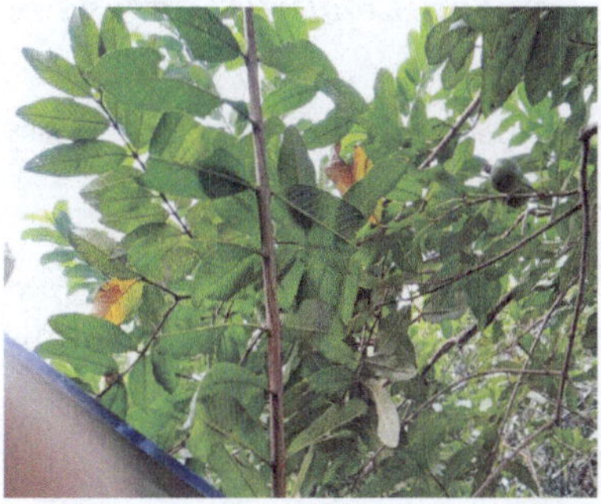

Scientific name : *Annona squamosa*

Common name: Custard apple, sugarapple, sweetsop

Distribution: Indian Subcontinent

Parts used: root, bark, leaf, flower, and fruit

Bioactive principles: Annonaine, Benzyltetrahydro- isoquinoline, Camphene, Camphor, Higemamine, Isocorydine, Limonine

Remark: Exhibits nephroprotective effects by modulating oxidative stress and maintaining normal levels of serum creatinine and urea.

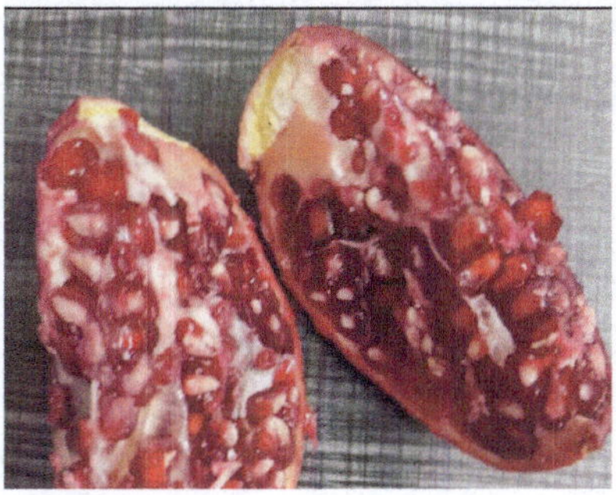

Scientific name: *Punica granatum*

Common name: Pomegranate

Distribution: Indian Subcontinent

Parts used: Fruit pulp, seeds, pulverized flower buds, Peels

Bioactive principles: Punicalin, Pedunculagin, Punicalagin, Gallic and ellagic acid

Remark: Rich in antioxidants like punicalagin that prevents kidney damage by reducing oxidative stress and lipid peroxidation

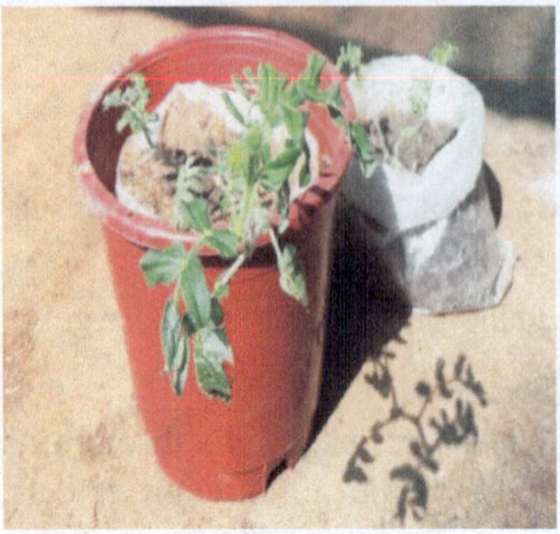

Scientific name: *Tribulus terrestris*

Common name: Gokshur/ Gokharu

Distribution: Indian Subcontinent

Parts used: Whole herb

Bioactive principles: Steroidal saponins (terrestrosins), Flavonoids, Glycosides, Alkaloids, Tannins

Remark: Enhances kidney function by reducing urinary crystallization, acting as a diuretic and preventing renal stone formation.

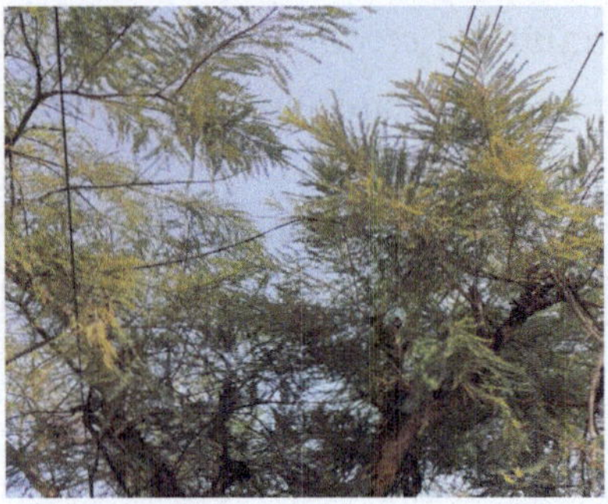

Scientific name: *Emblica officinalis/* Phyllanthus emblica

Common name: Amla, Indian Goose berry

Distribution: Indian Subcontinent

Parts used: Leaf, flower and fruit

Bioactive principles: Gallic acid, chebulinic acid, quercetin and tannin

Remark: Provides renal protection through its high vitamin C content, scavenging free radicals and mitigating oxidative damage in kidney tissues

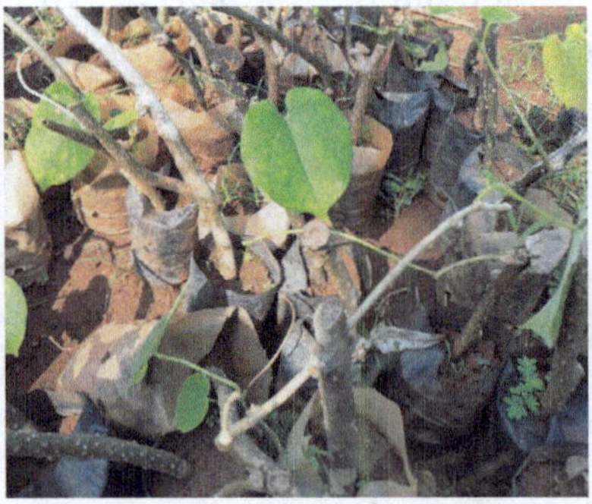

Scientific name: *Tinospora cordifolia/ Tinospora sinensis/ Tinospora malabarica*

Common name: Gado/ Galo/ Giloy/ Guduchi/ Amrita

Distribution: Indian Subcontinent

Parts used: Stem, root, leaf

Bioactive principles: Tinosporaside, Tinosporide, Berberine, Choline, Palmatine, Tembetarine, Tinocordiside, Tinocordifolioside

Remark: Exhibits anti-inflammatory and antioxidant activities, protecting renal cells from toxins and oxidative damage

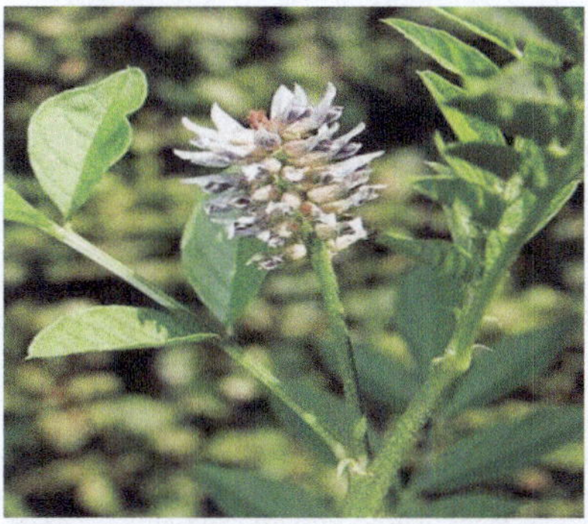

Scientific name: *Glycyrrhiza glabra*

Common name: Liquorice

Distribution: Southern Europe, India and portions of Asia

Parts used: Root

Bioactive principles: Glycyrrhizinm, Liquiritin, Isoliquiritin, Licuraside

Remark: Glycyrrhizin reduces oxidative stress and inflammation, supporting renal function and preventing nephrotoxicity

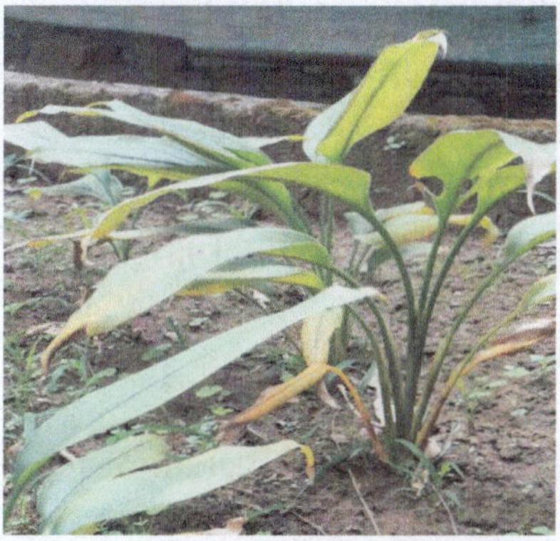

Scientific name: *Curcuma longa*

Common name: Turmeric

Distribution: Indian Subcontinent

Parts used: Rhizomes

Bioactive principles: Curcumin, dimethoxycurcumin, bis-dimethoxycurcumin,

Remark: Curcumin protects kidneys by reducing inflammation, fibrosis and oxidative stress in renal tissues

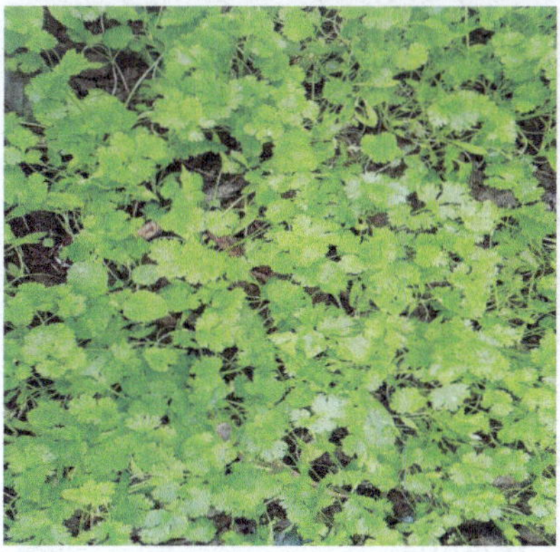

Scientific name: *Coriandrum sativum*

Common name: Coriander, Chinese parsley

Distribution: Southern Europe, Northern Africa and Southwestern Asia

Parts used: Seed and leaves

Bioactive principles: Glycosides, Kaempferol 3-O-rutinoside, Ferulic acid glucoside and p-Coumaroylquinic acid

Remark: Act as diuretic, reduces oxidative stress and helps in the excretion of toxins

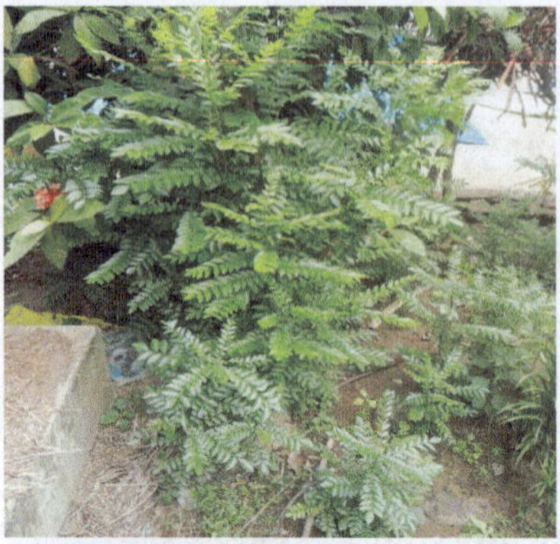

Scientific name: *Murraya koenigii*

Common name: Curry leaf

Distribution: Indian Subcontinent

Parts used: Leaves and bark

Bioactive principles: Flavonoids, Terpenoids and Polyphenols

Remark: Exhibits antioxidant and anti-inflammatory activities, reducing renal damage and improving kidney function.

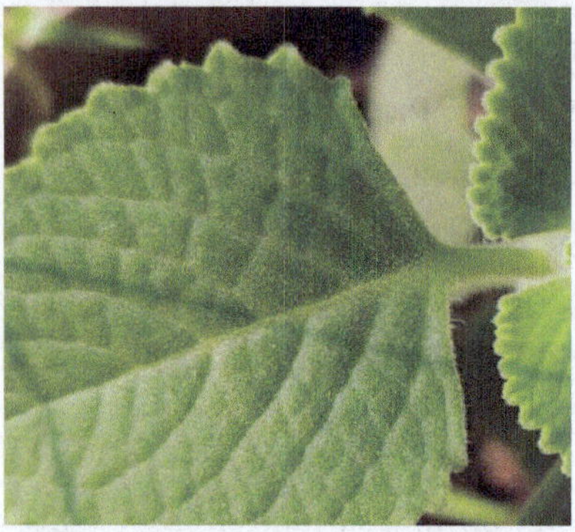

Scientific name: *Mentha piperita*

Common name: Peppermint/ Mint

Distribution: Indian Subcontinent

Parts used: Leaves

Bioactive principles: Menthol, Menthone, Menthyl acetate, Pulegone, Phenolic acids, Flavonoids

Remark: Renoprotective effect is due to antioxidant activity and regulation of renal oxidative stress markers

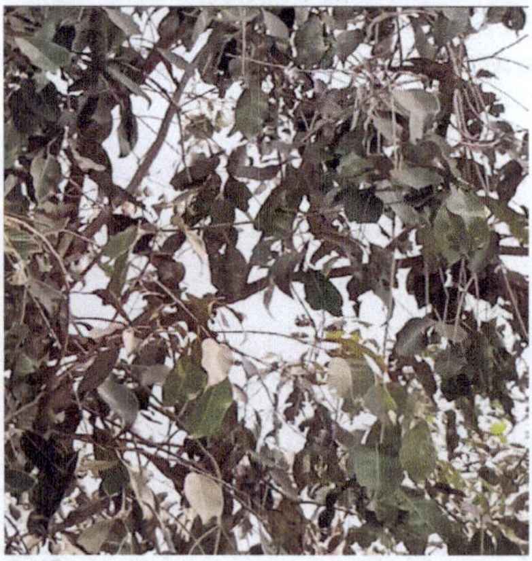

Scientific name: *Syzygium cumini*

Common name: Malabar plum/ Purple plum/ Jamun/ Indian blackberry/ Black plum/ Java plum/ Portuguese plum/ Jamaica/ Damson plum

Distribution: Indian Subcontinent

Parts used: Leaves, bark, flowers, root, fruits

Bioactive principles: Jambosine, Jambolin, Sugar, Minerals, Vitamin C, Oxalic acid, Gallic acid, Tannins

Remark: Protect kidneys by reducing oxidative stress, inflammation and preventing renal damage produced by toxins

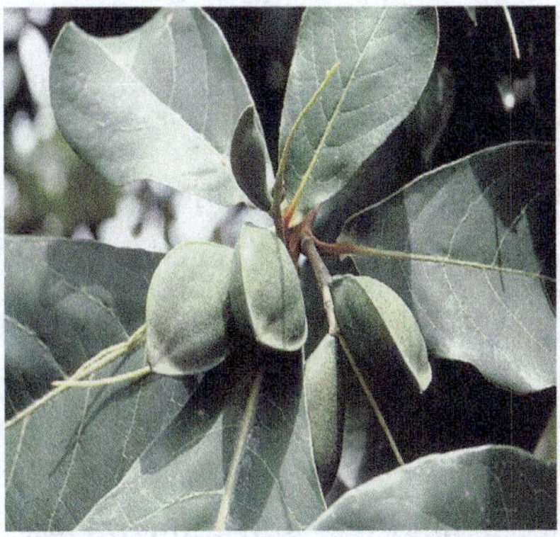

Scientific name: *Terminalia bellirica*

Common name: Bahera/ Beleric Bhaira/ Bastard myrobalan/ Belliric Myrobalan/ Beach almond/ Bedda nut tree

Distribution: Indian Subcontinent

Parts used: Bark, fruit (seed), leaf

Bioactive principles: Belleric acid, Bellericosides , Bellericanin, Gallic acid, Sugar

Remark: Contains tannins and other antioxidants that protect kidneys from oxidative stress and nephrotoxic agents

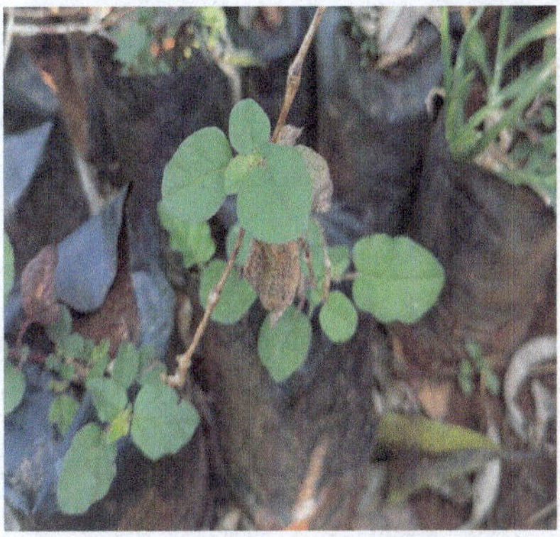

Scientific name: *Boerhavia diffusa*

Common name: Common Hogweed, Punarnava

Distribution: Indian Subcontinent

Parts used: Root, seed, leaf, flower, and fruit

Bioactive principles: Rotenoids, Flavonoids, Lunamarine, Ascorbic acid

Remark: Known for its diuretic and antioxidant properties, it prevents renal fibrosis and promotes toxin excretion

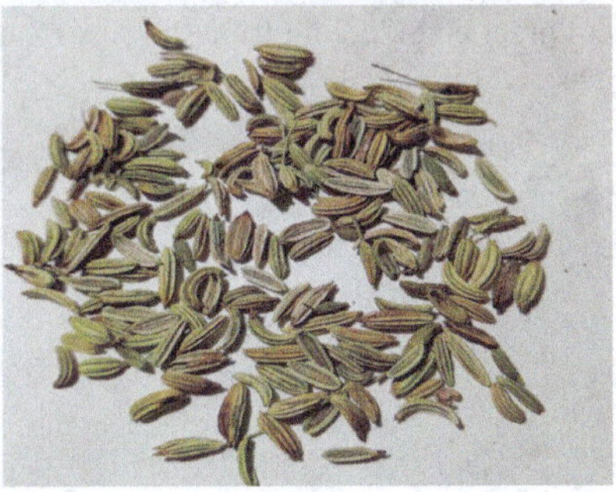

Scientific name: *Foeniculum vulgare*

Common name: Sweet fennel/ Fennel/ Florence fennel

Distribution: Indian Subcontinent

Parts used: Roots, leaves, fruit (seeds)

Bioactive principles:
Transanethole, Estragole, Fenchone, Neochlorogenic acid, Chlorogenic acid, Gallic acid

Remark: Protect kidneys by acting as a diuretic, reducing oxidative damage and enhancing renal detoxification

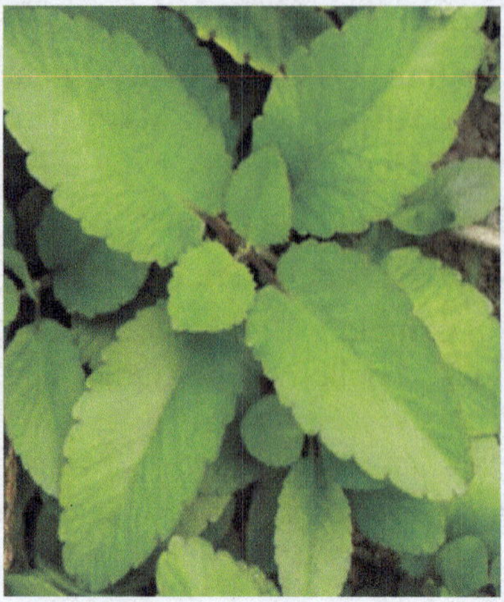

Scientific name : *Bryophyllum pinnatum*

Common name: Patharchatta, Kalanchoe Pinnata, Panfuti

Distribution: Indian Subcontinent

Parts used: Leaves

Bioactive principles: Bryophyllins A, Bufadienolides, Stigmasterols, anthocyanins, phenylpropanoids

Remark: Protects renal tissue by its antioxidant and anti-inflammatory properties, reduce nephrotoxicity and oxidative stress

References

Aggarwal D, Dumka V, Saini S, Sharma M. Abamectin induced toxicity and its amelioration by Aegle marmelos in rats. J Pharm Innov. 2022 Dec 21;11(1):1074-81.

Ali BH, Al ZM, Adham SA, Yasin J, Nemmar A, Schupp N. Therapeu*t*ic e*f*fect of chrysin on adenine-induced chronic kidney disease in rats. Cell Physiol Biochem. 2016 Jan 20;38(1):248-57.

Deshmukh AB, Patel JK. Aqueous extract of Annona squamosa (L.) ameliorates renal failure induced by 5/6 nephrectomy in rat. Indian J Pharmacol. 2011 Nov;43(6):718-21.

Dwivedi J, *Singh M, Sharma* S, Sha*r*ma S. Antioxidant and nephroprotective potential of Aegle marmelos leaves extract. *J Herbs Spices* & Med Plants. 2017 Nov 22;23(4):363–77.

Kore KJ, Shete RV, Jadhav PJ. RP-HPLC method of simultaneous nephroprotective role of Aegle marmelos extrac. Int J Res Pharm Chem. 2011; 1(3):617-23.

Qaseem *A, Hopkins RH*, Sweet DE, Star*k*ey M, Shekelle P. Screening, monitoring, and treatment of stage 1 to 3 chronic kidney disease: a clinical practice guideline from the American Co*llege of Physici*ans. Ann Intern Medi. 2013 Dec 17;159(12):835-47.

14

Medicinal Plants Effective in Central Nervous System Disorders in Animals

Nisha A R, Varsha B, Archana A, Sudhakar S and Pooja Krishna

Department of Veterinary Pharmacology and Toxicology,
College of Veterinary and Animal Sciences, Mannuthy, Thrissur 680 651, Kerala

Nervous system Disorders in Domestic Animals

Nervous system disorders in domestic animals encompass a range of conditions that affect the brain, peripheral nerves, and spinal cord. These disorders can result in a variety of clinical signs, depending on the area of the nervous system involved. Infectious disorders like rabies, canine distemper, toxoplasmosis, listeriosis. Congenital and developmental disorders like hydrocephalus, cerebellar hypoplasia and chiari-like malformation can cause these disorders. Traumatic and degenerative disorders like Intervertebral Disc Disease. Degenerative myelopathy, metabolic and toxic disorders like hepatic encephalopathy, hypocalcemia, lead poisoning, organophosphate toxicity, autoimmune and inflammatory disorders like meningitis and meningoencephalitis may also lead to nervous system disorders. Some tumours associated with nervous system like meningiomas and peripheral nerve sheath tumours also cause nervous system disorders.

Nervous System Disorders Induced in Lab Animals

Nervous system disorders induced in laboratory animals are often used in research to study the mechanisms, treatment options, and prevention strategies for neurological diseases in humans. These disorders are typically created using a variety of methods, such as chemical exposure, genetic manipulation, or physical injury. Below are some common examples of nervous system disorders induced in lab animals.

1. Neurodegenerative Diseases

Alzheimer's Disease: Transgenic animal models, particularily in mice, are engineered to express mutant genes.

Parkinson's Disease: Animal models are created by using neurotoxins like MPTP (1-methyl-4-phenyl-1,2,3,6-tetrahydropyridine) to damage dopaminergic neurons, mimicking Parkinson's disease.

Huntington's Disease: Genetic models with a mutant Huntington gene (HTT) are created to study the progressive motor dysfunction and cognitive decline associated with the disease.

2. Multiple Sclerosis (MS)

This is the most common animal model for studying MS. It involves immunizing animals (usually mice or rats) with myelin proteins to induce inflammation and demyelination of the central nervous system.

3. Epilepsy

Kindling Model: Repeated stimulation of specific brain regions (such as the amygdala or hippocampus) in animals induces seizures. This model is useful for studying the pathophysiology of epilepsy.

Pentylenetetrazol (PTZ) Model: PTZ is a chemical that, when administered to animals, induces convulsive seizures. This model helps in testing anticonvulsant drugs.

4. Traumatic Brain Injury (TBI)

Traumatic brain injury is commonly induced in animals through controlled mechanical impact, such as cortical impact injury or fluid percussion injury. These models are used to investigate the brain's response to trauma and potential therapeutic approaches.

5. Stroke

Ischemic Stroke Model: This is often induced by occlusion of a blood vessel (e.g., middle cerebral artery) in rodents. This model mimics ischemic stroke and is used to test neuroprotective agents.

Hemorrhagic Stroke Model: Hemorrhagic stroke is induced by the rupture of blood vessels, typically using collagenase injection into the brain.

6. Autism Spectrum Disorders (ASD)

Animal models of autism are often generated through genetic mutations or through prenatal exposure to chemicals. These models aim to replicate behaviours such as social withdrawal, repetitive behaviors, and communication deficits.

7. Peripheral Neuropathy

This condition can be induced by methods such as ligating the sciatic nerve or through exposure to neurotoxic substances like vincristine, which causes damage to peripheral nerves, mimicking symptoms of peripheral neuropathy.

8. Anxiety and Stress Disorders

Elevated Plus Maze: This is a behavioural model in which rodents are exposed to an elevated maze with open and closed arms to assess anxiety levels.

9. Drug-Induced Neurological Disorders

Certain drugs or toxins can induce neurological symptoms in lab animals, which can be used to study substance-induced disorders, such as dopamine depletion (similar to Parkinson's) or caused by neurotoxins like MPTP or the use of phencyclidine (PCP) to induce symptoms similar to schizophrenia. Drugs used to treat nervous system disorders are often classified based on the type of disorder they are meant to address. These drugs can include those for treating pain, seizures, mood disorders, neurodegenerative diseases, and others. Analgesics like non-steroidal anti-inflammatory drugs, opioids like morphine, oxycodone, hydrocodone. Anticonvulsants like gabapentin, pregabalin. Antidepressants like Selective Serotonin Reuptake Inhibitors also used to treat anxiety and depression . Mood stabilizers are used in bipolar disorder to prevent mood swings. Examples are lithium, valproate, antipsychotics like clozapine, olanzapine, risperidone, anticonvulsants like valproic acid, carbamazepine, levetiracetam, lamotrigine, cognitive enhancers, dopaminergic drugs, muscle relaxants, cholinesterase inhibitors, anxiolytics and NMDA antagonists like memantine are frequently used in the treatment of nervous system disorders.

Herbal treatment in nervous system disorders

Herbal treatments for nervous system disorders have been used since centuries in traditional medicine systems like Traditional Chinese Medicine (TCM), Ayurveda, and others. While some herbal remedies may offer benefits for various nervous system conditions, it's important to approach them with utmost care.

Medicinal Plants used in Nervous System Disorders

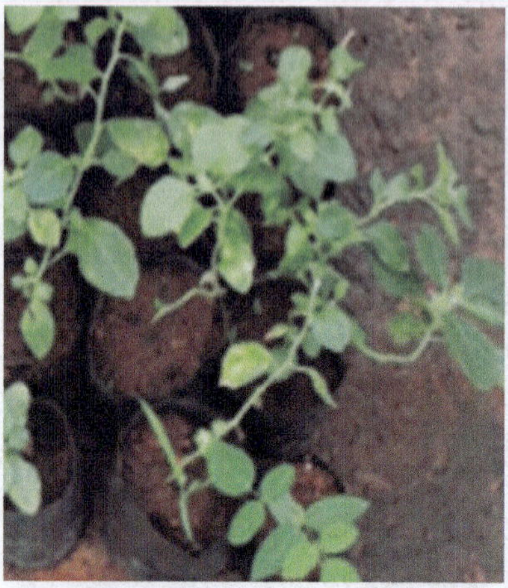

Scientific Name: *Withania somnifera*

Common Name: Ashwagandha, Indian Ginseng

Distribution: Native to India, North Africa, and the Middle East

Part Used: Root

Bioactive Principles: Withanolides, Alkaloids, Saponins

Remarks: Known for its adaptogenic properties, Ashwagandha is used to reduce stress, improve cognitive function, and treat anxiety, depression, and insomnia.

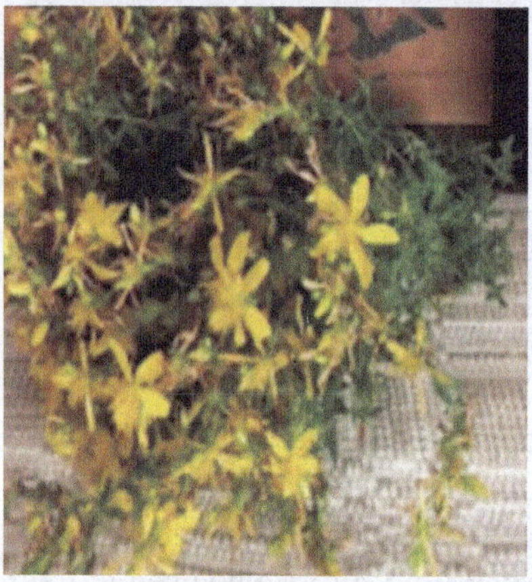

Scientific Name: *Hypericum perforatum*

Common Name: St. John's Wort

Distribution: Native to Europe, North America, & parts of Asia

Part Used: Flowering tops

Bioactive Principles: Hypericin, Hyperforin, Flavonoids, Tannins

Remarks: St. John's Wort is widely used as a treatment for mild to moderate depression & anxiety. It may interact with other medications and is contraindicated in some conditions.

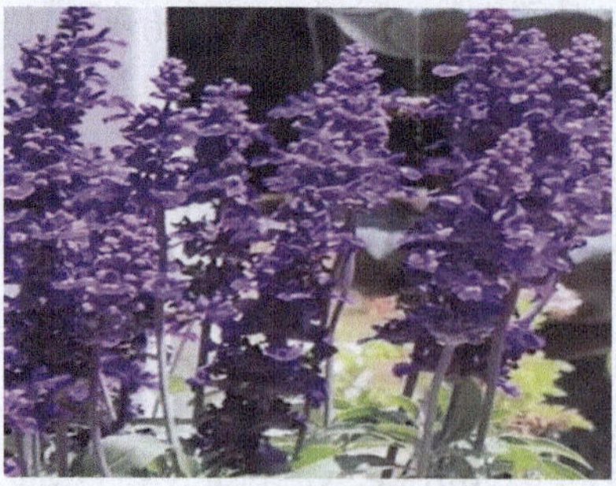

Scientific Name: *Lavandula angustifolia*

Common Name: Lavender

Distribution: Native to the Mediterranean region, widely cultivated in temperate climates

Part Used: Flowers and essential oil

Bioactive Principles: Linalool, Linalyl acetate, Camphor, Tannins

Remarks: Lavender is used for its calming effect to reduce anxiety, insomnia, and stress. The essential oil is commonly used in aromatherapy.

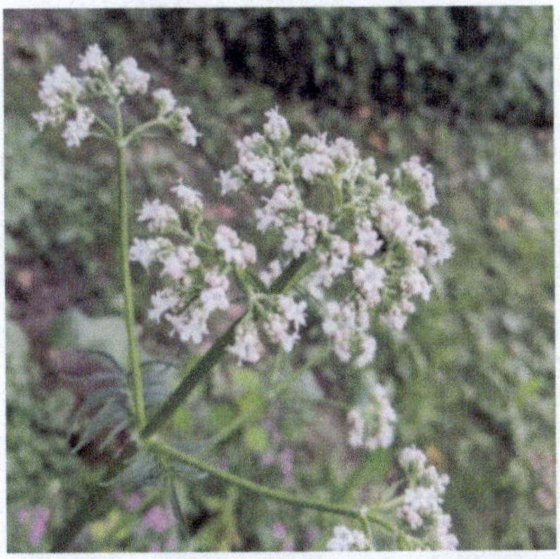

Scientific Name: *Valeriana officinalis*

Common Name: Valerian

Distribution: Native to Europe and Asia, now found in North America

Part Used: Root

Bioactive Principles: Valerenic acid, Valepotriates, Alkaloids

Remarks: Used as a mild sedative and anxiolytic, Valerian is often employed to treat insomnia, anxiety, and nervous agitation.

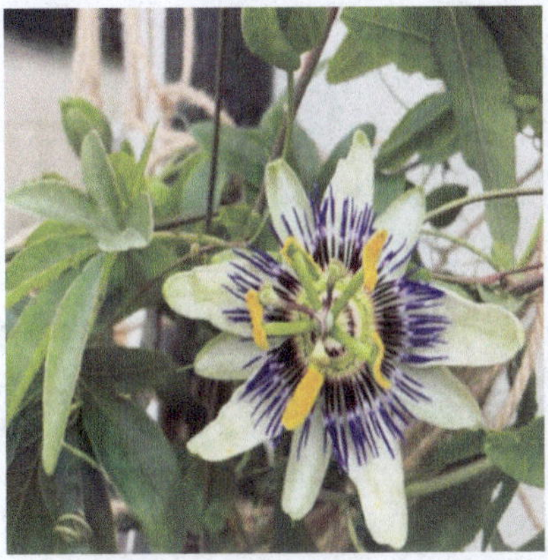

Scientific Name: *Passiflora incarnata*

Common Name: Passionflower

Distribution: Native to the southeastern United States, Central and South America

Part Used: Aerial parts

Bioactive Principles: Flavonoids, Alkaloids, Glycosides

Remarks: Passionflower is used to treat anxiety, insomnia, and stress. It has a mild sedative effect and is often used in combination with other calming herbs.

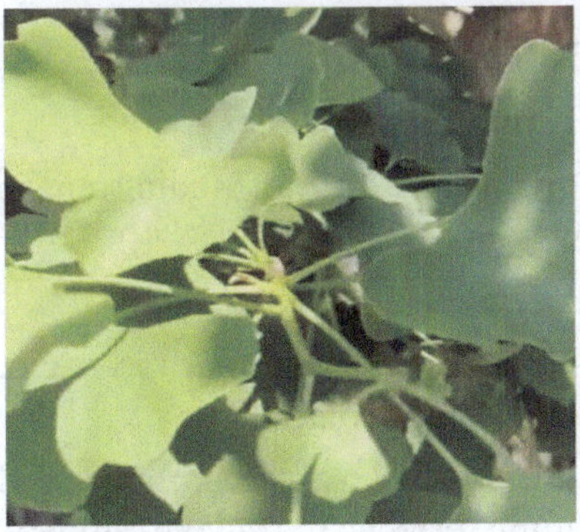

Scientific Name: *Ginkgo biloba*

Common Name: Ginkgo

Distribution: Native to China, now widely cultivated worldwide

Part Used: Leaves

Bioactive Principles: Ginkgolides, Bilobalide, Flavonoids, Terpenoids

Remarks: Known for improving memory and cognitive function, Ginkgo biloba is often used to treat dementia, Alzheimer's disease, and to enhance mental clarity.

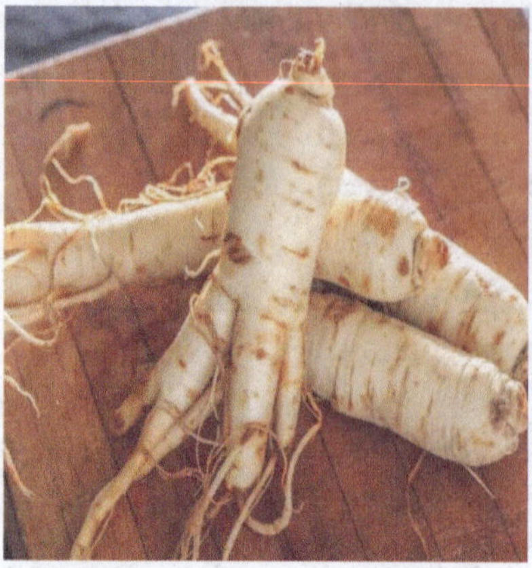

Scientific Name: *Panax ginseng*

Common Name: Ginseng

Distribution: Native to East Asia, particularly Korea, China, and Siberia

Part Used: Root

Bioactive Principles: Ginsenosides, Polysaccharides, Peptides

Remarks: Ginseng is known for its adaptogenic properties, enhancing physical and mental performance, reducing fatigue, and supporting overall nervous system health.

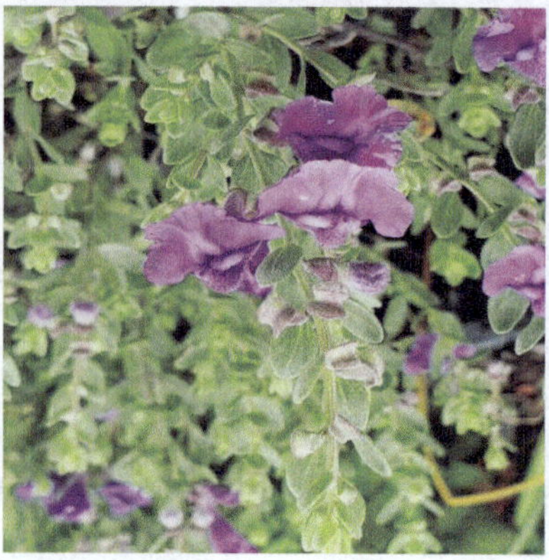

Scientific Name: *Scutellaria lateriflora*

Common Name: Skullcap

Distribution: Native to North America

Part Used: Aerial parts

Bioactive Principles: Baicalin, Baicalein, Scutellarin

Remarks: Skullcap is used as a calming herb for anxiety, nervous tension, and insomnia. It has mild sedative and neuro*protective properties.*

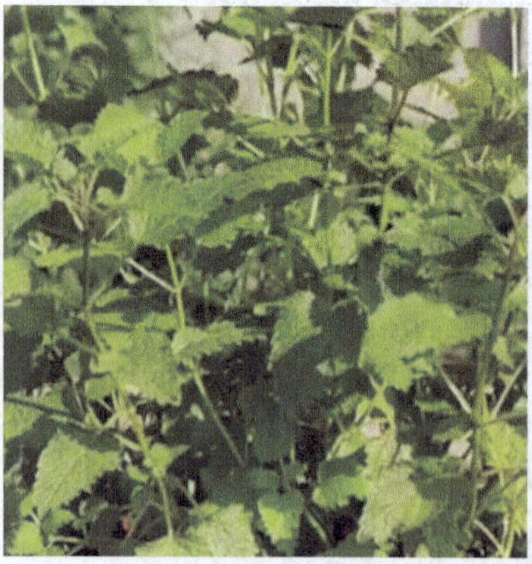

Scientific Name: *Melissa officinalis*

Common Name: Lemon balm

Distribution: Native to the Mediterranean region, now widely cultivated

Part Used: Leaves

Bioactive Principles: Rosmarinic acid, Tannins, Flavonoids, Volatile oils

Remarks: Lemon balm is commonly used for its calming effects to relieve anxiety, improve mood, and aid digestion. It is often used in combination with other calming herbs.

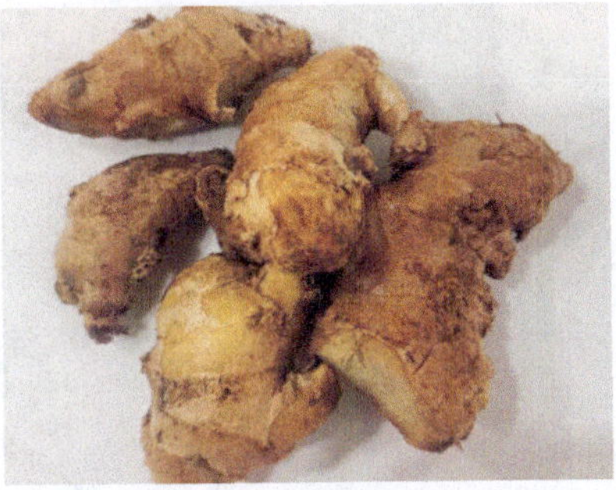

Scientific Name:*Zingiber officinale*

Common Name: Ginger

Distribution: Native to Southeast Asia, widely cultivated in subtropical and tropical regions

Part Used: Rhizome

Bioactive Principles: Gingerol, Shogaol, Zingiberene

Remarks: While primarily known for digestive health, ginger also has anti-inflammatory and antioxidant properties that support the nervous system, reduce stress, and improve circulation.

References

Awuchi, C.G., 2023. Plants, phytochemicals, and natural practices in complementary and alternative system of medicine for treatment of central nervous system disorders. International Journal of Food Properties, 26(1), pp.1190-1213.

Carlini, E.A., 2003. Plants and the central nervous system. Pharmacology Biochemistry and Behavior, 75(3), pp.501-512.

Castañeda, R., Cáceres, A., Velásquez, D., Rodríguez, C., Morales, D. and Castillo, A., 2022. Medicinal plants used in traditional Mayan medicine for the treatment of central nervous system disorders: An overview. Journal of Ethnopharmacology, 283, p.114746.

Kumar, V., 2006. Potential medicinal plants for CNS disorders: an overview. Phytotherapy Research: An International Journal Devoted to Pharmacological and Toxicological Evaluation of Natural Product Derivatives, 20(12), pp.1023-1035.

Osarobo, B.A., Aigbogun, I.E. and Azure, I.E., A Review on the Central Nervous System (CNS): Neurological Disorders and Plants with Therapeutic Effects on the CNS.

Ravi, Y., Suryakant, K.V., Sudharani, N., Gokavi, N., Sunilkumar, M.K. and Akshay, K.R., 2015. Importance of medicinal plants in the treatment of central nervous system disorders-A review. Research in Environment and Life Sciences, 9(2), pp.140-142.

Sahoo, S., 2018. Medicinal uses of plants for nervous disorders. Adv Complement Alt Med, 3, pp.1-6.

Vaidya, A.D., 1997. The status and scope of Indian medicinal plants acting on central nervous system. Indian journal of pharmacology, 29(5), pp.340-343.

15

Medicinal Plants Effective in Skin Disorders of Animals

***KK Sardar*[1*], *Satyajita Sadangi*[2], *SK Abdul Rashid*[1]**

[1]*Department of Veterinary Pharmacology & Toxicology, College of Veterinary Science & Animal Husbandry, Orissa University of Agriculture & Technology, Bhubaneswar- 751003, Odisha, India*

[2]*College of Veterinary Science & Animal Husbandry, Orissa University of Agriculture & Technology, Bhubaneswar- 751003, Odisha, India*

Introduction

Serving as the primary biological barrier, the skin aids in immunological responses and provides protection against environmental pollutants and microorganisms, dehydration, and mechanical harm. The skin's epidermis is made up of stratified and multilayered epithelial cells that, via a strictly controlled balance between terminal differentiation and cell proliferation, undergo lifelong self-renewal. One of the main causes of a wide range of skin conditions is the upset of this equilibrium.

Mycoses in humans and animals are prevalent worldwide. These diseases can arise as a result of a number of physiological and environmental factors, such as the effectiveness of the immune system of the recipient and the amount of fungi in the environment. Companion animal dermatoses rank among the most common reasons for clinic visits in day-to-day veterinary practice.

Skin disorders in Animals

- **Seborrhea -** Common dermatological conditions that affect seborrheic parts of the body include dandruff and seborrheic dermatitis (SD). SD causes flaking, scaling, irritation, and pruritus on the scalp, face, upper chest, and retro-auricular region. Sebaceous secretions, fungal colonization of the skin's surface, individual vulnerability, and interactions all have an impact on both disorders. Though their geography and severity vary, both illnesses react similarly to therapy.

- **Alopecia** - Alopecia presents itself as a frequent complaint of pet owners. The partial or total absence of hair in locations where it normally grows is known as Alopecia. It may be inherited or acquired. Congenital alopecia is non-inflammatory conditions that appear at or soon after birth due to lack of hair follicle development. When an animal with tardive alopecia sheds its juvenile coat or matures into a young adult, it may experience localized or universal hair loss. These animals are born with normal coats. The most common kind is called acquired alopecia. The most frequent cause of alopecia is Inflammatory Acquired Alopecia. The development of acquired alopecia occurs when an illness damages the hair shaft or follicle, prevents hair or wool from growing, or causes the animal to experience discomfort (such as pain or itching), which results in self-trauma and hair loss.
- **Pruritus** - Pruritus is characterized by an uncomfortable skin sensation that makes one want to scratch. In both small and large animals, it is the most prevalent dermatological issue. Clinical manifestations of hair loss, scaling, hair-piercing scales, odor, and/or oily seborrhea are frequently brought on by infectious causes of pruritus. Animals with concurrent bacterial and yeast infections frequently exhibit facial rubbing and marked pedal pruritus.
- **Urticaria** - Localized areas of red, swollen, and typically itchy skin are known as hives or urticaria. They frequently emerge and then abruptly vanish. After being exposed to the causal factor for a few minutes or hours, the wheals (eruptions) start to occur. In extreme situations, a fever, lack of appetite, or dullness precedes the skin eruptions. Although they can appear anywhere on the body, they most frequently do so on the legs, back, neck, eyelids, and flanks. They can appear on the nasal, conjuctival mucous membranes eye lining, rectum, and vagina in more severe cases. Hives typically go away as quickly as they form, generally in a matter of hours.
- **Dermatitis**- Dermatitis, the general term for the skin's reaction to injury, can include multiple manifestations of itching, scaling, abnormal redness, thickness, excessive pigmentation, atypical odor, excessive oil, and hair loss. This skin illness typically develops with a deeper trigger those results in blisters, scabs, boils, or scales.

Diagnosis of Skin Problems

A thorough history, physical checkup, and the right diagnostic tests are necessary for an accurate diagnosis of the etiology of a skin condition.

Specialized skin testing, blood and urine tests, cultures of skin swabs or hair, microscopic examination of the skin scrapings and hair, and even biopsies may be recommended.

- **Physical Examination** - To aid in the diagnosis of a skin condition, an in-depth physical exam should always be conducted. A detailed dermatological examination necessitates a comprehensive study of the skin and hair coat in bright light; huge animals' skin may require flashlights. Some primary lesions include macules, papules, wheals, nodules etc. while secondary lesions include scars, calluses, ulcers etc.
- **Skin scrapping** - A skin-scraping spatula is used to do skin scrapings, which are mostly used to detect the presence or absence of mites. Skin scrapings come in 2 forms - superficial and deep. Information is obtained from the epidermis' surface by superficial scrapings, which do not result in capillary bleeding while the substance is taken from inside the hair follicle by deep skin scrapings; capillary haemorrhage showing that the sampling was sufficiently deep.
- **Bacterial & Fungal Cultures** - To cultivate intact pustules, rupture the lesion and use a sterile culture swab to swab the area. If there isn't an intact pustule, wet the tip of the swab and turn it 360 degrees. Skin biopsies are the most effective way to cultivate deep pyodermas. It is recommended to avoid topical and systemic agents for 72 hours prior to sampling**.** Dermatophyte infections can be identified using fungal culture on dermatophyte test medium or Sabouraud agar. Inoculated plates are preferred, and animals are sampled using a toothbrush. Incubation is at room temperature.
- **Biopsy** - In any situation that seems severe, out of the ordinary, or does not improve with the right treatment, a skin biopsy is recommended. Animal skin disorders must be examined by a pathologist who is knowledgeable in biopsy specimens. As samples might shrink up to 50% in formalin, a 6-mm or 8-mm biopsy punch should be employed. Others methods employed for diagnosis of skin conditions include cytological tests, hair trichograms & intradermal skin testing techniques.

Treatment of Skin Problems

Treatment protocol followed is based on the confirmatory diagnosis made by the clinician. Animals are usually administered Antihistamines (to alleviate allergic symptoms). Medicated shampoos are used to improve fur coat & glossiness. Skin Supplements which include various vitamins & minerals and essential fatty acids such as Fish Oils are advised. Antibiotic therapies are also administered to treat the underlying infective condition. Antiparasitic drugs are prescribed if the etiology is confirmed to be of parasitic origin. Many times, systemic ailments lead to skin disorders; for such cases hormonal therapies are also administered.

Herbal Treatment of Skin Problems

Conventional medications replaced natural remedies in veterinary care until in the late nineteenth century. The majority of treatment protocols for dogs, cats, horses, and ruminants are based only on clinical experience or research data gathered from work with people and laboratory animals, despite the fact that there is substantial scientific backing for the use of herbs in veterinary medicine. More herbal therapy techniques might eventually be investigated scientifically and applied to animal care.

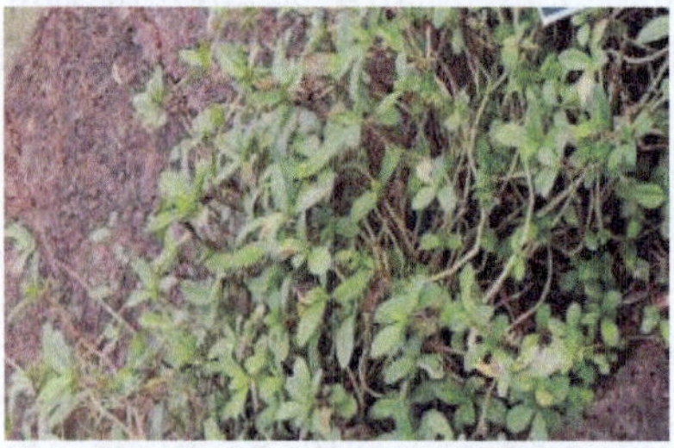

Scientific Name: *Eclipta alba*

Common Name: Bhrungaraj

Distribution: widely distributed throughout India especially in Assam, Bihar, Uttar Pradesh, and Manipur

Parts Used: Leaves

Bioactive Principles: Coumestans

Remarks: Causes Prominent follicular hypertrophy in the basal epidermal and matrix cells thus supporting growth of hair in cases of hair loss due to abnormal keratinization.

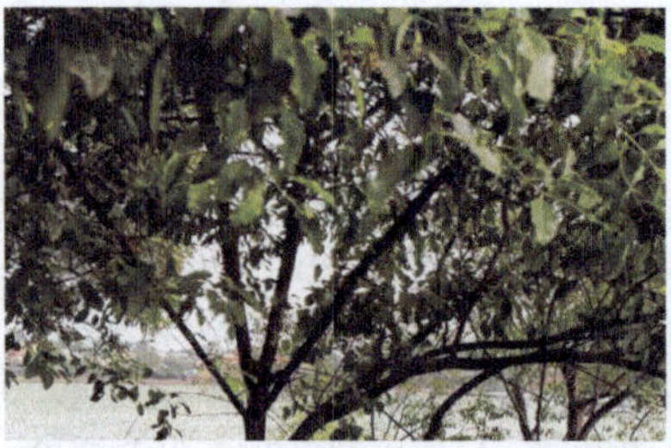

Scientific Name: *Santalum album*

Common Name: Indian Sandalwood

Distribution: The majority of Karnataka and the nearby districts of Andhra Pradesh, Tamil Nadu, and Maharashtra

Parts Used: Timber

Bioactive Principles: α-Santalol

Remarks: cooling, calming, and skin-hydrating. mostly used to treat dry skin disorders brought on by irritation and moisture loss. It can be used to treat acne and greasy skin, as well as to relieve psoriasis and eczema.

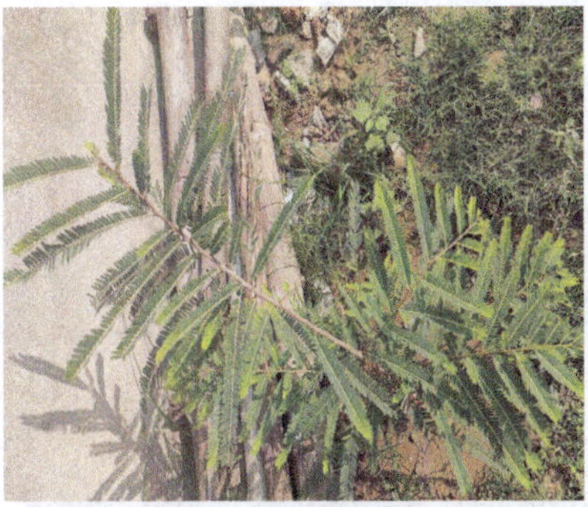

Scientific Name: *Phyllanthus emblica*

Common Name: Indian Gooseberry

Distribution: Tamil Nadu, UP,HP, MP, Rajasthan, Punjab

Parts Used: Fruit

Bioactive Principles: Flavonols & Phenolic Acids

Remarks: Protects against aging process, boosts antioxidants

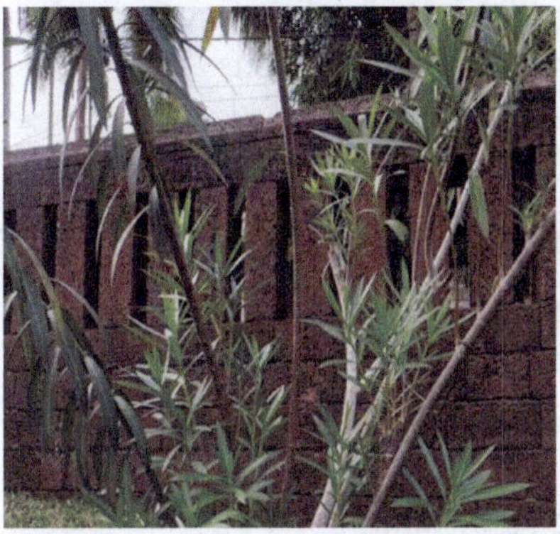

Scientific Name: *Nerium oleander*

Common Name: Indian Oleander

Distribution: Found throughout India, commonly in tropical and subtropical regions, especially in gardens and as road dividers in states like Tamil Nadu, Kerala, and Karnataka.

Part Used: Leaves, flowers, and bark

Bioactive Principles: Oleandrin, neriin, and flavonoids

Remark: Known for its antimicrobial and anti-inflammatory properties, oleander is traditionally used for treating skin conditions such as eczema and fungal infections. However, it is toxic and should be used cautiously.

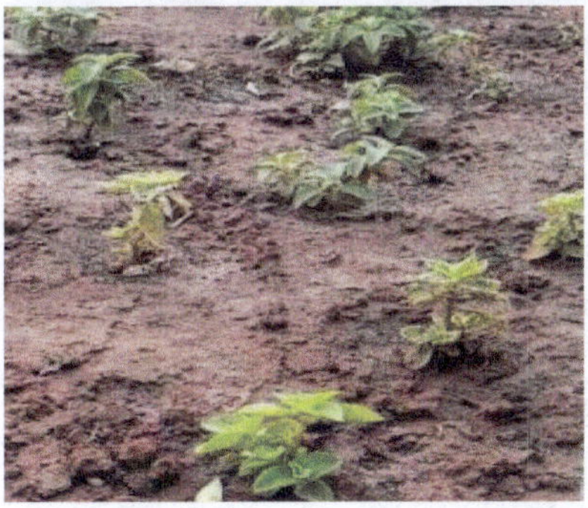

Scientific Name: *Coleus barbatus*

Common Name: Rukuna Hatapocha

Distribution: Found in the southern states of India, especially Karnataka, Kerala, and Tamil Nadu, in rocky areas and dry soil.

Part Used: Roots

Bioactive Principles: Forskolin and essential oils

Remark: Coleus is known for its anti-inflammatory and antimicrobial effects. It is used in Ayurveda for treating skin disorders and promoting wound healing.

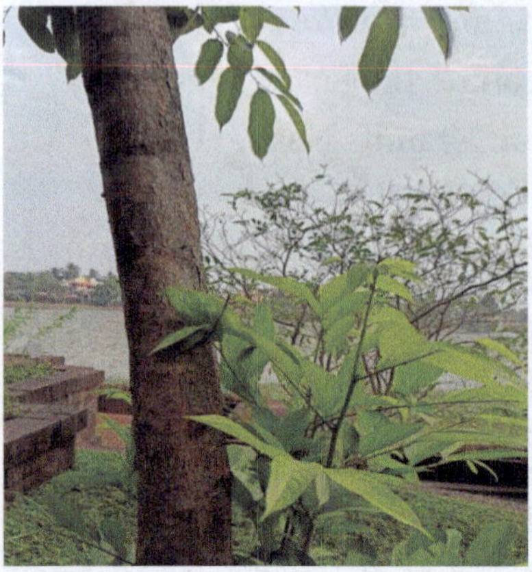

Scientific Name: *Hydnocarpus wightianus*

Common Name: Chalamogra

Distribution: Native to the Western Ghats, found in Kerala, Karnataka, and Maharashtra.

Part Used: Seeds and oil

Bioactive Principles: Hydnocarpic acid, chaulmoogric acid, and flavonoids

Remark: The oil extracted from seeds is used for treating leprosy, eczema, and other chronic skin conditions due to its antibacterial properties.

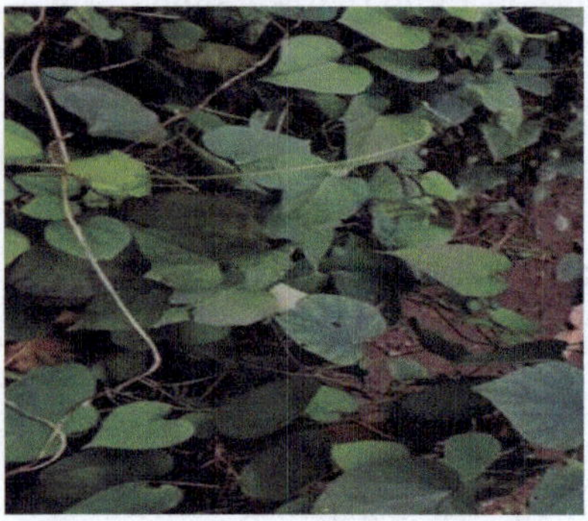

Scientific Name: *Stephania hernandifolia*

Common Name: Akanabindhi

Distribution: Found across India, especially in the northeastern states, Bihar, and Odisha, growing in forested and rocky regions.

Part Used: Roots and tubers

Bioactive Principles: Stepharine, alkaloids, and flavonoids

Remark: Known for its anti-inflammatory and soothing properties, it is used in traditional medicine for skin rashes and ulcers.

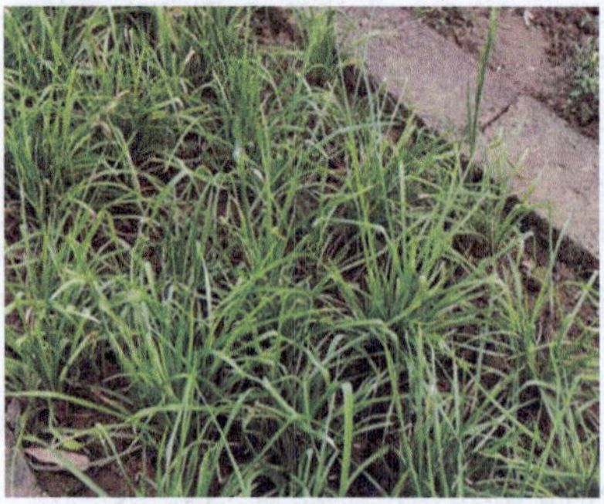

Scientific Name: *Polianathes tuberrose*

Common Name: Rajnigandha

Distribution: Cultivated in several states, including Uttar Pradesh, Karnataka, and West Bengal, for ornamental and aromatic purposes.

Part Used: Flowers

Bioactive Principles: Benzyl acetate, methyl benzoate, and eugenol

Remark: Tuberose oil is known for its soothing and anti-inflammatory properties and is often used in skin rejuvenation therapies.

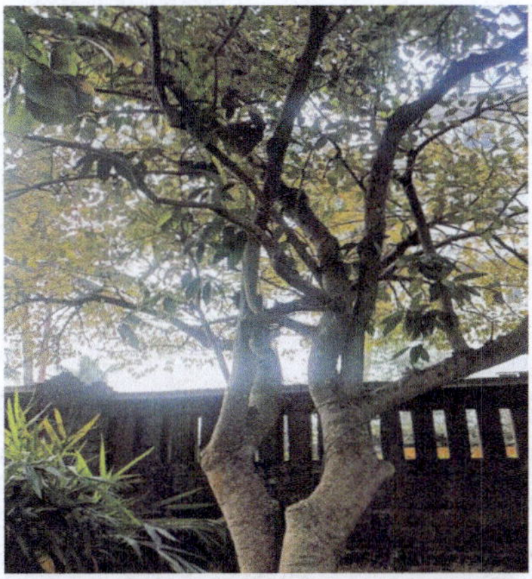

Scientific Name: *Cratev religiosa*

Common Name: Barun

Distribution: Found in moist and semi-moist regions, especially in states like Odisha, West Bengal, and Uttar Pradesh.

Part Used: Bark and leaves

Bioactive Principles: Lignans, saponins, and flavonoids

Remark: Known for its antimicrobial and healing properties, it is used in treating boils, ulcers, and other skin ailments.

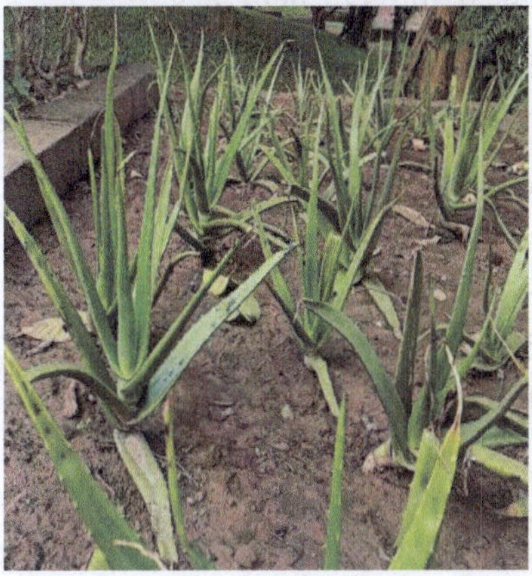

Scientific Name - *Aloe barbadensis*

Common Name - Aloe vera

Distribution: Tropical and subtropical regions of India.

Part Used: Leaves (gel and latex)

Bioactive Principles: Aloin, aloesin, emodin, saponins, and polysaccharides

Remark: Aloe vera gel is used for its soothing, moisturizing, and healing properties in skin infections and burns. It promotes wound healing and has antibacterial and anti-inflammatory effects.

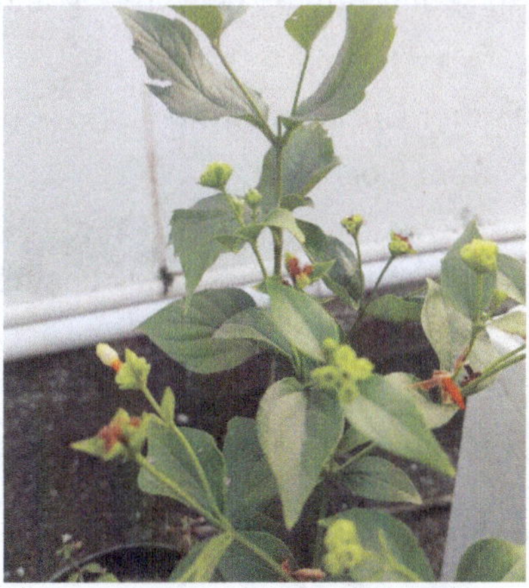

Scientific Name: *Nyctanthes arbortristis*

Common Name: Shiuli

Distribution: Found throughout India, commonly in states like West Bengal, Assam, and Odisha, in gardens and forests.

Part Used: Leaves, flowers, and bark

Bioactive Principles: Iridoid glycosides, tannins, and flavonoids

Remark - Parijat is used for its anti-inflammatory and antimicrobial effects to treat fungal infections, wounds, and skin rashes.

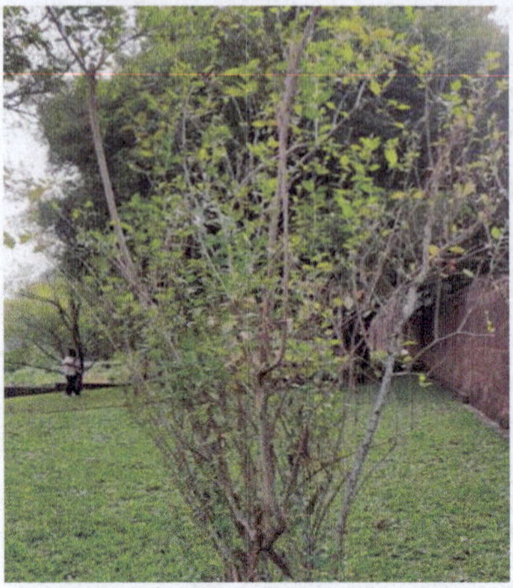

Scientific Name: *Lawsonia inermis*

Common Name: Henna

Distribution: Widely grown in Rajasthan, Gujarat, Madhya Pradesh, and Uttar Pradesh for its dyeing and medicinal properties.

Part Used: Leaves

Bioactive Principles: Lawsone, tannins, and flavonoids

Remark: Henna is widely used for its antimicrobial properties, treating dandruff, skin irritation, and fungal infections, and promoting skin and hair health.

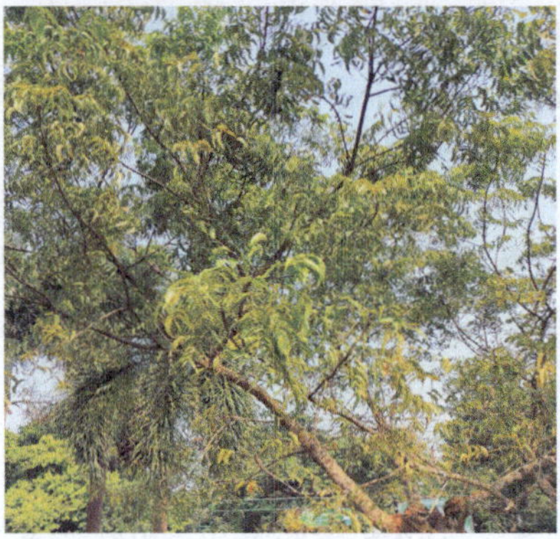

Scientific Name: *Azadirachta indica*

Common Name: Neem, Indian Lilac

Distribution: Indian subcontinent, Southeast Asia, and parts of Africa

Part Used: Leaves, bark, seeds, and oil

Bioactive Principles: Azadirachtin, nimbin, nimbidin, nimbolide, and quercetin

Remark: Neem is renowned for its antibacterial, antifungal, and anti-inflammatory properties. It is used in treating various skin infections, acne, eczema, and psoriasis. Neem oil and paste also aid in wound healing and help maintain overall skin health by detoxifying and purifying the skin.

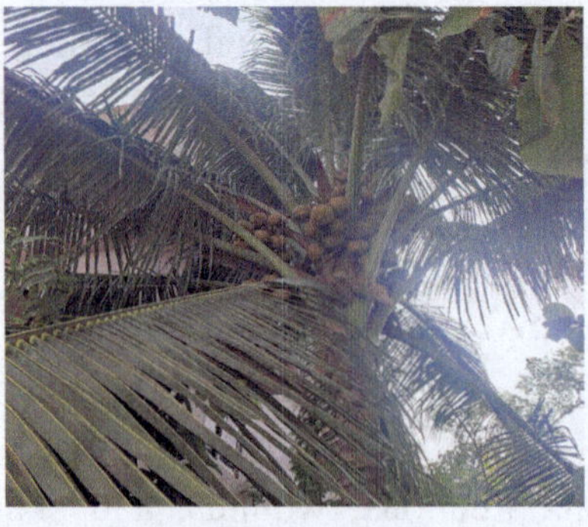

Scientific Name: *Cocos nucifera*

Common Name: Coconut

Distribution: Tropical regions worldwide, especially in Southeast Asia, the Pacific Islands, India, and the Caribbean.

Part Used: Fruit (oil, water, and flesh)

Bioactive Principles: Lauric acid, capric acid, caprylic acid, phenolic compounds, and tocopherols

Remark: Coconut oil is widely used for its antimicrobial, moisturizing, and wound-healing properties. It is effective in treating dry skin, eczema, and minor skin infections. The phenolic compounds also provide antioxidant benefits, promoting healthy and glowing skin.

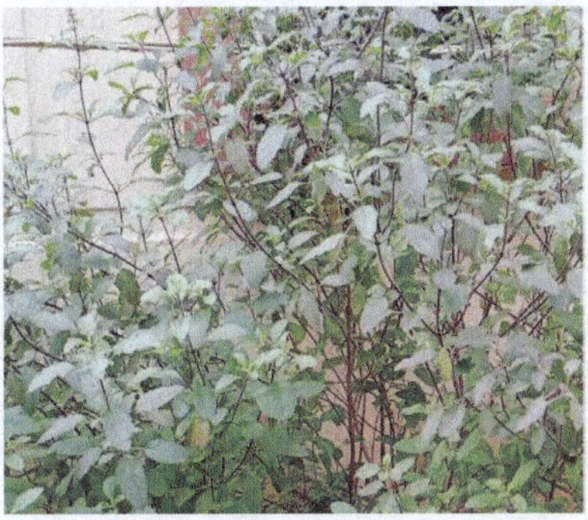

Scientific Name: *Ocimum sanctum*

Common Name: Holy Basil, Tulsi

Distribution: Widely grown across India, especially in Uttar Pradesh, Bihar, Madhya Pradesh, and Karnataka, commonly in household gardens and temples.

Part Used: Leaves, seeds, and roots

Bioactive Principles: Eugenol, ursolic acid, flavonoids, and rosmarinic acid

Remark: The antibacterial, anti-inflammatory, and antioxidant qualities of tulsi are well known. In addition to promoting wound healing and general skin health, it is used to treat rashes, acne, and skin infections. Additionally, it aids in skin detoxification and oxidative stress reduction.

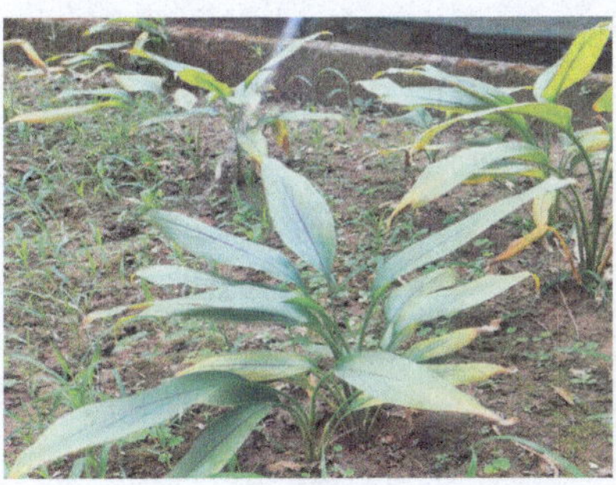

Scientific Name - *Curcuma longa*

Common Name - Turmeric

Distribution - India, Southeast Asia, and China

Part Used - Rhizome

Bioactive Principles - Curcumin, demethoxycurcumin, and essential oils (turmerone)

Remark - Turmeric is widely used for its anti-inflammatory, antimicrobial, and antioxidant properties. It is effective in treating acne, scars, and hyperpigmentation and promotes skin healing and glow.

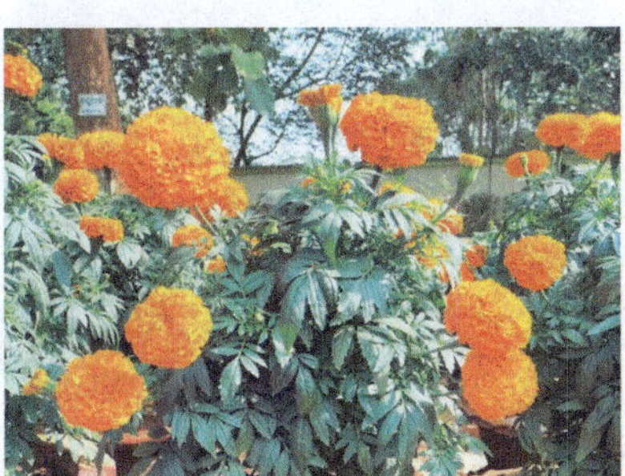

Scientific Name: Tagetes spp. (e.g., Tagetes erecta, Tagetes patula)

Common Name: Marigold

Distribution: Grown for decorative, therapeutic, and religious purposes all over India, but particularly in Karnataka, Tamil Nadu, West Bengal, and Maharashtra.

Part Used: Flowers, leaves, and essential oil

Bioactive Principles: Lutein, carotenoids, thiophenes, and flavonoids

Remark: Marigold's antibacterial and anti-inflammatory qualities make it valuable. It aids in lowering inflammation and promoting skin healing and is used to treat wounds, ulcers, and infections of the skin. Because of its calming and protecting properties, the plant's extract is often utilized in skincare products.

References

Borda LJ, Wikramanayake TC. Seborrheic dermatitis and dandruff: a comprehensive review. Journal of clinical and investigative dermatology. 2015 Dec;3(2).

Dworecka-Kaszak B, Biegańska MJ, Dąbrowska I. Occurrence of various pathogenic and opportunistic fungi in skin diseases of domestic animals: a retrospective study. BMC veterinary research. 2020 Jul 17;16(1):248.

Jha, Umang & Singh, Miss & Baghla, Amandeep Singh. (2022). Phytochemical and pharmacology activity of Bhringraj: A review. International journal of health sciences. 11113-11125. 10.53730/ijhs.v6nS3.8560.

Kumari I, Kaurav H, Chaudhary G. Eclipta alba (bhringraj): a promising hepatoprotective and hair growth stimulating herb. Asian Journal of Pharmaceutical and Clinical Research. 2021 May 31;14(7):16-23.

Kumar R, Anjum N, Tripathi YC. Phytochemistry and pharmacology of Santalum album L.: a review. World Journal of Pharmaceutical Research. 2015 Aug 4;4(10):1842-76.

Mecklenburg L. An overview on congenital alopecia in domestic animals. Veterinary dermatology. 2006 Dec;17(6):393-410.

MSD Veterinary Manual

Prananda AT, Dalimunthe A, Harahap U, Simanjuntak Y, Peronika E, Karosekali NE, Hasibuan PA, Syahputra RA, Situmorang PC, Nurkolis F. Phyllanthus emblica: a comprehensive review of its phytochemical composition and pharmacological properties. Frontiers in pharmacology. 2023 Oct 26;14:1288618.

Zhang JY. Animal Models of Skin Disorders. In Animal Models for the Study of Human Disease 2017 Jan 1 (pp. 357-375). Academic Press.

16

Medicinal Plants Effective in Infertility in Bovines

Anil Kumar Nahak[1], Jagyaseni Meher[1], M Sudhakar Reddy[1] Samapika Mahapatra[2] and Ritun Patra[3]

[1]Department of Animal Reproduction, Gynaecology and Obstetrics
[2]Veterinary Dispensary, Balugaon, Khordha, Odisha
[3]Department of Veterinary Anatomy and Histology
College of Veterinary Science and Animal Husbandary, OUAT, Bhubaneswar, Odisha

Introduction: The phenomenon of reproduction is an important aspect, which needs special attention in livestock farming to achieve optimum productivity and increase the economic status of the farmers. Various gynaecological problems like anestrus, repeat breeding, endometritis, retention of placenta, etc reduce thereproductive performance in farm animals. Besides indirect reducing the milk yield, it also creates financial burden on the farmers due to high cost of therapeutic drugs prescribed for their treatment. The use of various hormonal preparations and antibiotics has been critical in treating these disorders inthe farm animals. However, herbal treatments render a holistic approach to manage the reproductive problems with minimalcost and no side effects.

1. Name of the condition: Anestrous

About the condition/definition: Anestrus is a reproductive cycle dysfunction in which an animal does not display the obvious symptoms of estrus. It is one of the major limiting factor in achieving better reproductive performance in farm animals.

Etiology and pathogenesis: Expression of estrus is controlled by secretion of reproductive hormones. Any disturbance in their secretion due to the effect of either ofSeason, stress, uterine diseases, poor management techniques, inadequate nourishment, etc., delays the process.The animals with smooth non-functional ovary are said to true anestrous, whereas absence of estrus due to retained CL on ovary due to uterine pathology are false anestrous.

Symptom: Delay in attaining puberty, non-return to estrous for a prolonged period of time after parturition or sudden cassation of estrus in non-pregnant animals. It increases the inter-calving period and hence causes reduced treatment costs, replacement expenses, and lifetime milk yield.

General treatment: With differing degrees of efficacy, numerous hormonal and non-hormonal substances have been utilized widely. To boost the animal's health, deworming and adding a high-quality mineral mixture to the diet are recommended.

Herbal treatment

Plant-based heat inducers, which are abundant in vitamins and minerals and some of which have inherent estrogenic qualities, have been used to treat anestrus in animals. Numerous plants including *Leptadenia reticulate*, *Abroma augusta* (Ulatkambal), *Carica papaya*, *Trigonellafoenum graecum* (Methi), *Murraya koenigii* (curry leaves), *Aegle marmelos*, *Saraca asoca* (Ashoka),*Bambusa aruninacea*, *Asparagus recemosus*, *Courupita guianesis*, *Semecarpus anacardium*, *Nigella sativa* (kalonji), and *Pergulacia daemia* have been given to anoestrous animals either alone or in combination with diverse reactions to oestrus induction.

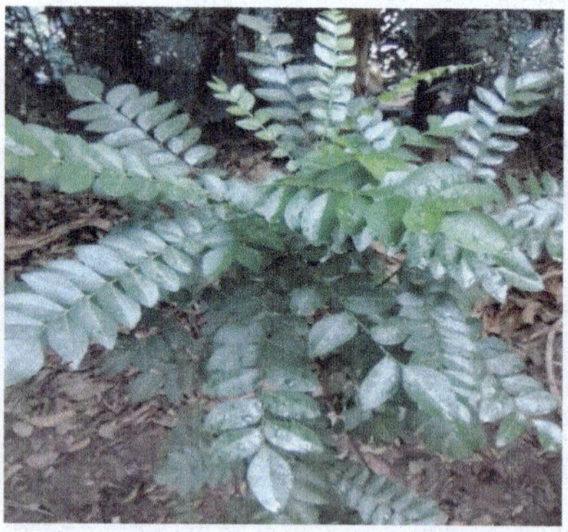

Scientific name: *Murraya koenigii* (L.)

Common name: Curry leaves

Distribution: India

Part used: Leaves

Bioactive principle: Triterpenoid alkaloids, crystalline glycosides, cyclomahanimbine, tetrahydromahanimbine, girinimbin, koenine, koenimbine, koenidine, protein, iso-mahanimbin, carbohydrate, minerals, fiber, nicotinic acid, vitamin C, vitamin A, oxalic acid, carotene, calcium, carbazole alkaloids as well as koenigin; Amino acids like Asparagines, glutamic acid, glycine, serine, and aspartic acid.

Remarks: The antibacterial, antioxidant, and anti-inflammatory qualities of plant leaves also contribute to their notable benefits in the treatment of endometritis. Supplementation of curry leaves at the dose rate of 100 gm/day orally daily for 30 days induces oestrus in anestrus cows.

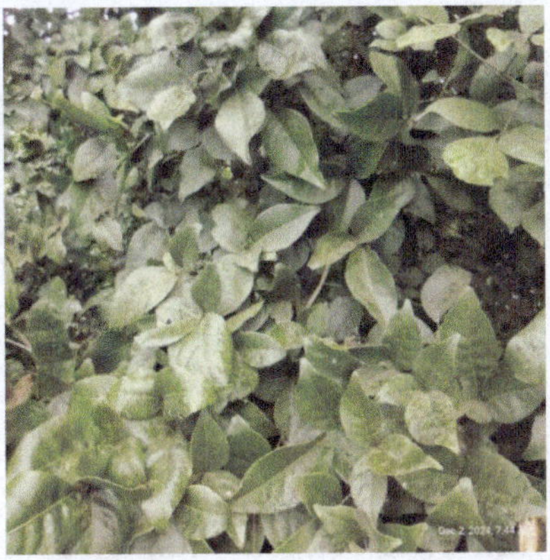

Scientific name: *Aegle marmelos* (L.) Correa.

Common name: Bael

Distribution: Central plains and eastern ghats of India

Part used: Leaves

Bioactive principle: Aeglin, β-sitosterol, Cineol, Citral, Euginol, γ-sitosterole, Lupeol, O-isopentenyl, Mameline, Skimmianine, Hallordiol, Rutin, Citronellal, Cuuminaldehydephenylethylecinnamamides, Marmesinin, Aegelin, Flavone, Glycoside

Remarks: Supplementation of bael leaves at the dose rate of 100 gm/day orally daily often with curry leaves (100 gm/day) for 30 days induces oestrus in anestrus cows.

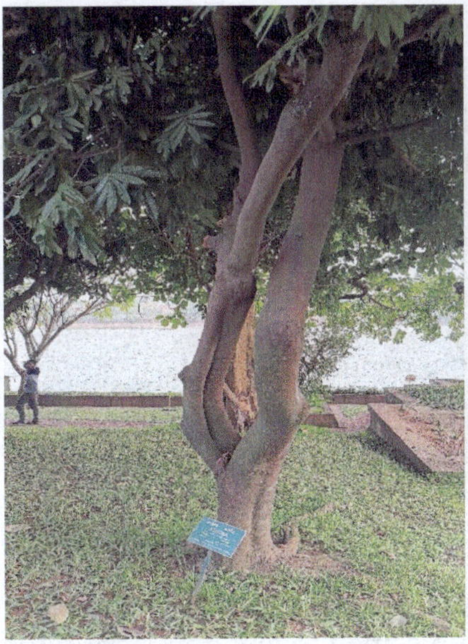

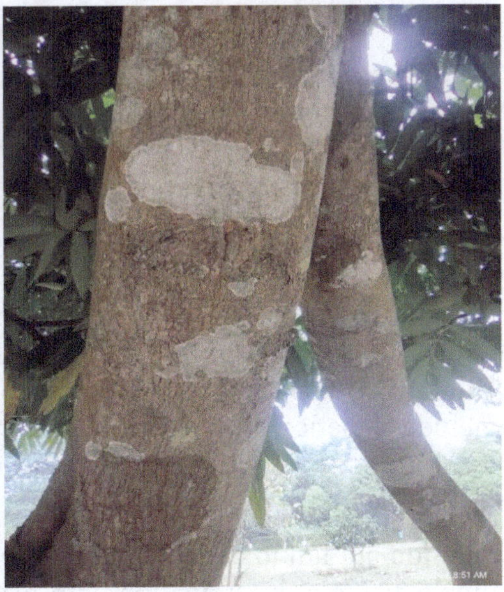

Scientific name: ***Saraca asoca*** Roxb. wild (Fabaceae)

Common name: Ashoka

Distribution: India

Part used: Stem bark

Bioactive principle: Leucocyanidin, leucopelargonidin, epicatechin, procyanidin, leucocyanidin, 11'-deoxyprocyanidin B, and catechin. Other elements found in the tree's powered bark include silica, calcium, iron, magnesium, phosphate, potassium, sodium, aluminum, strontium, and calcium.

Remarks: This medication is given as an aqueous suspension for 21 days without interruption.

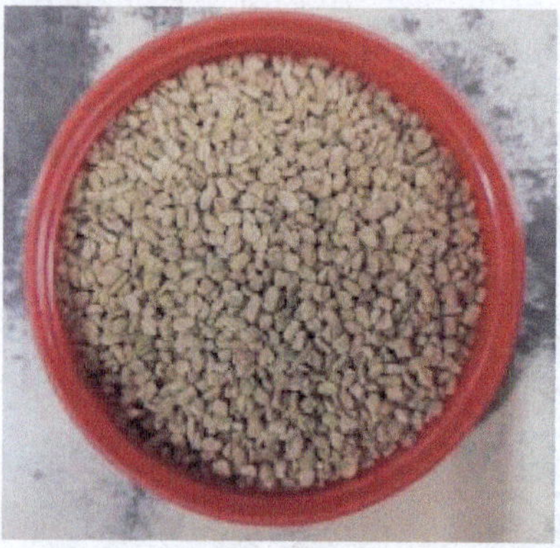

Scientific name: *Trigonella foenum-graecum* L.

Common name: Greek Hay, Fenugreek, Methi, Mutti

Distribution: India

Part used: Seed

Bioactive principle: saponins, tannins, alkaloids, amino acids, flavonoids, phenolic acid derivatives

Remarks: feeding dairy cows at the dose rate of 1gm/kg body weight improves reproductive performance. Dairy cows when supplemented fenugreek seeds along with jaggery, linseed oil results onset of estrus a well as enhance conception rate.

2. Repeat Breeding

About the condition/definition: Repeat breeding in cattle is defined as the failure to conceive after three or more regularly spaced services.

Etiology and pathogenesis: Some potential causes of repeat breeding include Genetics, age, uterine infection, congenital defects of the genital tract, improper ovarian function, nutrition, artificial insemination.

Symptom: Cows coming to estrus in normal interval and exhibit normal duration but fail to conceive even after three times of natural mating or timely artificial insemination with fertile semen, maintaining optimum thawing and handling protocols.

General treatment: Dewarming, nutritional supplement, intra-uterine administration of antiseptic solutions and hormonal treatments are often followed. Buserelin acetate, a GnRH analogue used along single insemination. Double insemination at a 24-hour interval, or any of the oestrous synchronisation protocols are also widely used to treat repeat breeding.

Herbal treatment

1. Garlic extract and Ashwagandha powder

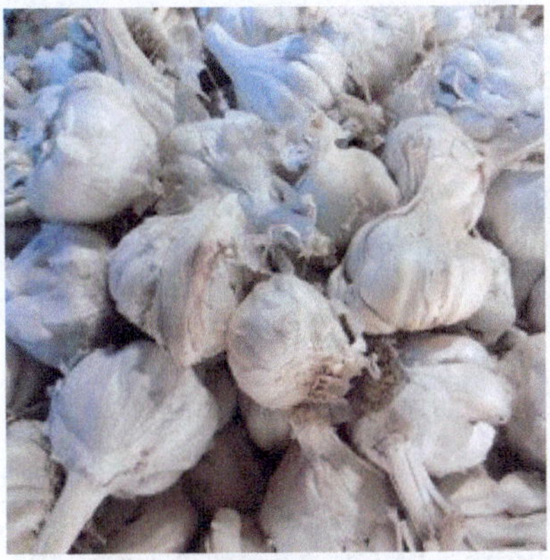

Scientific name: *Allium sativum* L.

Common name: Garlic

Distribution: Central Asia, South Asia and North eastern Iran

Part used: bulbs/cloves

Bioactive principle: thiosulphinates such as allicin. Aged Garlic Extract contain S-allylcysteine, S- allylmercaptocysteine, N-(alpha) fructosyl arginine, etc.

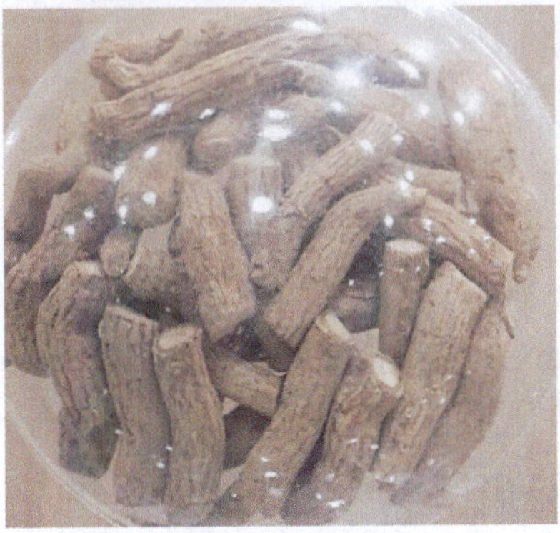

Scientific name: *Withania somnifera* (L.) Dunal

Common name: Ashwagandha

Distribution: Asia, Africa

Part used: Root

Bioactive principle: Withanolides, withaferin A, alkaloids and other compounds like flavonoids, carbohydrates, glycosides,saponins, tannins, terpenoids and coumarin

Remarks: In infectious cause of repeat breeding, Garlic extract @10µg in 30 ml PBS administered by intrauterine route in mid-estrus stage and Ashwagandha powder @15 gm administered orally with concentrates for 5 days for enhancing conception[6].

2. Combination of radish, moringa leaves, aloe vera, Cissus quadrangularis stem, and curry leaves

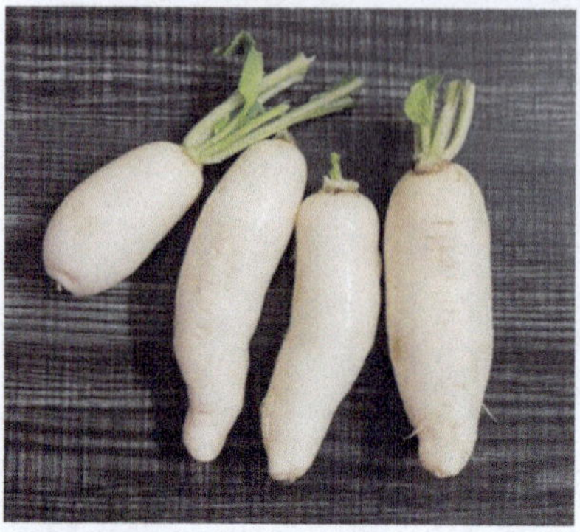

Scientific name: *Raphanus sativus* L. (Brassicaceae)

Common name: Radish, Muli, Mula

Distribution: Tropical and Temperate zone

Part used: Whole rhizome

Bioactive principle: Flavonoids, non-flavonoid polyphenols, terpenes and derivatives, glucosinolates, hydrocarbon, pyrogallol, Vanillic acid, Epicatechin, Coumaric acid, Glucoraphasatin

Remarks: 100g of whole rhizome fed orally daily in case of post partm anestrus

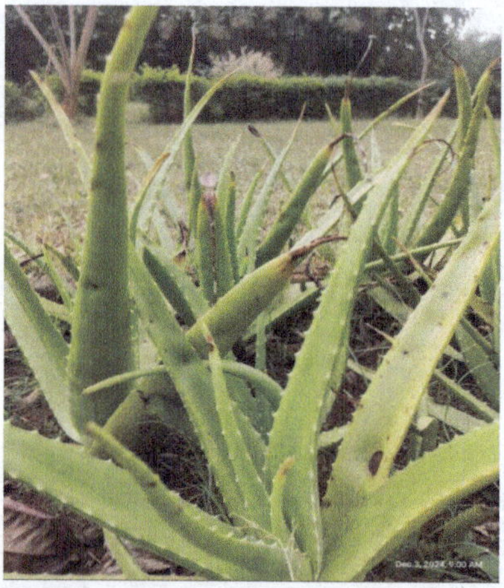

Scientific name: *Aloe barbadensis miller* (Liliaceae)

Common name: Aloe vera, Ghritkumari, Barbados aloe, Cape aloe, Indian aloe, burn aloe, etc.

Distribution: Tropical and sub-tropical regions including India, Africa, America & Australia

Part used: succulent leaves

Bioactive principle: Anthraquinones, salicylic acid, lignin, saponins , carbohydrates, inorganic compounds, hormones (auxins and gibberellins) vitamins, enzymes, minerals, fatty acids (lupeol and campesterol),

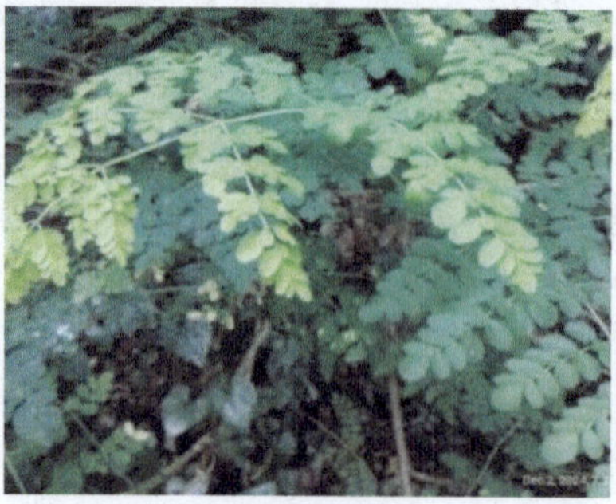

Scientific name: Moringa oleifera Lam.

Common name: Drumstick, Munga, Sajana, Sahjan

Distribution: Tropical and Temperate zone

Part used: Leaves, fruit

Bioactive principle: Flavonoids, carotenoids, phenolic acids, alkaloids,

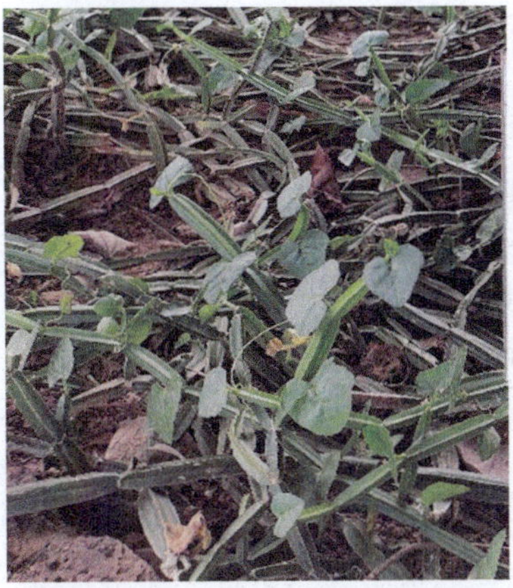

glucosinolates, tannins, isothiocyanates

Scientific name : *Cisuss quadrangularis* L.

Common name : Veld grape, Devil's Backbone, Hadjod (Hindi), Hadabhanga (Odia)

Distribution : India, Srilanka, Malaysia, Indonsia, Philipines, Tropical Africa, USA, Islands of Indian & pacific ocean

Part used : Nodes

Bioactive principles: α-amyrin, β-amyrin, β-sitosterols, friedelin, quercetin, genistein, diadzenin

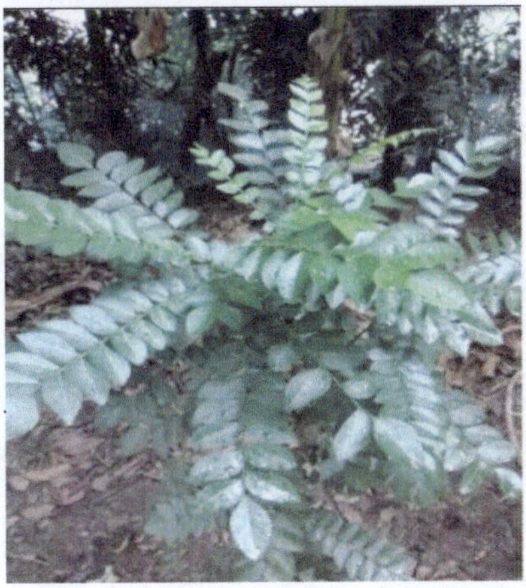

Scientific name: *Murraya koenigii* L.

Common name: Curry leaves

Distribution: India

Part used: Leaves

Bioactive principle: Triterpenoid alkaloids, cyclomahanimbine, iso-mahanimbin, tetrahydromahanimbine, crystalline glycosides, girinimbin, , koenine, koenimbine, koenidine

Combination of Bael leaves and Curry leaves.

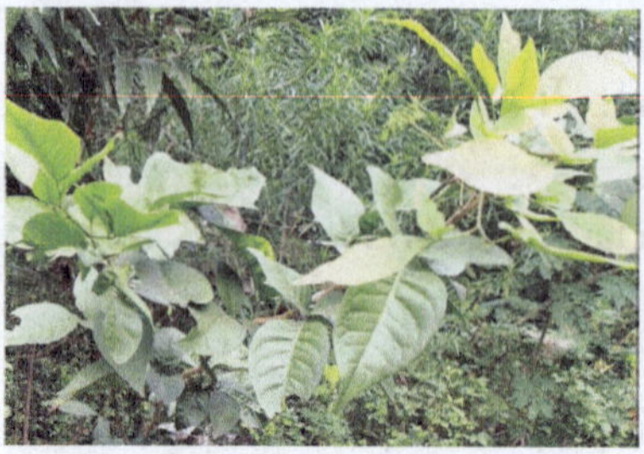

Scientific name: ***Aegle marmelos*** (L.) Correa.

Common name: Bael

Distribution: Eastern Ghats and central plains of India

Part used: leaves

Bioactive principle: Aeglin, β-sitosterol, Cineol, Citral, Euginol, γ-sitosterole, Flavone, Lupeol, Mameline, Skimmianine, Hallordiol, Rutin, Citronellal, O-isopentenyl, Aegelin, Cuumin aldehyde phenyl ethyle cinnamamides, Marmesinin, Glycoside

Remarks: herbal mixture containing 100g of shade dried powdered Bael leaves (A. marmelos) and 100g of shade dried powdered Curry leaves (M. koenigii) mixed at 1:1 ratio and fed at a dose rate of 200g/day/animal for 5 days from the day of estrum.

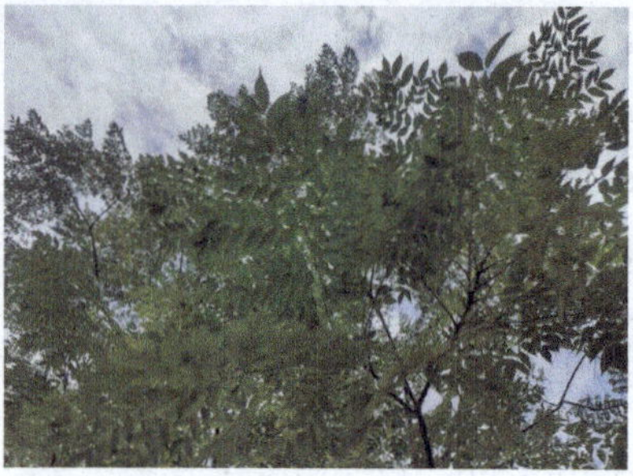

Melia leaves

Scientific name : ***Melia azedarach*** L.

Common name: Chinaberry, Cape lilac, Bakain(Hindi) , Ghora-neem (Asamese), Mahanimbah (Sanskrit)

Distribution : Sub-tropical regions of whole world including India, Africa, America & Australia

Part used : Leaves

Bioactive principles: Azadirachtins, TRiterpenoids, limonoids, steroids, flavonoids, phenolics

Remarks : Leaves @ 150-250g orally daily for 10 days after insemination [3].

3. Endometritis

Endometritis is the localized inflammation of the mucosal lining of the uterus i.e. the endometrium. The condition is mostly caused by various pathogenic bacteria that invade uterus after parturition (calving) when the uterus is vulnerable.

Etiology: Bacterial Infection like *Escherichia coli (E. coli), Arcanobacterium pyogenes, Fusobacterium necrophorum, Trueperella pyogenes, Streptococcus* spp, *Clostridia* spp., etc., mechanical trauma during calving or artificial insemination, Postpartum Uterine Involution Issues, Poor Hygiene, Delayed or Incomplete Placental Expulsion, etc.

Clinical signs : Cows may show variable amount of white or whitish yellow mucopurulent vaginal discharge and its quantity usually increases during estrus when cervix dilates. Systemic illness seldom occurs. However, milk yield and appetite may slightly reduce occasionally.

Infertility: Endometritis can interfere with the cow's ability to conceive, causing delayed estrus cycles or failure to become pregnant.

Diagnosis: Clinical signs: Observation of discharge and other symptoms.

Vaginal examination: Manual or digital rectal exams help identify inflammation in the uterus.

Cytology: of uterine discharge to detect the presence of bacteria or inflammatory cells.

Culture: Bacterial culture of uterine discharge helps identify specific pathogens.

Ultrasound: Ultrasound can be used to evaluate uterine health and check for thickening of the uterine lining or fluid accumulation.

Treatment: Common antibiotics like cephalosporins, penicillin, or tetracyclines; Prostaglandins if CL is present: aids uterine involution and expel any remaining placental material; Oxytocin: Stimulates uterine contractions and helps clear out the infection. Non-Steroidal Anti-Inflammatory Drugs (NSAIDs); Uterine lavage such as lugol's iodine or povidone iodine, etc.

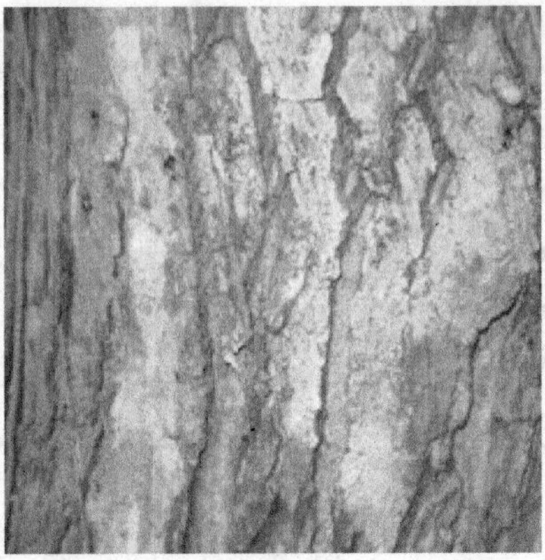

Scientific name: *Azadirachta indica A.* Juss.

Common name: Neem ,Margosa, Indian lilac

Distribution: India, Pakistan, SriLanka, Thailand, Malaysia, indonesia, Fiji, Mauritius, Central & South America, African Countries

Part used: Neem bark

Bioactive principles: Azardichtin, Nimbin, Nimbidine, Nimbolide and other limonoids

Remarks: Endometritic cows are treated thrice at 24 hrs. interval with intrauterine alcoholic extract of neem bark dissolved in 30 ml of Normal Saline @ 7.5mg/ml.

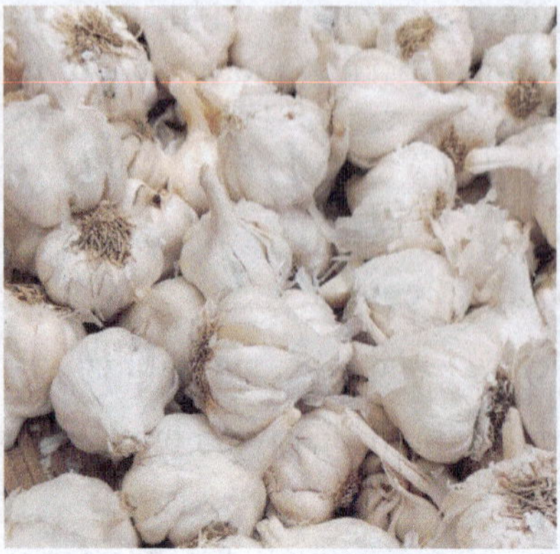

Scientific name: Allium sativum L.

Common name: Garlic, Lahsun (hindi), Rasuna (odia)

Distribution: China, India, Bangladesh,Korea, Egypt, Kazakhstan, Kyrgyzstan, Uzbekistan, North & South American countries

Part used: Garlic cloves

Bioactive principles : Allicin, Alliin, Diallyl sulphide

Remarks: Endometritic cows are treated thrice at 24 hrs. interval with intrauterine alcoholic extract of garlic cloves dissolved in 30 ml of Normal Saline @ 20mg/ml.

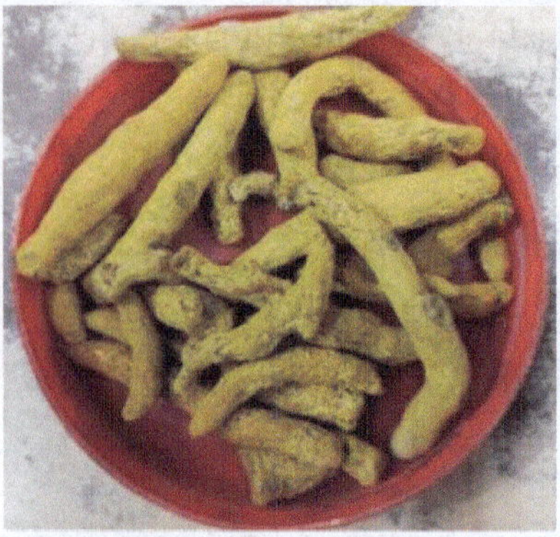

Scientific name: *Curcuma longa* L.

Common name: Turmeric, Haldi

Distribution: India, China, Indonesia, Malaysia, East Africa

Part used: Rhizome

Bioactive principles: Curcumin

Remarks : Endometritic cows are treated thrice at 24 hrs. interval with intrauterine alcoholic extract of neem bark dissolved in 30 ml of Normal Saline @ 20mg/ml.

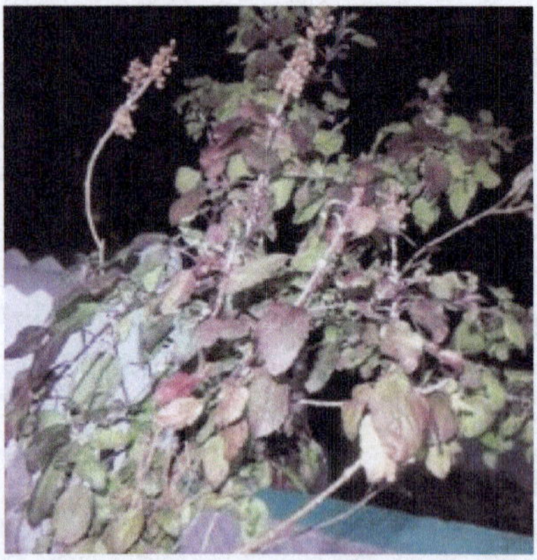

Scientific name: *Ocimum tenuiflorum* L.

Common name: Tulsi

Distribution: South east Asian Tropical & subtropical countries, Australia, Western Pacific

Part used : Leaves

Bioactive principles: Eugenol, methyl eugeol, cirsilineol, circimaritin, isothymusin, apigenin, rosameric acid, orientin and advincentin

Remarks: Endometritic cows are treated thrice at 24 hrs. interval with intrauterine alcoholic extract of neem bark dissolved in 30 ml of Normal Saline @ 65mg/ml.

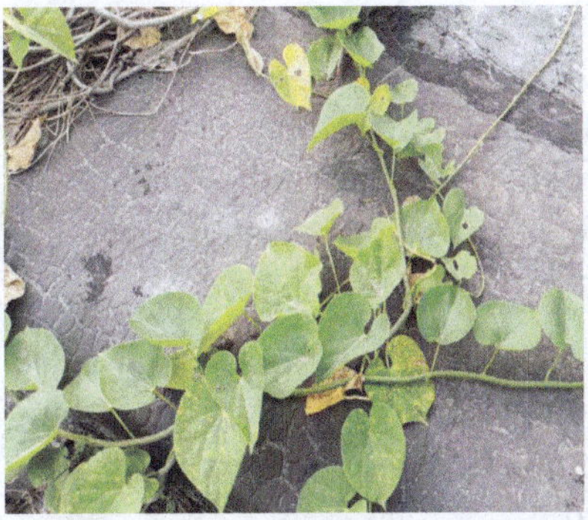

Scientific name: *Tinospora cordifolia* (Willd.) Miers

common names: Indian quinine, heart-leaved moonseed, Gulvel, guduchi and giloy.

Distribution: tropical areas of India, China, Myanmar and Sri Lanka.

Bioactive principles: alkaloids, steroids,lignans, diterpenoid lactones,tinosporic acid, tinosporone, cordifolisides A to E, aliphatics, picrotene, bergenin and glycosides have been isolated from the different parts of the plant body, including root, stem, and whole plant.

Remarks: 50ml (3000 mg total dose) of aqueous extracts of giloy is to be administered for 3 consecutive days.

Giloy has an immunomodulator, antibacterial, anti-infective & anti-inflammatory properties which is very effective in infective repeat breeder cows.

Scientific name: ***Tinospora cordifolia*** (Willd.) Miers

Common names: Indian quinine, heart-leaved moonseed,Gulvel,guduchi and giloy.

Distribution: tropical areas of India, China, Myanmar and Sri Lanka.

Bioactive principles: alkaloids, steroids,lignans, diterpenoid lactones,tinosporic acid, tinosporone, cordifolisides A to E, aliphatics, picrotene, bergenin and glycosides have been isolated from the different parts of the plant body, including root, stem, and whole plant.

Remarks: 50ml (3000 mg total dose) of aqueous extracts of giloy is to be administered for 3 consecutive days.

Giloy has an immunomodulator, antibacterial, anti-infective & anti-inflammatory properties which is very effective in infective repeat breeder cows.

4. Retention of Placenta

About the condition/definition: Retention of placenta is said to occur in farm animals when there is failure inexpelling the fetal membranes or placenta from the uterus of mother even after 24 hr of parturition.

Etiology and pathogenesis: Delay in the separation of the caruncle and cotyledon due to any mechanical or inflammatory event or improper time of delivery lead to edema formation that locks the placenta into the uterus. This grip persists until detachment occursdue to necrosis of the devitalised placenta. The leukocytes migrate from caruncle into placenta surface hastens necrosis, sometimes bacteria may enter and lead to systemic illness.

Symptom: Small part of discoloured and rotting membrane from vulval opening, may or may not be visible, foul- smelling discharge may come in long standing. Reduced appetite, sometimes accompanied by elevated body temperature is observed when placenta is retained.

General treatment: Oxytocin, Collagenase, methyl ergometrine are often used. Herbal ecbolic preparations are also administered orally for expulsion of uterine debris and accelerating the process of involution.

Herbal treatment

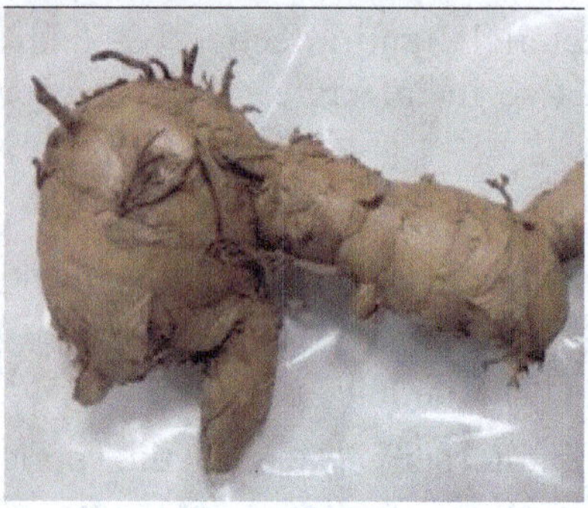

Scientific name: ***Curcuma amada*** *Roxb.*

Common name : Mango ginger, Aam adrak, Amba haldi

Distribution : Tropical countries of Africa, Asia and Australia

Part used : Rhizome

Bioactive principles: β-myrcene, epicurzeronone, squalene,α-acaridial, β-pinene, tetramethyl-hexadeca-pentaene and aromadandrene

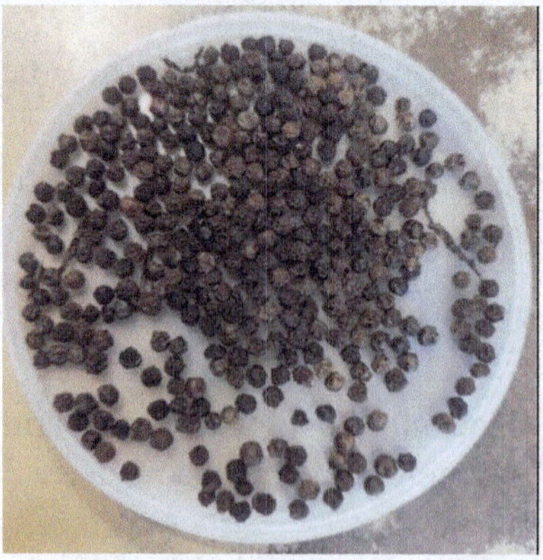

Scientific name: *Piper nigrum L.*

Common name: Black pepper, Chavyam (Sanskrit), Kalimirch (Hindi), Golamaricha (Odia)

Distribution: India, Indonesia, Malaysia, Brazil, Sri Lanka, Cambodia

Parts used: Fruit (dried)

Bioactive principles: amides, piperidine, pyrrolidines, safrole

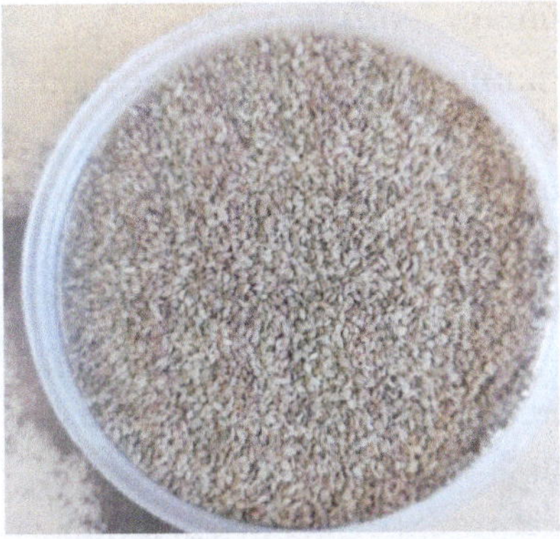

Scientific name : *Trachyspermum ammi* (L.) Sprague ex Turrill

Common name : Thymol seed, Carom seed, Ajwain (Hindi), Juani(Odia)

Distribution : India, Iran, Afghanistan, Iraq, Parts of northen Africa

Parts used : Fruit

Bioactive principles: Monoterpenes, Thymol, Cumene, Terpene, α & β- pinene, Para-cymene, limonene

Remarks: A mixture of 100gm of dried rhizome of aam adrak, 100 gm of ajwain seeds, 100 gm of kalimirch, 250 gm of Jaggery,100gm ghee and black salt is given orally one time in a day for fast placental expulsion.

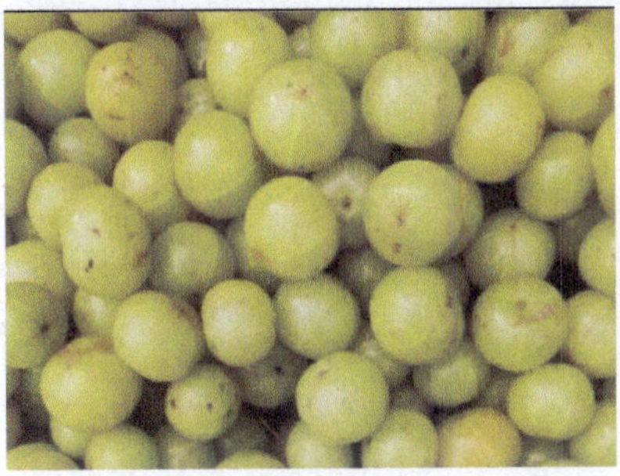

Scientific name :***Phyllanthus emblica*** L.

Common name : Indian gooseberry, amlaki, amla, Dhatri

Distribution : India and Southeast Asia

Part used : fruit

Bioactive principles: phytochemicals, including polyphenols like ellagic acid, gallic acid, chebulinic acid, and quercetin, Vitamin C and other nutrients

Remarks : 200g of dried alma powder orally daily for 5 days (total of 1 kg) to hasten placenta removal.

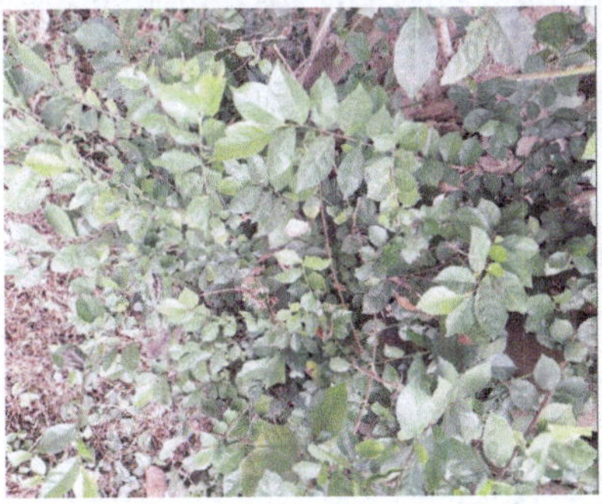

Scientific name: *Streblus asper* Lour.

Common name: Siamese rough bush, Serut, khoi, Dahia (hindi) , Sahada (odia), Toothbrush tree

Distribution: India, Srilanka, Malaysia, Philipines,Thailand

Part used : Leaf

Bioactive principles : volatile oils, flavonoids

Remarks : Leaves are given as feed after delivery to hasten removal of placenta.

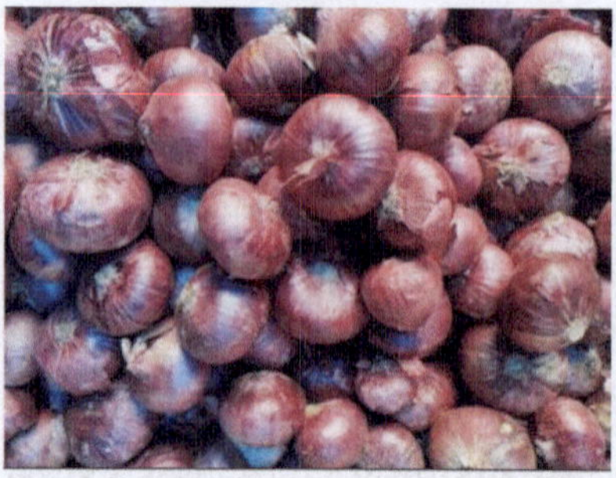

Scientific name: ***Allium cepa L.***

Common name: Onion , Pyaz (hindi), Piaza (odia)

Distribution : China, India, Unites states, Turkey, Japan , Australia, South America

Part used: Bulbs

Bioactive principles: flavonoids like fisetin, quercetin, polyphenolic substances, phenolic acids, ascorbic acid and sulphur compounds

Remarks : Bulbs are fed orally along with fodders to expel retained placenta[3].

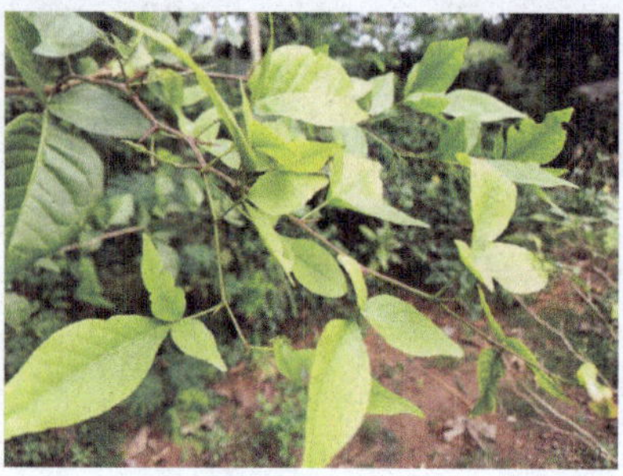

Scientific name: ***Aegle marmelos (L.) Correa.***

Common name: Stone apple, Bengal Quince, Golden apple, Sirphal, Bel, Bilawa, Wood apple

Distribution: Bangladesh, Myanmar, Vietnam, India, Cambodia, Sri Lanka, Thailand, Pakistan, Malaysia, Egypt, Surinam, Trinidad, and Florida

Part used : Leaves

Bioactive principles: Aeglin, β-sitosterol, Cineol, Citral, Euginol, γ-sitosterole, Lupeol, O-isopentenyl, Glycoside, Skimmianine, Hallordiol, Rutin, Citronellal, Cuuminaldehydephenylethylecinnamamides, Mameline, Marmesinin, Aegelin, Flavone,

Remarks: Leaves of *Aegle marmelos* (Bel), *Trachyspermum ammi* (Ajwain), *Vitex negundo* (Nirgudi)and seeds of *Sesasum indicu*m (Til) are boiled in water and the aqueous extract is drenched orally to cattle with retained placenta[9].

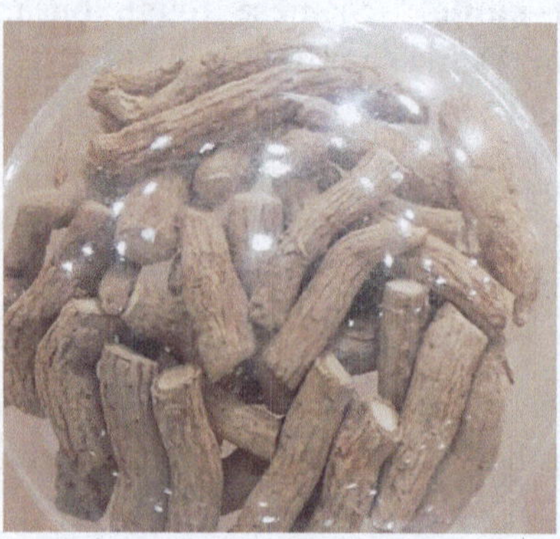

Scientific name : ***Withania somnifera*** (L.) Dunal

Common name : Ashwagandha, Inian ginseng, poison gooseberry, winter cherry

Distribution : India, Sri Lanka,Nepal, parts of Africa,

Part used : Roots

Bioactive principles : Withanolides, steroidal lactone, Alkaloids, Flavonoids,

Phenolics, Polysterols,Triterpenoids, Dulcitol, Withancil, Hentriacontane

Remarks : Root powder boiled in milk is given to animal to cure retained placenta. Or Crushed roots of aswagandha , dried rhizome of Zingiber officinale (ginger) mixed with jiggery and ghee together to form a bolus that is to administered PO twice a day.

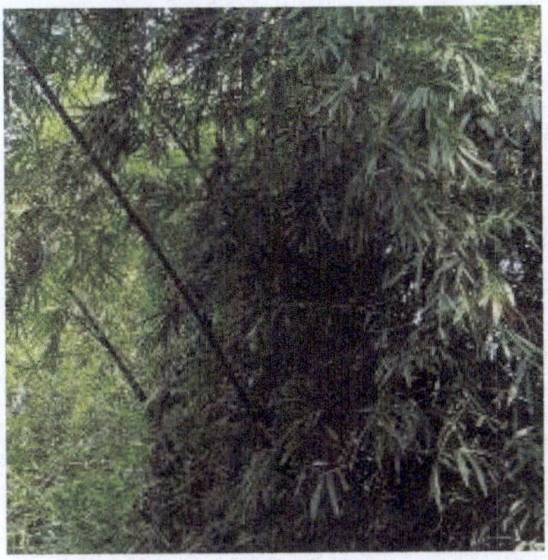

Scientific name: ***Bambusa tulda Roxb.***

Common name: Bengal Bamboo, Indian timber bamboo, Baans, Baunsa

Distribution: Indian subcontinent,China, Bhutan, Bangladesh, Nepal, Vietnam, Myanmar, ThailandColombia, Australia, Ecuador

Parts used : Young leaves

Bioactive Principles: Tannins, Polyphenols. Saponin glycosides, steroids, flavoniods, coumarin, triterpenoid

Remarks: Young leaves are given as fodder to cow or buffalo after delivery to hasten removal of placenta.

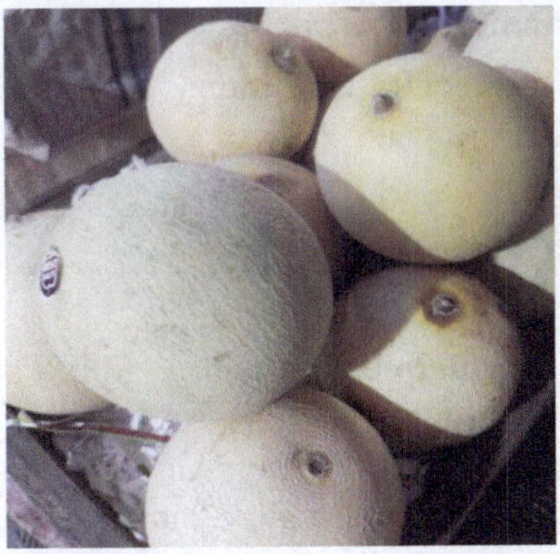

Scientific name: ***Cucumis melo L.***

Common name: American Cucumber, Honeydew, Muskmelon, Phoot, Kharbooj

Distribution: Tropical countries of whole world including India

Part used: Fruit

Bioactive principles: Vit-A, β-carotene,polyphenols, Carotenoids, folic acid, Vitamin C,dietary fibres, niacin

Remarks : Fresh fruits along with fodder is fed in placental retention cases.

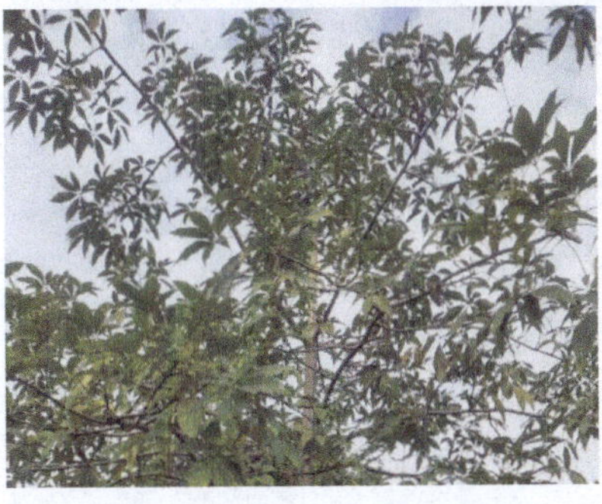

Scientific name: ***Bombax ceiba L.***

Common name: Red silk cotton, Semal (hindi) , Semak, Semalkand, Simili (Odia)

Distribution: India, south-east Asia, Tropical Africa, Queensland

Part used: Flower

Bioactive principles: Quercetin, Mangiferin, Amurenlactone A, Syringin, Ferulic acid, Perlargonidine, cyaniding, Hentriacontane, Bombalin, Naringenin,β-sitosterol, Kaempferol,Vicrnin

Remarks : Flowers of *Bombax ceiba* is mixed with powdered stem and bark of *Alangium salvifolium* (Ankol) are given to cattle for quicker removal of retained placenta.

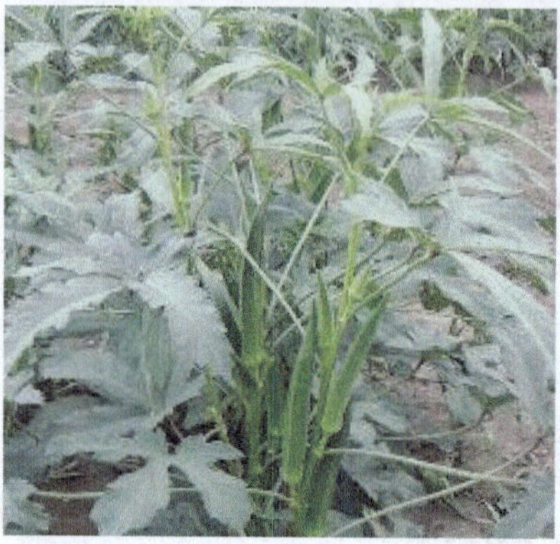

Scientific name: ***Abelmoschus esculentus (L.) Moench***

Common name: Okra , Lady's finger, Bhindi (hindi), Bhendi (odia)

Distribution: Asia, Africa, Southern Europe, Middle east & north Africa

Part used : Leaves

Bioactive principles: Tannins, Flavonol glycosides, polysachharides and phenolic compound

Remarks : Leaves are given as feed after delivery to hasten removal of placenta.

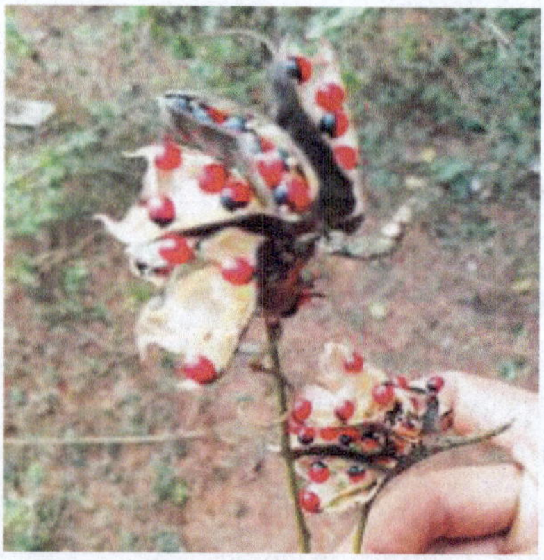

Scientific name: *Abrus precatorius L.*

Common name: Ratti, Jurang, Kaincha, Guraj and Rosary pea

Distribution: South-east Asia, Africa, South America

Part used : seeds

Bioactive principle: Abrin, Abralin, Flavonoids, steroids, Alkaloids, Anthocynin, Lecithin, lectins, Glycyrrhizin, Amino acids (alanin, serine, choline, valine and methyl ester)

Remarks : 10-12 seeds are made into a paste which is mixed with jaggery and fed orally to cattle for retention of placenta.

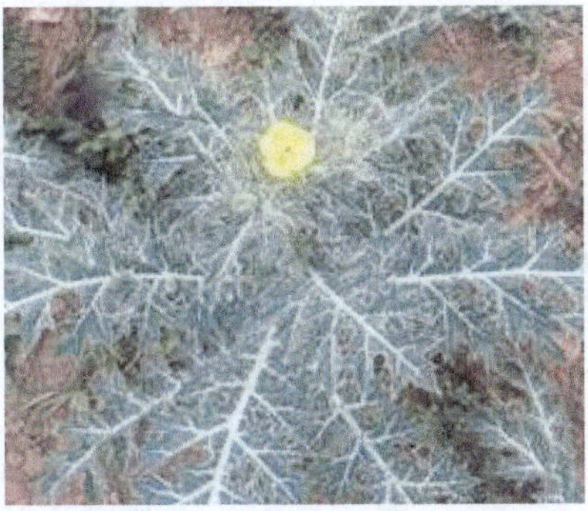

Scientific name: ***Argemone Mexicana L.***

Common name: Mexican Poppy, flowering thistle, Cardo, Pilikatari, Peela Kantasla, Satyanashi, Bhamadanti, Swarnaksheeri

Distribution: India, China, Bangladesh, Nepal, Pakistan, Nepal, Mexico, Costa Rica, USA, Australia, Bulgaria, Spain, Africa

Part used : Whole plant

Bioactive principles: Flavonoids

Remarks: Plant is given with fodders to feed on for early removal of placenta in cows after delivery[9].

Cervico-vaginal Prolapse

- **About the condition/definition:** When genital organs such as vagina, cervix are displaced distally and simultaneously everted out through vulva as a protrusion is called Cervico-vaginal prolapse, commonly occurs during late gestation.
- **Etiology :** Excessive relaxation of pelvic ligaments , vulva & vulvar spincture muscles due to increased concentration of estrogen and relaxin along with increased intrabdominal pressure during late gestation leads to such cases. Hypocalcemia, inadequate exercise, excessive fat deposition in perivaginal space, overdistention of abdomen due to bulky food are the predisposing factors. Feeding of estrogenic plants, exogenous estrogen administration and follicular cyst leading to rise in estrogen concentration and ultimately causes prolapsed genitalia.
- **Clinical signs :** Intitially vagina protrude through vulva only when animal sits and vaginal mucosa becomes little congested. If not treated at this stage, later vagina remains constantly protruded and gradually cervix also comes out along with vagina. Continuous exposure to outside environment make the mucosa congested, edematous, thickened and infected.
- **Treatment :** The prolapsed mass is usually washed with mild antiseptic solution(KMnO4), hygroscopic substances (Magnesium sulphate) are applied and repositioned manually under epidural anaesthesia.Along with that Fluid therapy, antibiotics, antihistaminic and calcium are administered. Surgical approaches like Buhner's suture is very common to prevent recurrence.

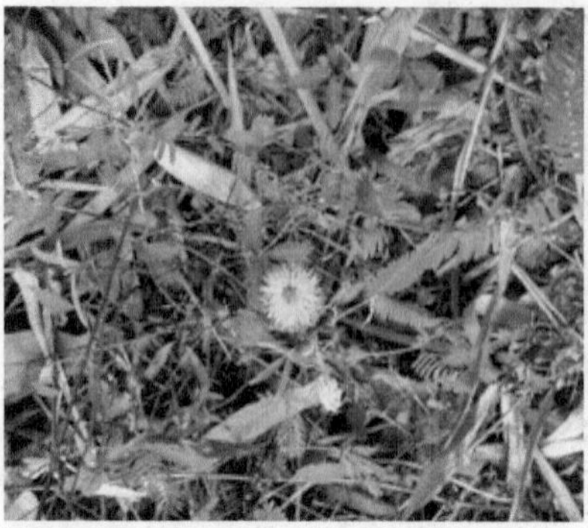

Scientific name: *Mimosa pudica* L.

Common name: Shame plant, sensitive plant, touch-me-not, Lajakuli (odia), Lajwanti, Lajjalu

Distribution : South east Asia, Ghana, Nigeria, Uganda, Pacific islands, USA

Plant part used : whole plant

Bioactive principle: Coumarins, Terpenoids, alkaloids, favonoids, quinines, glycosides, phenols, tannins and saponins

Remarks: 100g of whole plant is to fed orally for 3 days along with a suitable antibiotics[14]. (OR) After cleaning and disinfecting the prolapsed mass, mustard oil and leaves of Mimosa pudica are taken in equal amount and crushed together to form a paste. That paste is applied on prolapsed mass gently and then pushed inside with the palm gives better result [5].

References

Ahmed BM. Effect of fenugreek (*Trigonella foenumgraecum*) seeds as feed additive on production performance of dairy goats. PhD thesis submitted to NDRI, Karnal, 2009.

Baitule1, Mohan M., Gawande1 A.P., Kumar,Umesh, Sahatpure S. K., Patil Manoj S. and Baitule Mansi M. (2016). Effect of Aegle marmelos and Murraya koenigii in treatment of delayed pubertal buffaloes heifers. Veterinary World, 9: 1375-1380.

Balakrishnan, Nair M. N., Punniamurthy, N. and Kumar, S. K. (2017) Ethno-veterinary Practices for Animal Health and the Associated Medicinal Plants from 24 Locations in 10 States of India. RRJVS. 3(1): 25-34

Berhane M. Studies on feeding some indigenous galactopoeitic feed supplements on milk production in crossbred cows. MSc Thesis submitted to JNKVV, Jabalpur, 2000.

Kumar, R. and Kumar A.B. (2012) Folk veterinary medicines in Bareilly district of Uttar Pradesh, India. Indian Journal of Traditional Knowledge, 12(1): 40-46.

Lawange S.R., Markandeya, N.M. Kumawat, B.L. Sawale, A.G., Anbhule, R.S. and Kadam, P.D. (2019) Efficacy of garlic extract and ashwagandha for the treatment of infectious repeat breeding in cattle. Indian Journal of Animal Reproduction 40(1):31-34.

Mahour S. S., Nema S. P., Rajput N., Chhabra D., Karmore S. K., Kurechiya N. and Sikrodiya R. Therapeutic efficacy of ethanolic herbal extracts and ciprofloxacin in metritic crossbred cows . Journal of Entomology and Zoology Studies 2020; 8(5): 1221-1224

Panda, T., Mishra, N. (2016). Indigenous Knowledge on animal Health Care practices in Kendrapada District of Odisha, India. International letters of Natural Sciences. Vol.53 : 10-27

Parashar P. (2018) Ethnoveterinary studies of plants used in Retention of Placenta of cattle in Nimar region (M.P.) . International Journal of Scientific Research in Science and Technology. 4(1): 226-230

Rajkumar R, Srivastava SK, Varshney VP, Mahmood S. Effect of medicinal plants Saracaasoca and Trigonella foenum- graecum in anoestrus cows. Ind Vet J. 2008; 85:1281-1283.

Rautela Rupali, Das G.K, Khan F.A, Prasad Shiv, Kumar Avdesh, Prasad, J.K., Ghosh S.K., Dhanze, Himani, Katiyar Rahul, Srivastava, S.K.. (2018). Antibacterial, anti-inflammatory and antioxidant effects of Aegle marmelos and Murraya koenigii in dairy cows with endometritis. Livestock Science. 214: 142-148.

Satapathy, K. B. (2010) Ethnoveterinary practices in Jajpur district of Orissa. Indian Journal of Traditional Knowledge. 9 (2) : 338-343

Soundara Pandian, Satheshkumar. (2017). Estrus induction by supplementation of Murraya koenigii in anoestrus heifers. The Indian journal of Animal Reproduction. 30: 66-67.

Upadhyay A., Nema S.P., Shivhare M., Mehta H. K. and Kumar S. (2021) Effect of mimosa pudica (lajjalu) in cervico vaginal prolapse in buffaloes. Bufalo Bulletin. 40(1): 151-155.

17

Medicinal Plants Effective as Galactagogues

Pallavi Bhardwaj

Department of Veterinary Pharmacology and Toxicology, Dr. G.C. Negi College of Veterinary and Animal Sciences, CSKHPKV, Palampur, Himachal Pradesh

Herbal galactagogues are medicinal plants used to stimulate, sustain, and boost milk production. Several plants known for their galactagogue activity are being used traditionally in many cultures to stimulate milk production in animals. However, there is a knowledge gap regarding the safety and efficacy of these medicinal plants. Moreover, the mechanism of action of the herbal constituents present in these plants is not yet elucidated. Although, many herbal galactagogues have been reported as safe in domestic animals and can be used as food supplements in the dairy industry. Nowadays, the use of plant-derived supplements has increased in the dairy sector promoting a new trend of organic dairy farming. Traditional remedies being used for increasing milk production in animals often incorporate herbal treatments, mainly comprising of the following important herbs [1-8]:

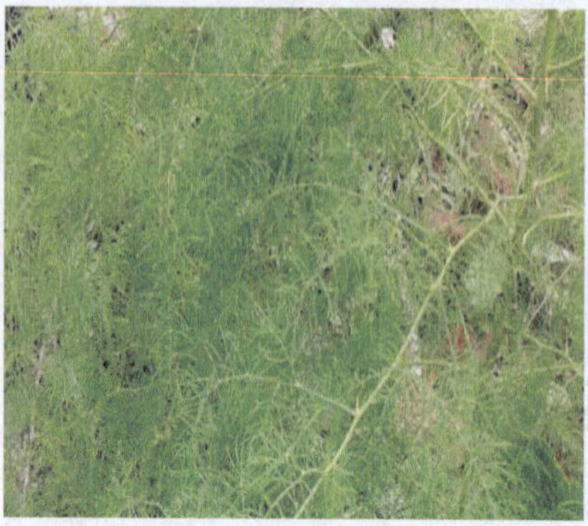

Scientific name: *Asparagus racemosus*

Common name: Shatawar, Sevariya, Satamuli, Shatavari

Distribution: The Himalayas, Sri Lanka, and India

Part used: Roots

Bioactive principles: Steroidal saponins (Shatavarins I-IV), flavanoids-Glycosides of rutin, quercitin, hyperoside, polycyclic alkaloid-Aspargamine A

Remarks: Ricalax tablet, a herbal formulation of *A. racemosus*, can increase milk production being oestrogenic, it may be stimulating milk production by increasing levels of prolactin. Also, it increases the weight of mammary glands during animal studies

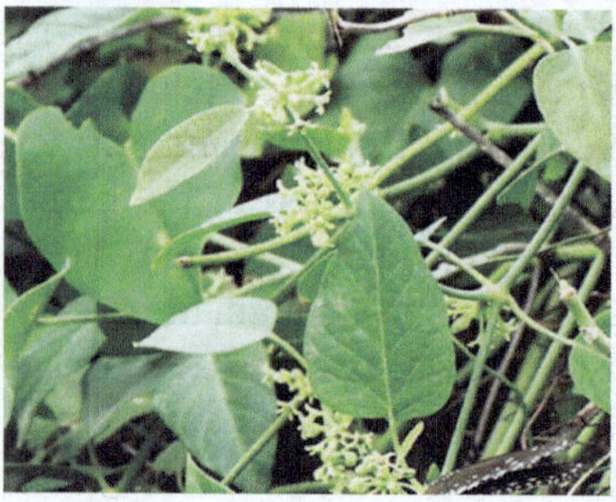

Scientific name: *Leptadenia reticulata*

Common name: Jeevanti, Jivanti, Jivaniya, Jivapushpa, Hemavati, Jivana

Distribution: The Himalayan ranges, Sikkim, Deccan Plateau, Karnataka, Khasi Hills, Konkan ranges, and Kerala up to an altitude of 2000 m

Part used: Whole plant

Bioactive principles: rutin, α-amyrin, β-sitosterol, diosmetin, β-amyrin, ferulic acid, luteolin, stigmasterol,hentricontanol, a triterpene alcohol simiarenol, leptaculatin, apigenin, reticulin, and deniculatin

Remarks: Leptaden tablet is a herbal formulation made from *L. reticulata that* is used for the milk yield enhancement

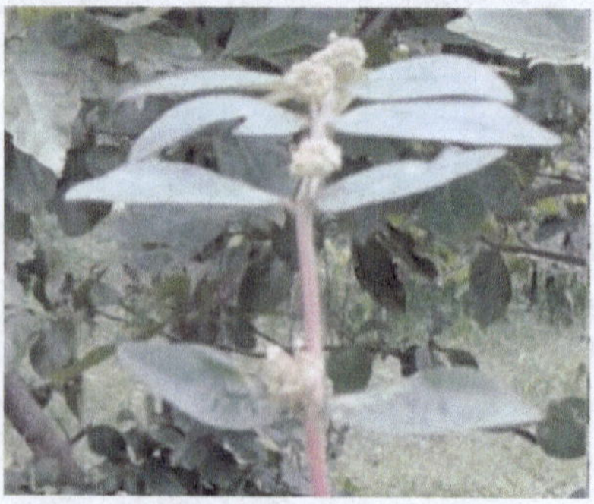

Scientific name: *Euphorbia hirta L.*

Common name: Thaur, Dudhai

Distribution: In the hotter parts of Australia and India

Part used: Leaves

Bioactive principles: Alkanes, amino acids, flavanoids, triterpenoids, alkaloids

Remarks: Crushed leaves are mixed with fodder administered to cattle to upsurge lactation in cattle

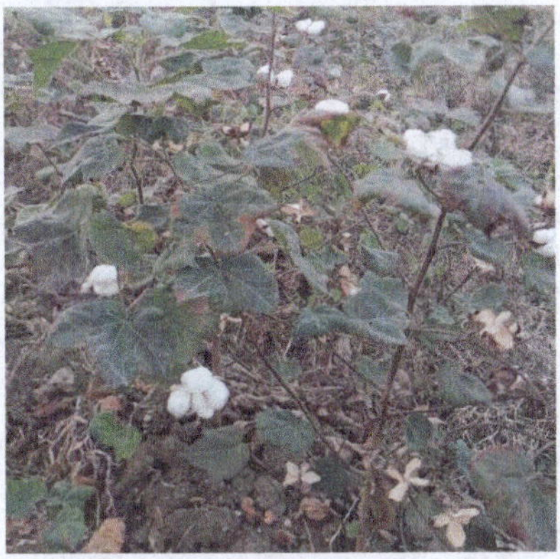

Scientific name: *Gossypium herbaceum L.*

Common name: Kapas, Levant Cotton

Distribution: Native to Africa and Asia

Part used: Seeds

Bioactive principles: carbohydrates, pectin alkaloids, flavonoids, glycosides, terpenoids, saponins, steroids, and tannins

Remarks: It stimulates prolactin in animals. It may be assisting the reflex of milk ejection.

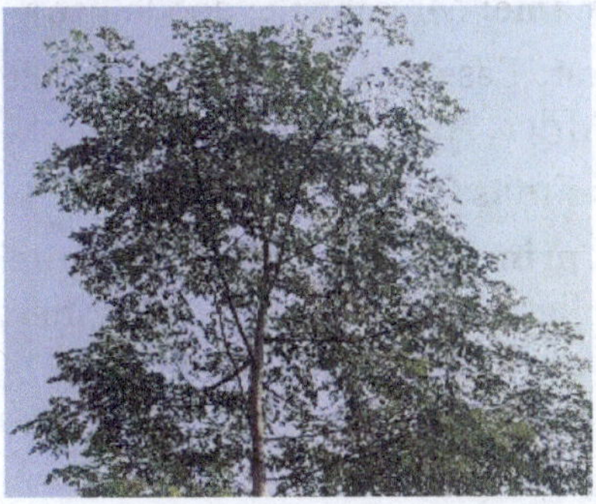

Scientific name: *Moringa oleifera*

Common name: Surjana, Sahjan, drumstick, kelor leave or malunggay

Distribution: Tropical and subtropical regions, origin is in India, Arabia, East Indies

Part used: Leaves, seeds

Bioactive principles: Arachidic acid (fatty acids) glucosinolates, tannins, flavonoids, sterols, carotenoids, phenolic acids, saponins alkaloids, and terpenes

Remarks: It increases prolactin, provides essential nutrients.

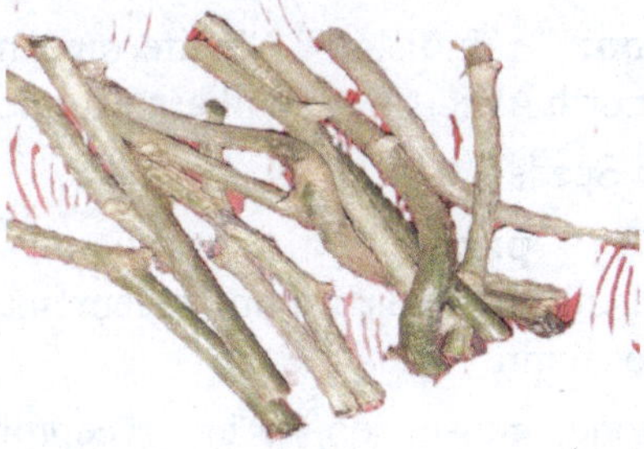

Scientific name: *Tinospora cordifolia*

Common name: Heart leaved Moonseed, giloy, guduchi

Distribution: Sub-tropical and tropical regions of Asia, Australia, and Africa

Part used: Stem, leaves

Bioactive principles: alkaloids, steroids, diterpenoid lactones, aliphatics, and glycosides

Remarks: The supplementation of ration with *Tinospora cordifolia* improves milk yield and stimulate milk secretion

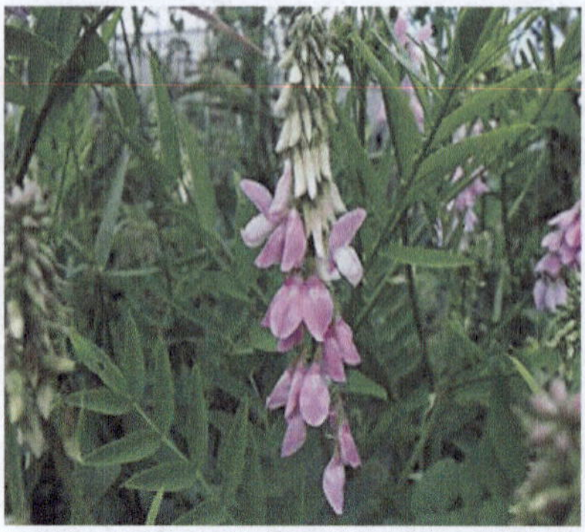

Scientific name: *Galega officinalis*

Common name: Goat's rue

Distribution: Northern Africa, western Asia and Europe

Part used: Aerial parts

Bioactive principles: Galegin, a precursor to metformin. flavonol triglycosides, kaempferol, quercetin, steroidal saponins.

Remarks: Stimulates mammary growth, increase milk yield and lactation persistency

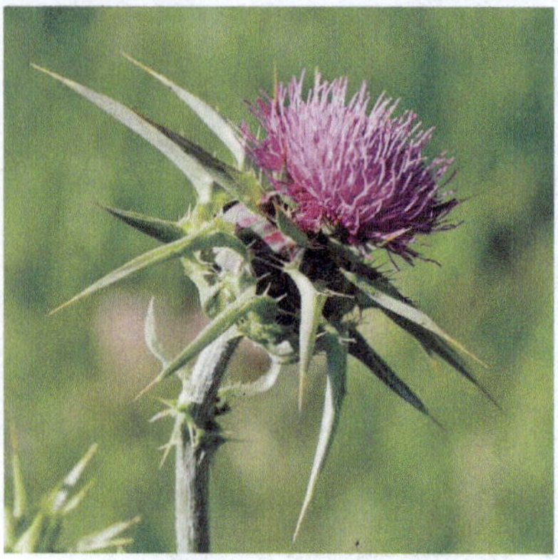

Scientific name: *Silybum marianum*

Common name: Milk thistle, doodh patra

Distribution: Eastern United States, South America, Africa, Australia and Asia

Part used: Fruits (seeds)

Bioactive principles: silymarin, mixture of flavonolignans, (silibinin, silycristine, silydianin, quercetin and taxifolin)

Remarks: Stimulate prolactin; possibly oestrogenic

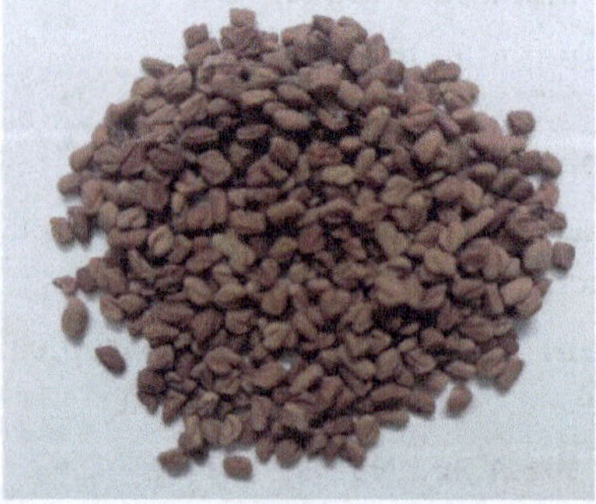

Scientific name: *Trigonella foenum-graceum L.*

Common name: Meithi, Fenugreek

Distribution: India, Mediterranean countries, north Africa, and southern Europe

Part used: Seeds

Bioactive principles: Saponins, phytoestrogens alkaloids, saponins, tannins, phenols diosgenin

Remarks: It stimulates the growth hormone, causes dopamine receptor antagonism that stimulate milk production. It posseses estrogen-like effects (phytoestrogens), mastogenic effect, oxytocic and anxiolytic effects that may contribute in milk ejection reflex for milk release efficiently.

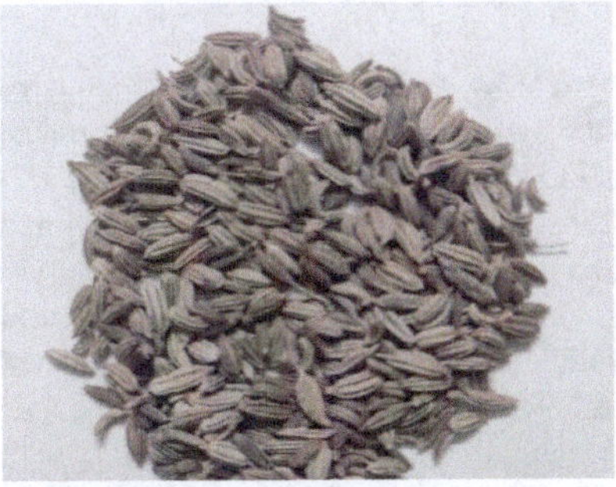

Scientific name: *Foeniculum vulgare*

Common name: Fennel

Distribution: Southern Europe, especially the Mediterranean coast, Temperate zones around the world

Part used: Fruit (seeds)

Bioactive principles: E2-like molecules, like estragole, anethole etc.

Remarks: It reduces the impact of dopamine on dopamine receptors, which indirectly stimulates prolactin through the trans-anethole. It may increase prolactin due to its oestrogenic qualities. By supporting the milk ejection reflex, it may also indirectly enhance milk production. Additionally, it has a mastogenic impact.

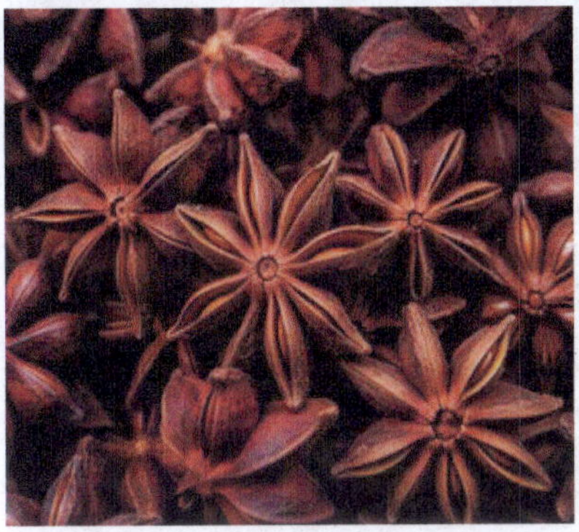

Scientific name: *Pimpinella anisum*

Common name: Anise or aniseed

Distribution: West Asia, Eastern Mediterranean, Mexico, and Spain

Part used: Fruit (seeds)

Bioactive principles: Trans-anethole, that is weakly oestrogenic

Remarks: The aromatic compound present in anise acts as a dopamine receptor antagonist

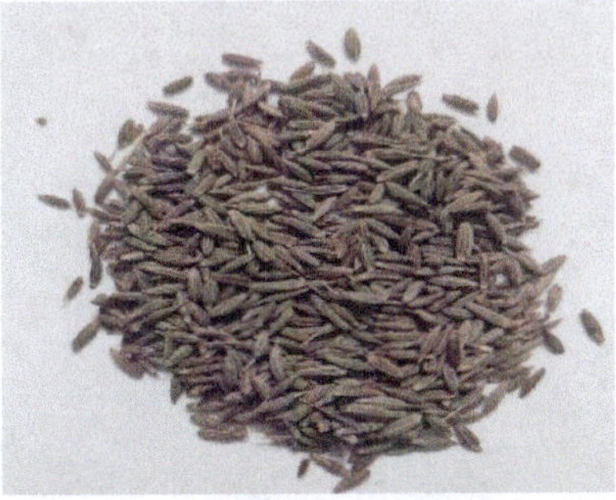

Scientific name: *Carium carvi*

Common name: Caraway, jeera

Distribution: Asia, Africa and Europe.

Part used: Seeds, fruit

Bioactive principles: Flavonoid glycosides, monoterpenoid glucosides, flavonoids, lignins, isoflavonoids, and alkaloids and other phenolic compounds.

Remarks: It is oestrogenic in nature

Caution: Herbal treatments should be taken under the guidance of a qualified practitioner to ensure safety and effectiveness

References

Alok S, Jain SK, Verma A, Kumar M, Mahor A, Sabharwal M. Plant profile, phytochemistry and pharmacology of Asparagus racemosus (Shatavari): A review. Asian Pac J Trop Dis. 2013 Jun;3(3):242–51. doi: 10.1016/S2222-1808(13)60049-3. PMCID: PMC4027291.

Drugs and Lactation Database (LactMed®) National Institute of Child Health and Human Development; 2006. U.S. Department of Health and Human Services

Foong SC, Tan ML, Foong WC, Marasco LA, Ho JJ, Ong JH., Oral galactagogues (natural therapies or drugs) for increasing breast milk production in mothers of non-hospitalised term infants. Cochrane Database of Systematic Reviews 2020, Issue 5. Art. No.: CD011505. DOI: 10.1002/14651858.CD011505.pub2.

Kumar S, Malhotra R, Kumar D. Euphorbia hirta: Its chemistry, traditional and medicinal uses, and pharmacological activities. Pharmacogn Rev. 2010 Jan;4(7):58-61. doi: 10.4103/0973-7847.65327. PMID: 22228942; PMCID: PMC3249903.

Mohanty SK, Swamy MK, Sinniah UR, Anuradha M. Leptadenia reticulata (Retz.) Wight & Arn. (Jivanti): Botanical, Agronomical, Phytochemical, Pharmacological, and Biotechnological Aspects. Molecules. 2017 Jun 19;22(6):1019. doi: 10.3390/molecules22061019. PMID: 28629185; PMCID: PMC6152761.

Parashar P and Ray S. Plants Used as Galactagogue in Nimar Region of M.P. Int.J.Curr. Microbiol.App.Sci. 2020, Special Issue-11: 1336-1341

Pareek A, Pant M, Gupta MM, Kashania P, Ratan Y, Jain V, Pareek A, Chuturgoon AA. Moringa oleifera: An Updated Comprehensive Review of Its Pharmacological Activities, Ethnomedicinal, Phytopharmaceutical Formulation, Clinical, Phytochemical, and Toxicological Aspects. Int J Mol Sci. 2023 Jan 20;24(3):2098. doi: 10.3390/ijms24032098. PMID: 36768420; PMCID: PMC9916933.

Penagos Tabares F, Bedoya Jaramillo JV, Ruiz-Cortés ZT. Pharmacological overview of galactogogues. Vet Med Int. 2014;2014:602894. doi: 10.1155/2014/602894. Epub 2014 Aug 31. PMID: 25254141; PMCID: PMC4165197.

18

Medicinal Plants as Growth Promoter of Livestock

Nibedita Nayak[1], Amiya Ranjan Sahu[1*] and Anuj Singh[2]

[1]ICAR-Central Coastal Agricultural Research Institute, Goa
[2]College of Veterinary and Animal Sciences, Kishanganj, Bihar

---

Feed additives like antibiotics, hormones are successfully employed in chicken production along with basic minerals, vitamins, and nutrients. Because of worries about antibiotic residues in animal tissues and the resulting development of bacterial resistance, the use of antibiotics as growth promoters (AGP) in cattle was outlawed in 2005. Given the rising concerns about antibiotic use and its involvement in antibiotic resistance, the use of plant-based chemicals in animal feed has become essential. Phytogenic feed additives, which are made from plants and their secondary metabolites, are becoming more and more popular as a result of the search for sustainable farming methods.

These natural growth promoters are seen as alternatives to synthetic chemicals, which are often associated with adverse environmental and health impacts. The usage of plant additions, also known as phytobiotics, have existed since the beginning of time, when people and farm animals were treated and prevented with herbs. The unique qualities of herbs and plant additions were effectively utilised by the ancient Greek, Egyptian, Roman, and Chinese civilisations. Phytogenic feed additives offer multiple benefits for livestock, including enhancing growth, improving immunity, supporting digestion, and promoting overall animal health. Water or alcohol extracts derived from plant additions, whether fresh or dried, fermented, or freeze-dried, can be used in poultry practices.

It is anticipated that the phytobiotics will improve nutrient absorption, help the body's detoxification, boost hunger, stimulate the release of bile and digestive enzymes, and control digestive processes. However, plant supplements can also have more targeted effects, such as preventing the growth of harmful microorganisms, controlling the gastrointestinal microbiome, boosting the immune, reproductive, and endocrine systems, having anti-inflammatory and antiallergic qualities, speeding up wound healing, increasing blood flow, reducing inflammation, encouraging intestinal villi and intestinal epithelial regeneration, and even improving the quality of eggs or meat.

The majority of plant-based active antioxidants are secondary metabolites that fall into the isoprene, flavonoid, and glucosinolate derivative families. Their qualities may also be used to influence the qualities of animal-based foods. Numerous plant materials have been effectively employed in practice to enhance meat quality, egg laying, and egg quality.

Consequently, because phytobiotics are natural, easily accessible, non-toxic, and residue-free, they are becoming more and more significant as potential substitutes for antibiotic growth promoters. Herbal extracts or plant parts (rhizomes, bark, roots, fruits, leaves, flowers, bulbs, stems, and seeds) that have the highest concentration of physiologically active compounds can be used as raw materials for phytobiotics. Alkaloids, essential oils, phenolic acids, phytosterols, glycosides, flavonoids, colours (primarily carotenoids and anthocyanins), and other isolated, pure bioactive compounds are also utilised.

The natural variability in the configuration of secondary metabolites of plant, their diversity, and the environment for plant growth, maturity, harvest time, and the method and duration of storage, conservation, or processing, can all lead to contradictory results when using plant additives. Furthermore, it is crucial to consider the analytical conditions needed to extract the bioactive substances from plants, the extraction process, potential synergism or antagonistic effects in mixtures of substances, presence of anti-nutritional and toxic components for a particular animal species, and microbiological infection of plant products.

The use of particular herbs to cure a particular ailment was made possible by several observations of the animals' reactions. Additionally, the usage of potentially toxic or hazardous plant species was eliminated. These days, the rapid advancement of analytical methods makes it possible to identify a wide variety of physiologically active compounds in plants that give them their advantageous properties.

Because biological indicators vary in vivo research, plants' anti-inflammatory, antiseptic, antibacterial, and anti-diarrheal qualities can also vary. It is crucial to remember that it will rely on the type of animal, the category of production, the surroundings, and the properties of the plant material utilised. Therefore, it is necessary to investigate several phytochemicals as growth boosters. The commercial use of these natural substances in the animal industry will grow more feasible as confirming studies demonstrate the beneficial benefits of different plants on cattle development and performance.

Herbal Growth Promoters

These plants improve the quality of growth and production of poultry and contribute to the sustainability of food systems by decreasing dependence on chemical interventions. The commercial application of promising phytochemicals as growth is given below.

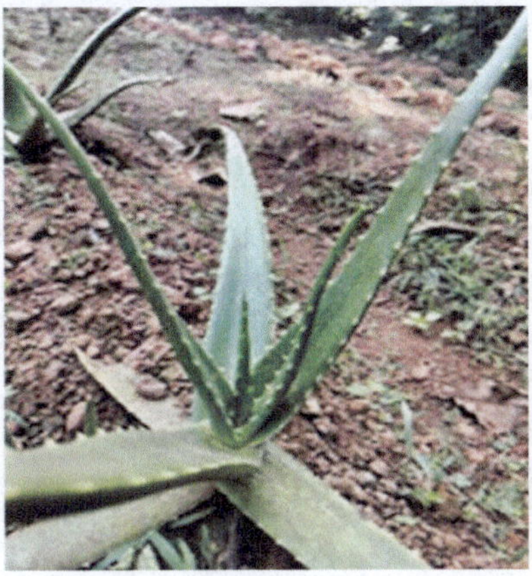

Scientific Name: *Aloe vera*

Common Name: Aloe vera, Ghritkumari

Distribution: Tropical and subtropical regions of India.

Part Used: Leaves (gel and latex)

Bioactive Principles: Aloin, aloesin, emodin, saponins, and polysaccharides

Remark: Aloe vera promotes growth by enhancing tissue regeneration and cellular repair through its rich polysaccharide and amino acid content. It aids in the growth of healthy skin and hair, making it a common ingredient in cosmetic products. Additionally, aloe vera supports digestive health and nutrient absorption, indirectly fostering bodily repair and overall development. Aloe vera polysaccharides enhance immune responses and tissue repair in broilers, promoting better growth performance.

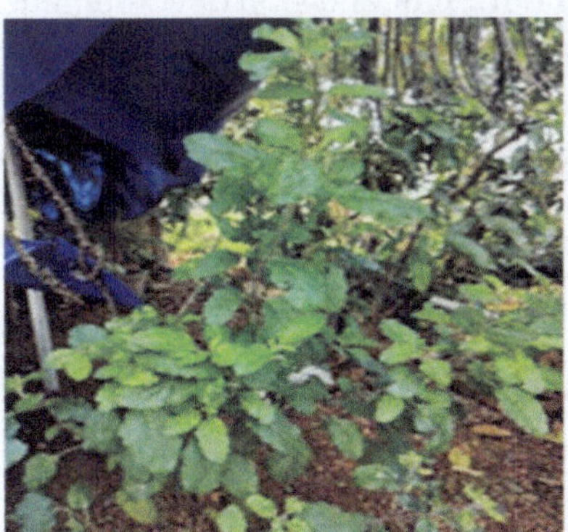

Scientific Name: *Ocimum* sp.

Common Name: Basil (Tulsi)

Distribution: India

Part Used: Leaves

Bioactive Principles: Eugenol

Remark: Basil acts as a natural growth promoter by boosting energy levels and metabolic efficiency through its adaptogenic properties. Its antioxidants protect cells from damage, supporting healthy tissue development. Furthermore, basil strengthens the immune system, allowing the body to allocate resources effectively toward growth and repair. A study by Maneesha et al. (2022) demonstrated that basil extract improves feed efficiency and metabolic activity in poultry.

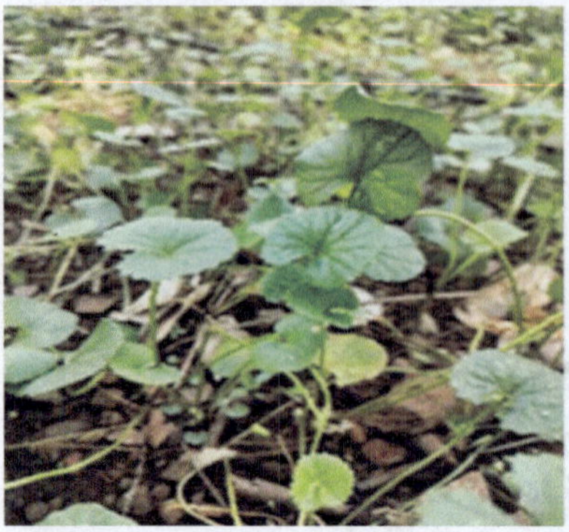

Scientific Name: *Centella asiatica*

Common Name: Centella (Ballari)

Distribution: India

Part Used: Leaves, whole plant extract

Bioactive Principles: Madecacoside, asiaticoside, aglycones

Remark: Centella is known to accelerate growth by stimulating collagen synthesis, which promotes skin and connective tissue regeneration. It also improves blood circulation, ensuring optimal nutrient delivery to growing tissues. Additionally, it enhances brain development and cognitive functions, contributing to mental growth.

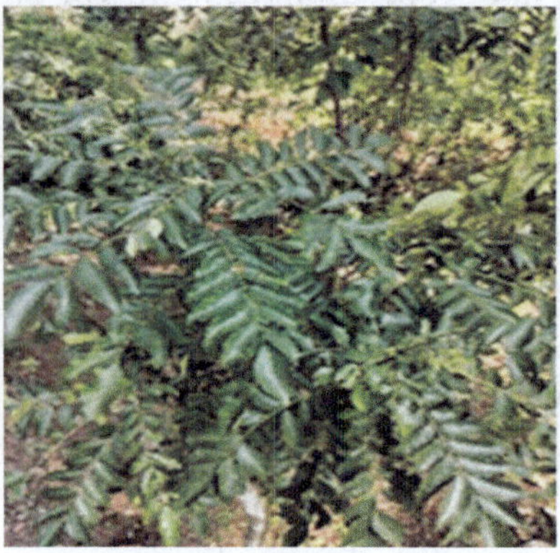

Scientific Name: *Murraya koenigii*

Common Name: Curry Leaf (Katnim)

Distribution: India

Part Used: Leaves

Bioactive Principles: Carbazole alkaloids

Remark: Curry leaves support growth by providing essential nutrients such as iron, which is vital for hair and skin development. Their antioxidant properties aid in cellular repair and overall tissue growth. By improving digestion and nutrient absorption, curry leaves play a key role in promoting physical development.

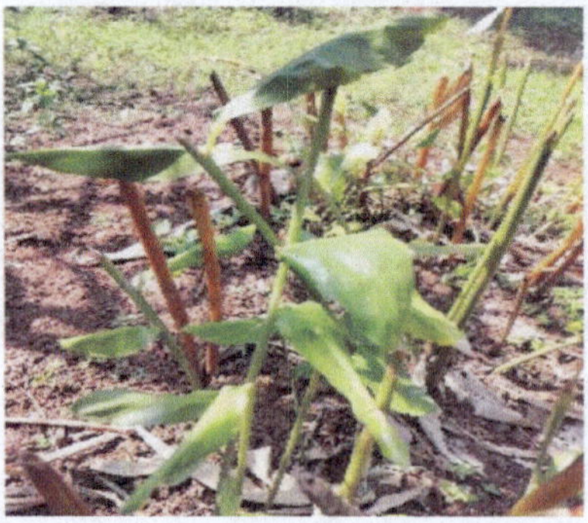

Scientific Name: *Costus speciosus*

Common Name: Costus

Distribution: India

Part Used: Rhizome

Bioactive Principles: Diosgenin, Dioscin

Remark: Costus enhances growth by improving insulin sensitivity, which helps regulate glucose metabolism. This supports cellular growth and energy production. Additionally, it promotes healthy skin and hair development by boosting circulation and nutrient transport.

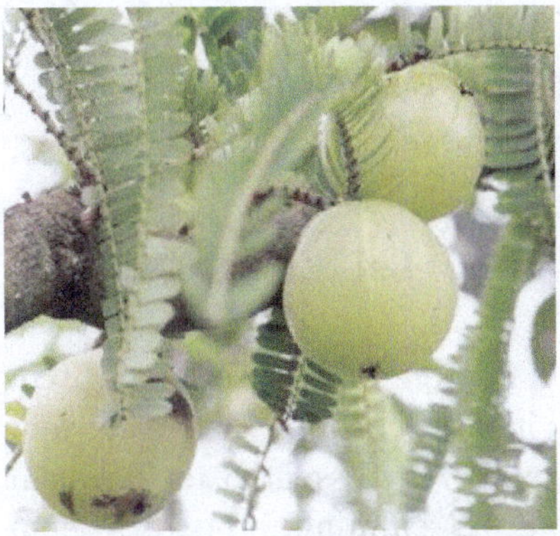

Scientific Name: *Emblica officinalis*

Common Name: Indian Gooseberry (Amla)

Distribution: India

Part Used: Fruits

Bioactive Principles: Ascorbic acid, Quercetin

Remark: Amla, or Indian gooseberry, is a powerhouse of vitamin C, which facilitates collagen production and tissue repair. It enhances hair and skin growth while strengthening the immune system, enabling the body to grow and recover effectively. Demir et al. (2003) found that Indian gooseberry (amla) serves as a potent antioxidant and supports collagen production, boosting tissue repair in livestock.

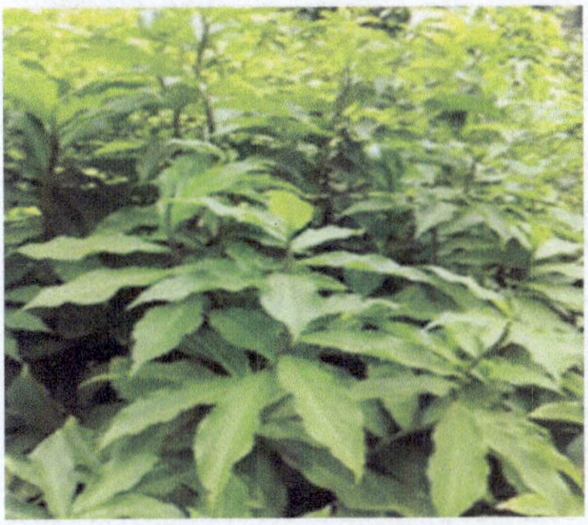

Scientific Name: *Costus igneus*

Common Name: Insulin Plant

Distribution: India

Part Used: Leaves

Bioactive Principles: Insulin precursor, Beta-carotene

Remark: The insulin plant supports growth by regulating blood sugar levels, reducing cellular stress, and promoting normal metabolic functions. Its antioxidant properties further assist in tissue repair and overall physical growth.

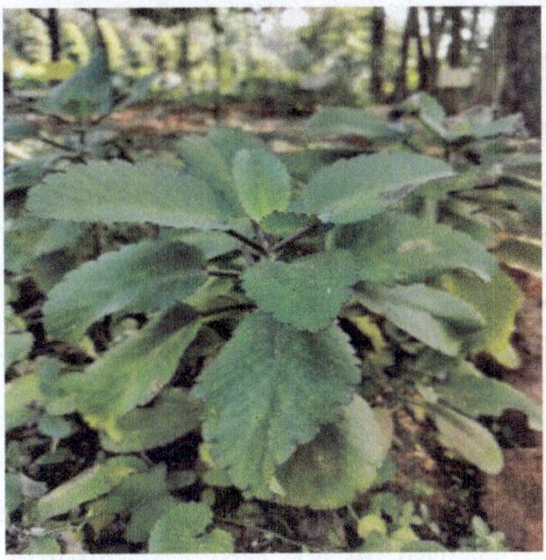

Scientific Name: *Bryophyllum pinnatum*

Common Name: Kalanchoe (Patherchutt)

Distribution: India

Part Used: Leaves

Bioactive Principles: Bufadienolides

Remark: Kalanchoe encourages growth by enhancing tissue regeneration and aiding in wound healing. It also supports respiratory health, ensuring better oxygenation of tissues, which is essential for development and repair.

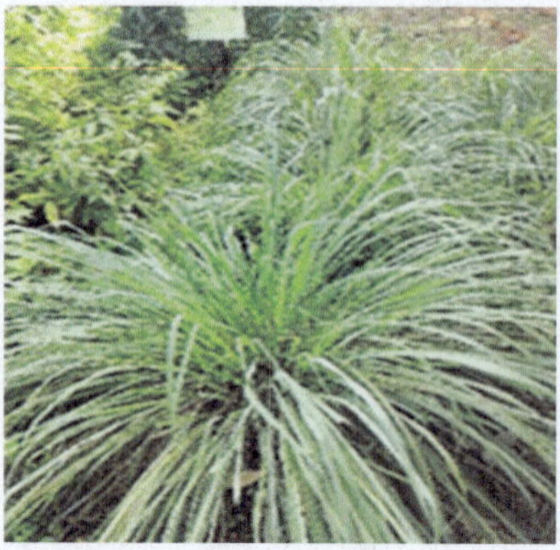

Scientific Name: *Cymbopogon citratus*

Common Name: Lemongrass

Distribution: India

Part Used: Leaves

Bioactive Principles: Citral, Limonene, Citronellol

Remark: Lemongrass aids growth by improving digestion and nutrient absorption, which are essential for physical development. Its calming properties help reduce stress, indirectly fostering an environment conducive to growth. Biswas et al. (2014) revealed that lemongrass improves nutrient absorption and reduces oxidative stress, fostering better growth in poultry.

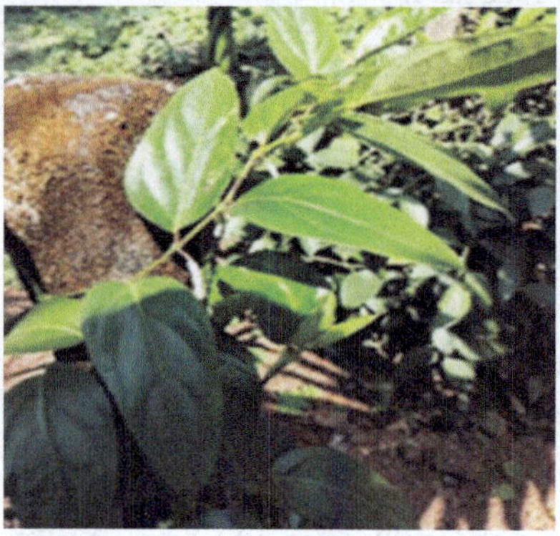

Scientific Name: *Piper longum*

Common Name: Long Pepper (Piplamul)

Distribution: India

Part Used: Fruits, Root

Bioactive Principles: Piperine, Piperethine

Remark: Long pepper acts as a growth promoter by stimulating metabolic activity, enhancing energy production, and supporting overall development. It also improves respiratory health, ensuring optimal oxygen delivery to tissues.

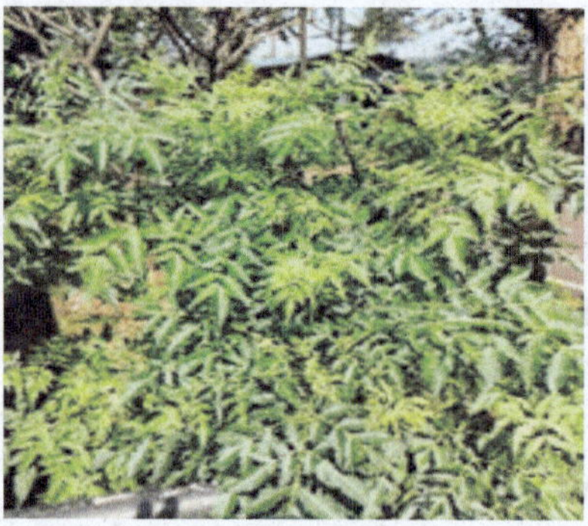

Scientific Name: *Azadirachta indica*

Common Name: Neem (Margosa Tree)

Distribution: India

Part Used: Leaves, Seeeds, Seed oil

Bioactive Principles: Azadirachtin

Remark: Neem purifies the blood, ensuring effective nutrient transport and cellular health. Its antimicrobial properties protect against infections, creating a supportive environment for tissue growth and repair . Attia YA et al. (2017) highlighted azadirachtin in neem as an effective immunomodulatory agent, reducing infections and improving livestock health.

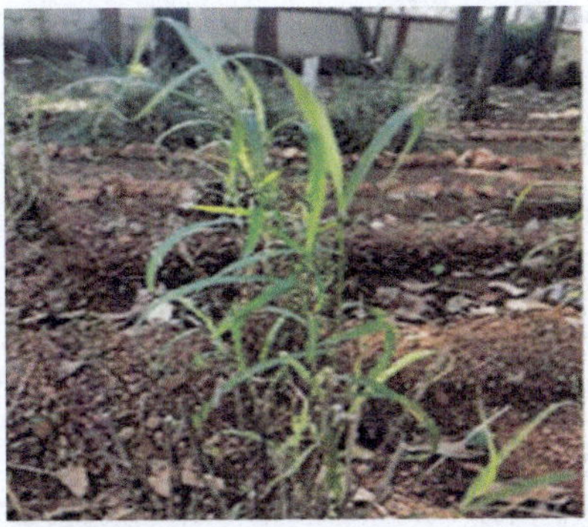

Scientific Name: *Cymbopogon martinii*

Common Name: Palmarosa

Distribution: India

Part Used: Leaves

Bioactive Principles: Geraniol

Remark: Palmarosa stimulates skin regeneration, promoting youthful growth. Its stress-relieving properties indirectly support development by encouraging relaxation and reducing growth-inhibiting stress.

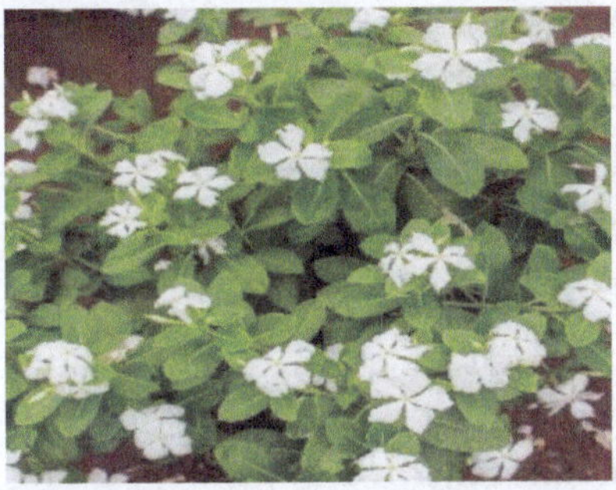

Scientific Name: *Catharanthus roseus*

Common Name: Periwinkle

Distribution: India

Part Used: Leaves, Roots

Bioactive Principles: Vinblastine, vincristine

Remark: Periwinkle promotes growth by supporting healthy cell division, essential for tissue repair. Its vascular-enhancing properties improve nutrient and oxygen delivery, facilitating physical development.

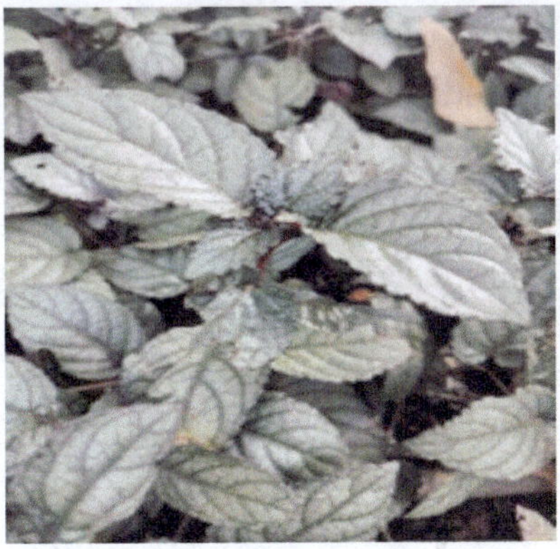

Scientific Name: *Hemigraphis colorata*

Common Name: Red Fame Ivy

Distribution: India

Part Used: Leaves

Bioactive Principles: Favonoids, polyphenols, tannins

Remark: This plant aids growth by promoting wound healing and skin regeneration through its antioxidant and anti-inflammatory effects. It supports healthy tissue development and repair.

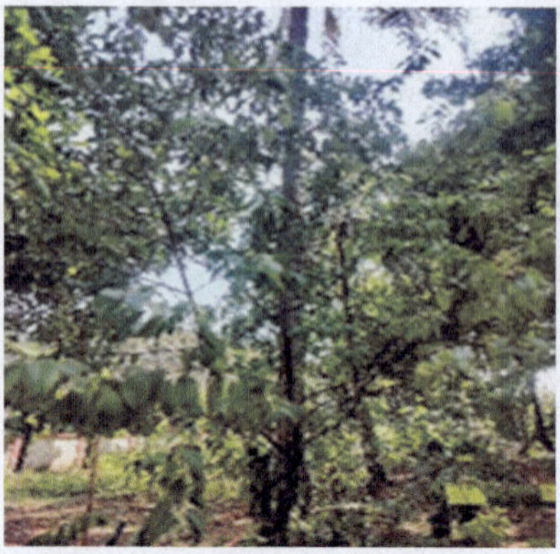

Scientific Name: *Santalum album*

Common Name: Sandalwood

Distribution: India

Part Used: Leaves, Wood

Bioactive Principles: Santalin

Remark: Sandalwood supports growth by improving skin health and reducing inflammation. Its calming properties also aid mental clarity and stress relief, indirectly fostering an environment for growth.

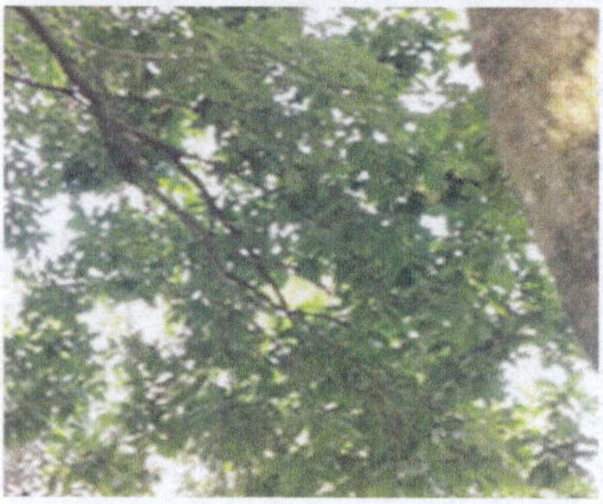

Scientific Name: *Sapindus trifoliatus*

Common Name: Soapnut Tree

Distribution: India

Part Used: Fruits, Leaves

Bioactive Principles: Saponins

Remark: Soapnut enhances scalp health, promoting strong and healthy hair growth. It is gentle on sensitive skin, supporting natural external growth without irritation.

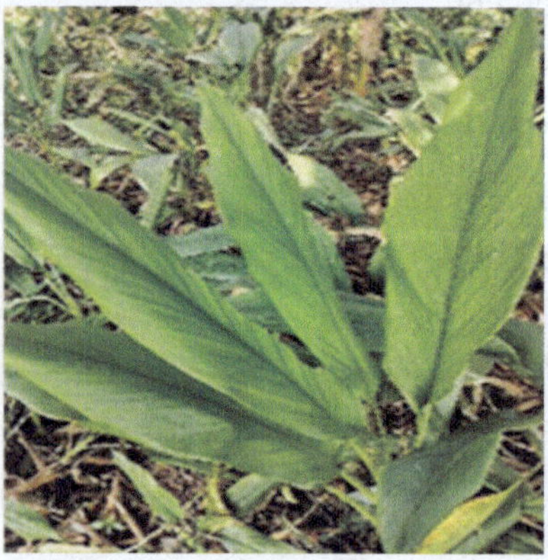

Scientific Name: *Curcuma longa*

Common Name: Turmeric

Distribution: India

Part Used: Rhizome

Bioactive Principles: Curcumin

Remark: Turmeric promotes growth through its active compound curcumin, which supports collagen synthesis and tissue repair. Its anti-inflammatory and antioxidant properties encourage healthy development. Attia YA et al. (2017) showed that curcumin in turmeric enhances antioxidant activity and promotes better growth and immune response in broilers.

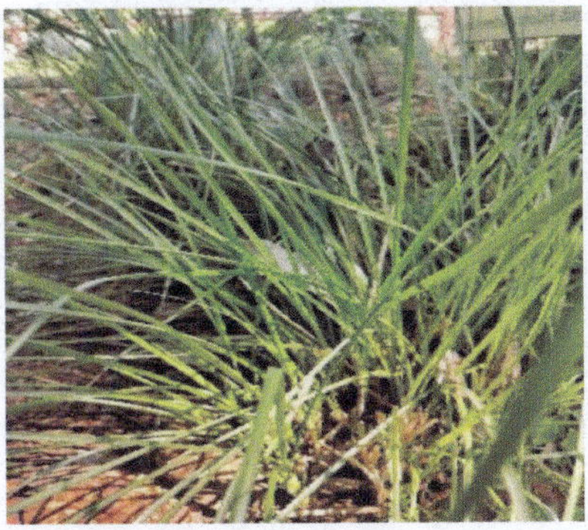

Scientific Name: *Vetiveria zizanioides*

Common Name: Vetiver

Distribution: India

Part Used: Roots, Leaves

Bioactive Principles: Vetiverol

Remark: Vetiver supports growth by promoting restful sleep, which is essential for both physical and mental development. Its calming properties enhance recovery and repair processes.

Conclusion

The use of phytogenic feed additives as growth promoters represents a significant shift toward more sustainable and eco-friendly agricultural practices. The diverse plants mentioned above, with their rich array of bioactive compounds, play crucial roles in enhancing growth, improving feed efficiency, and boosting overall animal health. These natural alternatives to antibiotics and synthetic growth promoters not only support the physical development of animals but also contribute to reducing the environmental footprint of agriculture. As the demand for natural and sustainable food production systems increases, the role of phytogenics will continue to grow, offering new opportunities for improving animal health and productivity. Further research into these plants and their mechanisms of action will help to refine their applications and expand their use in commercial animal production, ensuring a healthier and more sustainable future for both animals and humans. With the potential to reduce reliance on harmful chemicals and enhance the quality of livestock products, phytogenic feed additives represent a promising solution to many of the challenges facing modern agriculture.

References

Ali BH, Blunden G, Tanira MO, Nemmar A (2008). Some phytochemical, pharmacological and toxicological properties of ginger (Zingiber officinale). Food Chem Toxicol. 46(2): 409–420.

Attia YA, Al-Harthi MA, Hassan SS (2017). Neem (Azadirachta indica) as a phytogenic growth promoter alternative for antibiotics. Rev Mex Ciencias Pecuarias 8:11–21.

Attia YA, Al-Harthi MA, Hassan SS (2017). Turmeric (Curcuma longa Linn.) as a phytogenic growth promoter alternative for antibiotics. Rev Mex Ciencias Pecuarias 8:11–21.

Biswas P, Yadav AK, Sharma RP (2014). Effects of lemongrass oil on growth and antioxidant status in poultry. Indian J Anim Sci 84(3): 275–280

Biswas P, Yadav AK, Sharma RP (2014). Effects of lemongrass oil on growth and antioxidant status in poultry. Indian J Anim Sci 84(3): 275–280.

Demir E, Sarica Ş, Özcan MA, Suiçmez M (2003). Natural feed additives as alternatives for antibiotics in broiler diets. Br Poultry Sci 44:44-45.

Maneesha SR, Safeena SA, Solomon Rajkumar, Arunachalam V, Kumar P (2022). Plants of Dhanvantari Vatika - ICAR-CCARI, Goa, Technical Bulletin No: 72, pp. 1-88.

Part III
Special Topics

19

Medicinal Plants Effective in Wounds in Animals

Sushma Ghadigaonkar

Department of Veterinary Pharmacology & Toxicology, Maharashtra Animal and Fishery Sciences University Nagpur, Mumbai, India

Wound in Domestic Animals

A wound is defined as a break in the continuity of the skin, mucous membrane, or tissue surface that can result from physical, chemical, or biological agents. India has a diverse variety of livestock breeds, extensive countryside with vast grazing lands, and widespread use of livestock. The significant population of stray animals, including dogs, cats, and cattle, as well as the increase in pet ownership, make wounds in animals a commonly encountered condition. Wounds in animals can be a frustrating issue for both pets and productive animals, and this can also be a challenge for their owners. For instance, bleeding at the wound site from sudden cuts and bites can cause panic and distress among animal owners. Wounds can become complicated, as animals may lick, scratch, or otherwise irritate them, leading to infections, especially when they are soiled. Additionally, fly infestation and maggots, common in various temperate regions of India, further complicate the wound healing process. An unattended wound can quickly escalate to a severe microbial infection, which may lead to septicemia, maggot infestation, and can even become fatal for the animal. The cost of treating wounds in production animals, including expenses for antibiotics, can impose an economic burden on farmers. Common causes of wounds in domestic animals include penetrating injuries from horns, stamping injuries caused by mothers or other adult animals in tightly packed barns, tightened nose ropes, barbed wire injuries at the brisket region (in horses and cattle), and wet sores on the inner surfaces of the shoulder and groin in cattle due to friction and lack of air and sunlight exposure.

Wound Induced in Lab Animals

Lab animals can be used to model wounds in a variety of ways, including:

1. **Chronic wounds:** Induced by damaging the skin barrier, such as through cutting, burning, radiation, or mechanical pressure. Chronic wounds can also be created by inducing diabetes, ischemia, or reperfusion injury.
2. **Diabetic wounds:** Induced by injecting mice or rats with streptozotocin or alloxan to destroy insulin-producing cells in the pancreas. This causes hyperglycaemia, which can be followed by a cutaneous wound.
3. **Skin abrasion infections:** Induced by scratching, scraping, or other methods to create abrasions on the skin. Common bacterial species used to infect the wounds include S. aureus, P. aeruginosa, and C. albicans.
4. **Burn wounds:** Induced by placing a heated metal plate or bar on the skin of a guinea pig. The burns can be infected with a bacterial suspension
5. **Incisional wounds:** This model can be used for research on materials used in surgical incisions, including the deterioration of various suture threads and mechanical characteristics assessed by tensile strength. Incisional wounds can be categorised as either primary or secondary closure, and they can either be sutured right away or later. Due to a small degree of wound healing activity, primary closure or initial intention is an improved model for biomechanical analysis of wound strength than it is for histologic assessment of healing, evaluation of wound tissue biochemistry, or assessment of epithelialisation. When examining scarring at later stages (more than 65 days following incision), the secondary closure model of incisional wounds, also known as the second intention, can be useful.
6. **Excisional wounds**: These wounds are among the most widely used models for wound healing because they simulate acute clinical wounds, which need to heal by second intention—that is, without suturing the skin's borders together. The surgical excision of the animal's epidermis, dermis, and subcutaneous fat results in these wounds. Hemorrhage, granulation tissue development, inflammation, reepithelialization, angiogenesis, and remodeling can all be considered through this model.
7. **Drug induced wound**: a. Cadmium chloride: Wounds exposed to 1.0% cadmium chloride fail to heal within 7 days. b. Xylazine and fentanyl: The coadministration of these two drugs can lead to severe soft tissue injuries, including deep tissue necrosis and bone involvement.

Herbal treatment in wound healing

Herbal treatments for wound healing have been long used for ages in traditional medicine systems like Ayurveda, Traditional Japanese(TJM), Traditional Chinese Medicine (TCM), and others. While some herbal remedies may offer benefits for various wound conditions, it's important to approach them with utmost care.

Medicinal plants used in wound healing

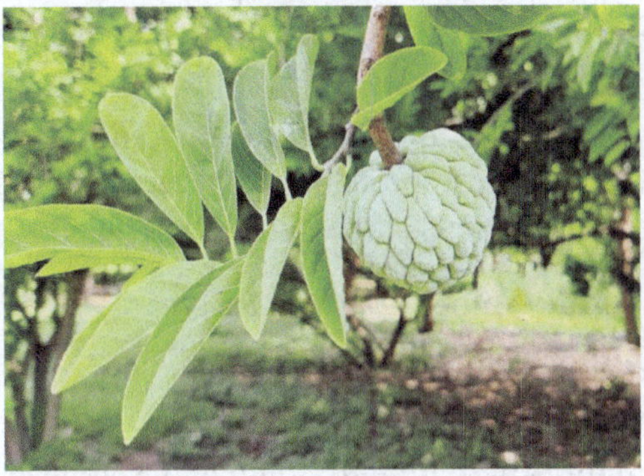

Scientific Name: *Annona squamosa*

Common name: Custard apple, Sitaphal

Part used: Leaves, seed, bark

Distribution: Native to tropical and subtropical regions around the world

Bioactive principles: tannin, Vitamin C, hydroxyproline, hexosamine, zinc, copper

Remarks: Known for its antibacterial properties that help prevent wound infections, which can lead to faster and safer healing. The leaves of the custard apple contain tannins, which can also promote wound healing

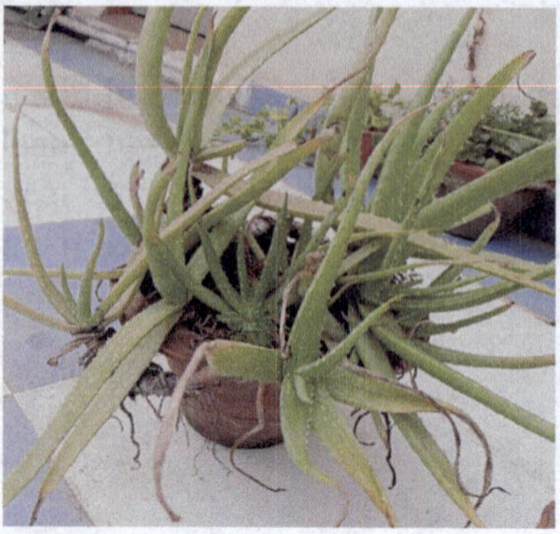

Scientific Name: *Aloe vera*

Common name: Aloe, korphad

Part used: leaves

Distribution: native to drier areas of Europe, North America, Africa, Asia, Indian states like Rajasthan, Andhra Pradesh, Gujarat, Tamil Nadu, Maharashtra

Bioactive principles: polysaccharides (Glucamannan and acemannan), carboxypeptidase,

Remarks: known for its healing properties, immunostimulant, and anti-inflammatory effects, antimicrobial properties, protetective effect against damage to skin through UV and gamma radiations and antidiabetic effect.

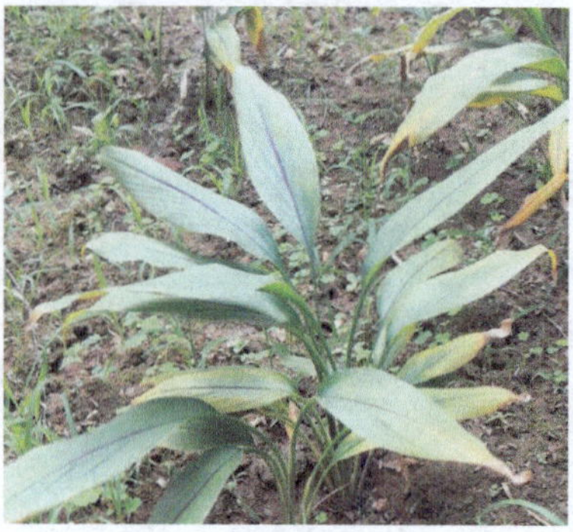

Scientific Name: *Curcuma longa*

Common name: Turmeric, Haldi

Part used: Rhizome, Leaves

Distribution: native to South and Southeast Asia

Bioactive principles: Terpenoids and phenolic constituents, with curcumin, demethoxycurcumin, and bisdemethoxycurcumin

Remarks: Curcumin has many properties that can help wounds heal, including: Anti-inflammatory, Antimicrobial, Stimulates growth factors, Enhances tissue formation with tissue remodeling, collagen deposition, and contraction of wound

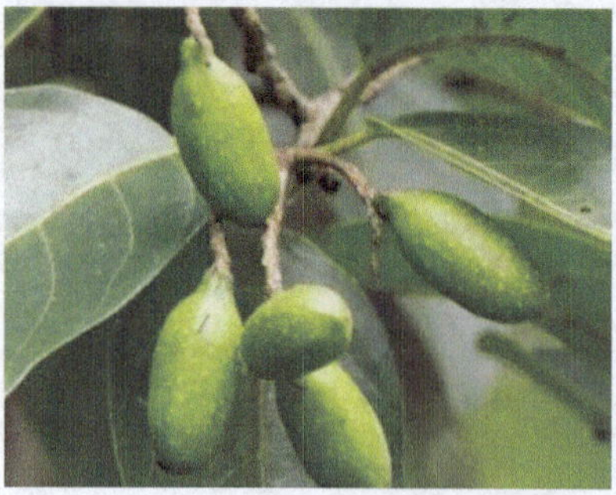

Scientific Name: *Terminalia chebula*

Common name: Black Myrobalan, Harad

Part used: bark, Fruit, Leaves

Distribution: native to southern Asia, from India and Nepal to Southwestern China

Bioactive principles: chebulanin, gallic acid, corilagin, chebulagic acid, chebulinic acid, chebulic acid, chebulanin, and ellagic acid

Remarks: known for its anti-carcinogenic, anti-inflammatory, hepatoprotective, cytoprotective and antiviral effects

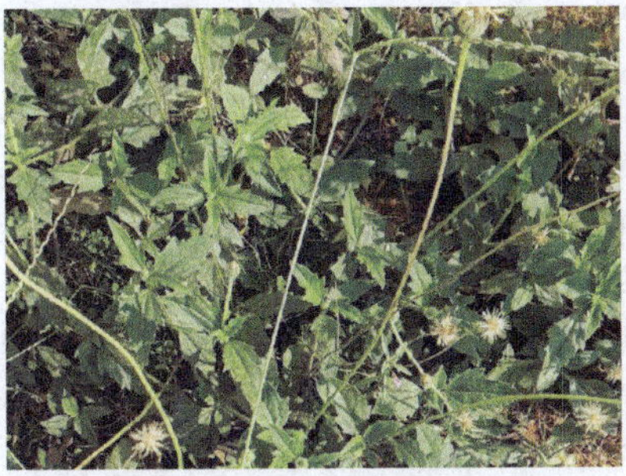

Scientific Name: *Tridax procumbens*

Common name: Coat buttons, Dagdi pala, Khal apala

Distribution: distributed throughout the tropical and subtropical regions. It is native to Mexico and tropical America

Part used: leaves

Bioactive principles: 6,8,3′- trihydroxy-3, 7, 4′- trimethoxyflavone; 8,3′-dihydroxy-3,7,4′ -trimethoxy-6-*O*- β-d-glucopyranosyl flavone, puerarincentaureidin, procumbetin, and centaurein,

Remarks : Tribal and rural populations in India use it as a nutritious vegetable. Leaves are used to cure fever, skin conditions, and wounds.

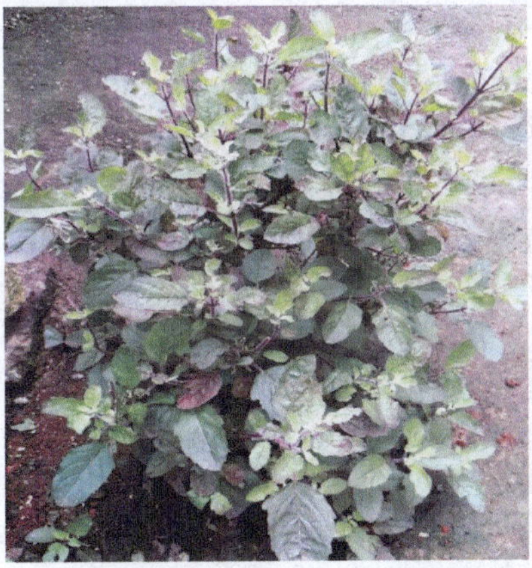

Scientific Name: *Ocimum sanctum*

Common name: Basil, Tulsi

Part used: Leaves

Distribution: Semitropical and tropical parts of India and world

Bioactive principles: camphor, eugenol, eucalyptol, alpha bisabolene, beta bisabolene, and beta caryophyllene

Remarks : Known to decrease free radicals, blood glucose, and myeloperoxidase while improving connective tissue production and antioxidant status to aid with wound healing.

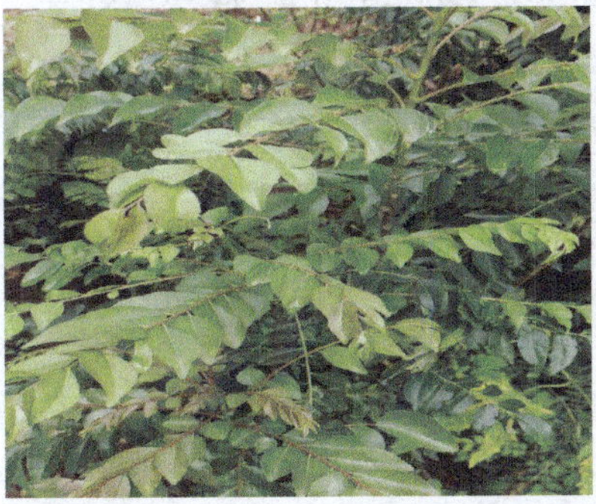

Scientific Name: *Murraya koenigii*

Common name: Curry leaves, kadhi pata

Part used: leaves

Distribution: native to the Indian subcontinent

Bioactive principles: Carbazole alkaloids, Terpenoids, Flavonoids and phenolics

Remarks: Curry leaves have anti-inflammatory and disinfectant properties that help with wound healing.

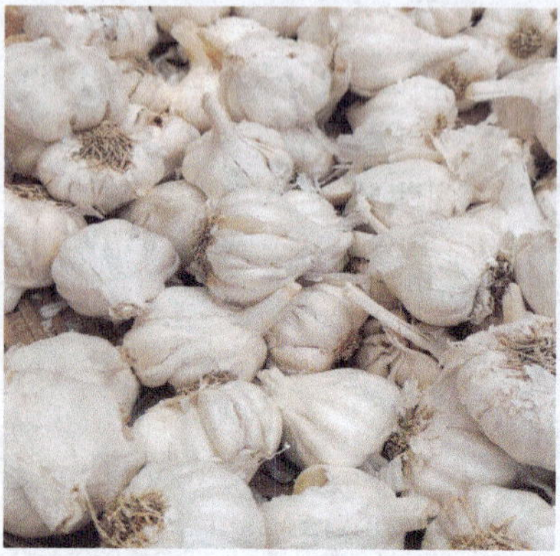

Scientific Name: *Allium sativum*

Common name: Garlic, Lasun

Part used: clove

Distribution: Central Asia (Kazakhstan, Turkmenistan, Kyrgyzstan, Tadzhikistan and Uzbekistan) and Iran

Bioactive principles: Alliin, Allicin, Ajoene

Remarks: Garlic contains allicin, a molecule that gives garlic its smell and has antibacterial and antifungal properties

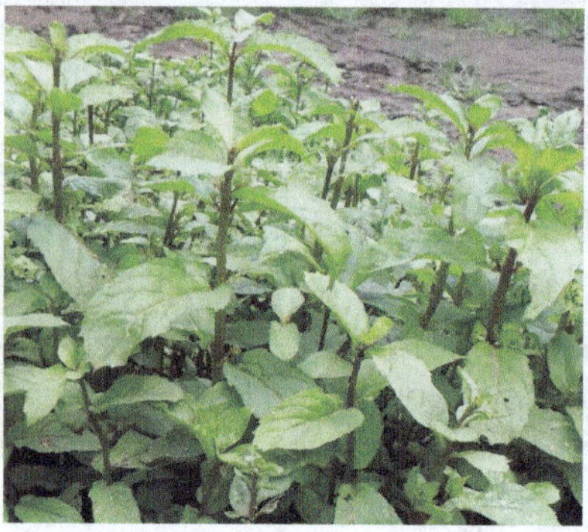

Scientific Name: *Mentha Arvensis*

Common name: Mentha, Pudina

Part used: leaves

Distribution: distributed in temperate areas of the world, Africa, Asia, Europe Australia, South America and North America

Bioactive prinicples: menthol, menthone, menthyl acetate, menthofuran, and other compounds

Remarks: The leaves of Mentha arvensis have anti-bacterial effects against multidrug resistant Acinetobacter baumannii. The essential oil from the leaves can stop the growth of several bacterial strains

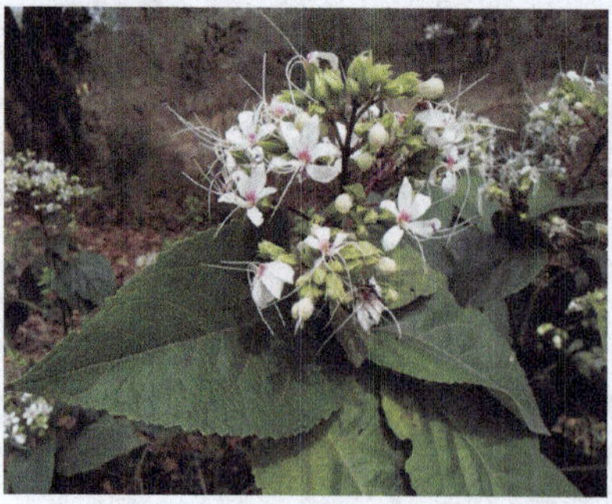

Scientific Name: *Cleodendrum infortunatum*

Common name: Bhat, hill glory bower

Part used: Leaves, root

Distribution: India and Sri Lanka

Bioactive principles: Acacetin 7-O-glucuronide, Apigenin 7-O-glucuronide, Clerosterol, acteoside, and isoacteoside,

Remarks: It has various effects such as anti-inflammatory, anticancer, antimicrobial, hypoglycemic anti-diarrheal, anti-nociceptive, memory enhancing, hepatoprotective, and hypolipidemic effects.

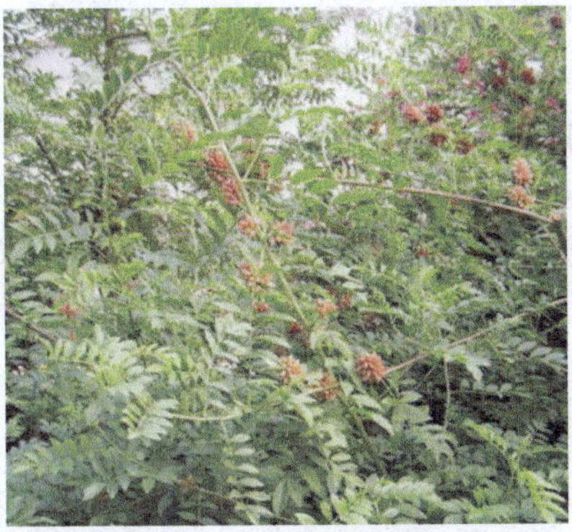

Scientific Name: *Glycyrrhiza glabra*

Common name: Sweet wood, Licorice

Distribution : globally distrubuted in tropical and semi-tropical regions, including Central Asia and Southern Europe

Part used : roots and rhizomes

Bioactive principles: Saponins like glycyrrhizic acid and glycyrrhitinic acid, flavones and flavonoids like glabridin, and volatile oils.

Remarks: Its antispasmodic, laxative, anti-inflammatory, anti-cancer, anti-hypertensive, anti-allergic, and antidepressant qualities are well-known. Furthermore, this plant has shown antiviral properties against a number of viruses, and more recently, it was confirmed to have potential efficacy against COVID-19.

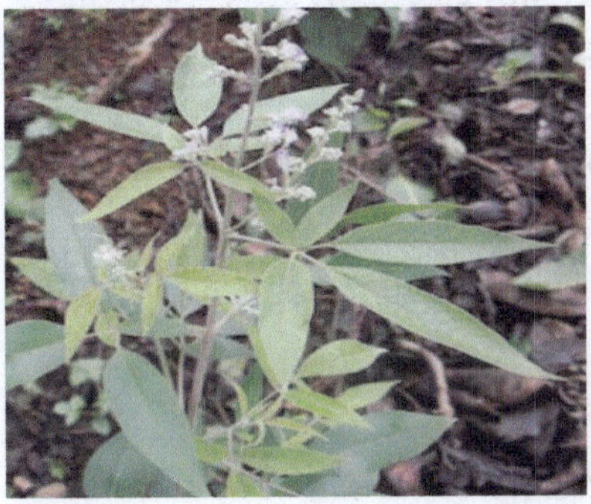

Scientific Name: *Vitex negundo*

Common name: Nirgudi, Chinese chaste tree, five-leaved chaste tree, or horseshoe vitex,

Distribution: widely distributed throughout India, China, Korea, Japan, Indonesia, the Philippines, and other Asian countries

Part used: leaves, flowers, twigs, roots, and seeds

Bioactive principles: Terpenoids, Flavonoids, Lignans, Alkaloids, Glycosides, Phenolic compounds, Phytosteroids, Iridoids, Essential oils

Remarks: Locals consume extracts of the leaves to treat coughs, colds, body aches, wounds, and snake bites. Traditional medicine has made use of *Vitex negundo* because of its ability to heal wounds.

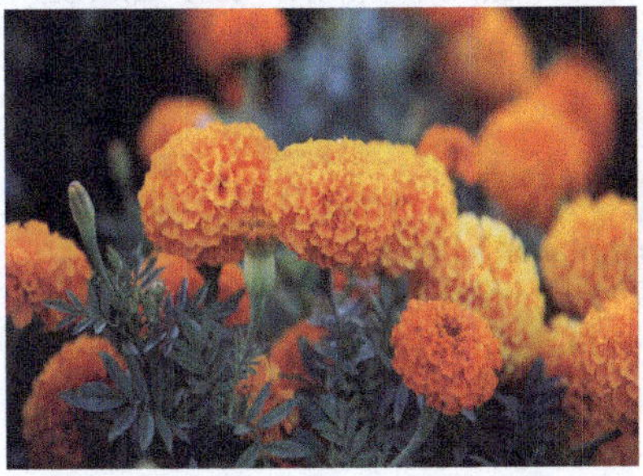

Scientific Name: *Calendula officinalis*

Common name: Marigold

Part used: Flowers, leaves

Distribution : Native or cultivated in North Africa, Europe, and Asia

Bioactive constituents: Terpenoids such as

triterpenoids, polyphenols (phenolic acids and flavonoids), polysaccharides, and carotenoids

Remarks: Through potential processes like decreased inflammation, enhanced blood flow, and antibacterial action, calendula aids in wound healing. Calendula contains flavonoids, such as quercetin, which have anti-inflammatory qualities that help reduce swelling and inflammation so the wound may concentrate on healing.

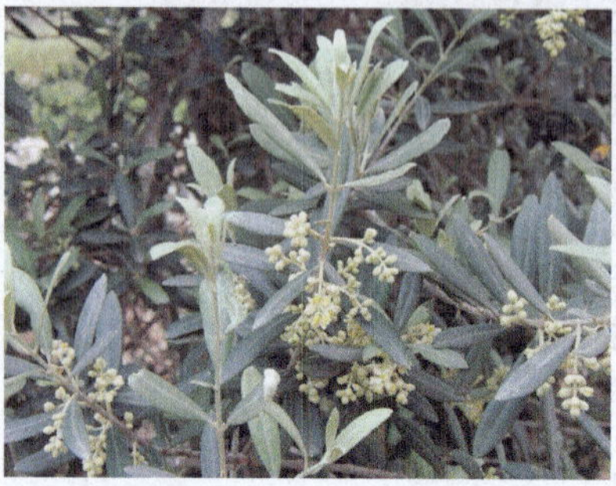

Scientific Name: *Olea europaea*

Common name: Indian Olive

Part used : leaves, wood, oil, fruits

Distribution : Native to northern Africa, southern Europe, and western Asia.

Bioactive principles:
Polyphenols: Oleuropein, oleuropein aglycone, elenolic acid, hydroxytyrosol, caffeic acid, and ligstroside Flavonoids: Apigenin, kaempferol, and luteolin Triterpenoids: Oleanolic acid, maslinic acid, and squalene

Remarks: Known for its Antioxidant and anti-inflammatory properties

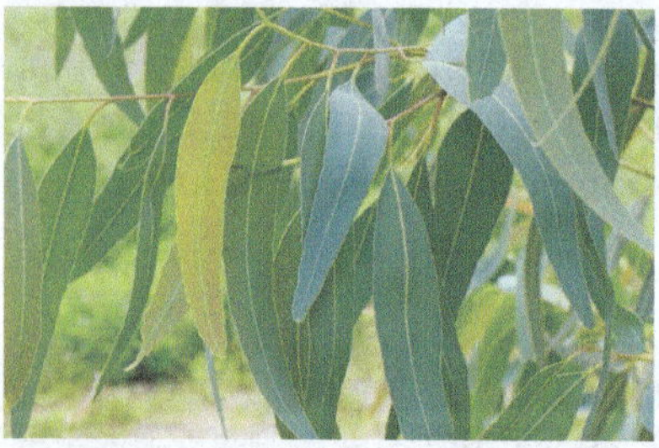

Scientific Name: *Eucalyptus globulus*

Common name: Nigiri, Tasmanian blue gum

Part used : leaves

Distribution: native to southeastern Australia

Bioactive principles: 1,8-cineole, p-cymene, limonene, terpineol, citronellal, α and β-pinene, citral, eudesmol, terpene-4-ol, and α-phellanderene.

Remarks: it reduces inflammation and pain linked with wounds. Capillary permeability: Intra-dermal administration of E. globulus oil can increase capillary permeability, which can help with wound healing

References

Albahri G, Badran A, Hijazi A, Daou A, Baydoun E, Nasser M, Merah O. The therapeutic wound healing bioactivities of various medicinal plants. Life. 2023 Jan 23;13(2):317.

El-Sherbeni SA, Negm WA. The wound healing effect of botanicals and pure natural substances used in in vivo models. Inflammopharmacology. 2023 Apr;31(2):755-72.

20

Medicinal Plants Effective in Different Toxicities

Sheen Tukra and Pawan Kumar Verma

Division of Veterinary Pharmacology & Toxicology
Faculty of Veterinary Sciences and Animal Husbandry, SKUAST-Jammu
RS Pura,181102, Jammu, J&K, India

Medicinal Plants for Arsenic Toxicity

Name of the Condition- Nephrotoxicity

About the condition/Definition- Intoxication of arsenic (arsenite or arsenate) result in renal impairment which is marked by a significant increase in the levels of creatinine, urea, uric acid and decline in levels of plasma protein profile especially albumin level in body.

Etiology- Nephrotoxicity results from arsenic damages mitochondria, which results in the excessive production of reactive oxygen species (ROS), a decline in ATP, and a suppression of respiratory activities along with dramatic alterations in the incidence of cellular growth. There is acute inflammation and the development of tubular necrosis, which lowers the glomerular filtration rate (GFR).

Symptoms- Phosphaturia (Fanconi syndrome), aminoaciduria, proteinuria and glycosuria along with progressive drop of renal function.

Pathogenesis- Arsenic produces renal damage by reducing mitochondrial complex function and elevating cellular ROS levels which directly damages renal cells. Membrane lipid peroxidation and protein oxidation by ROS, which results in complete loss of membrane potential and mitochondrial swelling.

General treatment- Acute arsenic intoxication can be counter by using chelating agents like DMSA, DMPS and BAL, fluid therapy, forced dieresis & dialysis.

Antibiotics- To counter any secondary infection.

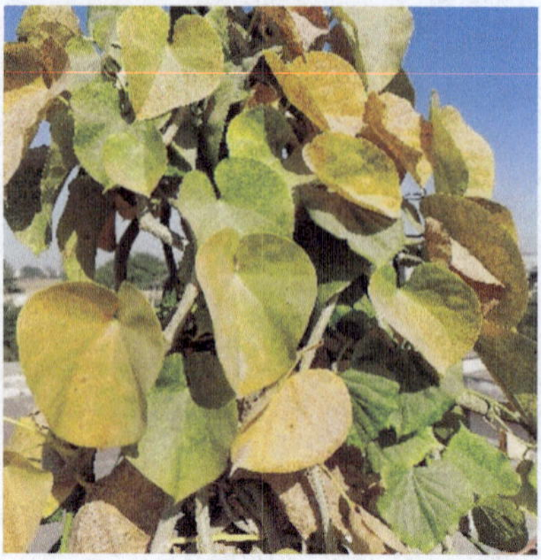

Scientific name: *Tinospora cordifolia*

Common name: Heart-leaved moonseed (English), amrita, guduchi (in Sanskrit), gurbel or giloy (Hindi).

Distribution: In India found in tropical and subtropical zones and other Asian countries like China, Bangladesh, Myanmar and Sri Lanka.

Part used: stems, leaves & roots

Bioactive principles: *Tinospora cordifolia* contains isoquinoline alkaloids like palmatine, magnoflorine and jatrorrhizine.

Remark: Ethanolic stem extract of 400 mg/kg body weight given in Charles Foster rats as a nephroprotective agent.

Name of the Condition- Hepatotoxicity

About the condition/Definition: Intoxication of Arsenic result in damage to hepatocytes which is reflected as significant increase in the levels of AST, ALT, LDH & ALP.

Etiology: Arsenic induces oxidative stress and mitochondrial dysfunction in hepatocytes.

Symptoms: Nausea, abdominal pain, vomiting, diarrhea & jaundice.

Pathogenesis: Arsenic causes oxidative stress by producing free radicals and reactive oxygen species (ROS). This causes harm to the liver cells (hepatocytes) proteins, lipids, and DNA. Oxidative damage can cause inflammation, fibrosis, and even cirrhosis over time, impairing liver function. Through modifications to mitochondrial respiration and a reduction in ATP synthesis, arsenic impairs mitochondrial function. Energy loss, membrane instability, and ultimately necrosis or apoptosis cause cell death as a result of this malfunction. Exposure to arsenic causes inflammatory pathways to become activated, which results in the release of pro-inflammatory cytokines (such as TNF-α and IL-6). Fibrosis and liver scarring are caused by chronic inflammation, which also encourages the activation of hepatic stellate cells and the deposition of extracellular matrix.

General treatment- Chelating agents like DMSA (dimercaptosuccinic acid), dimercaprol (BAL) and unithiol.

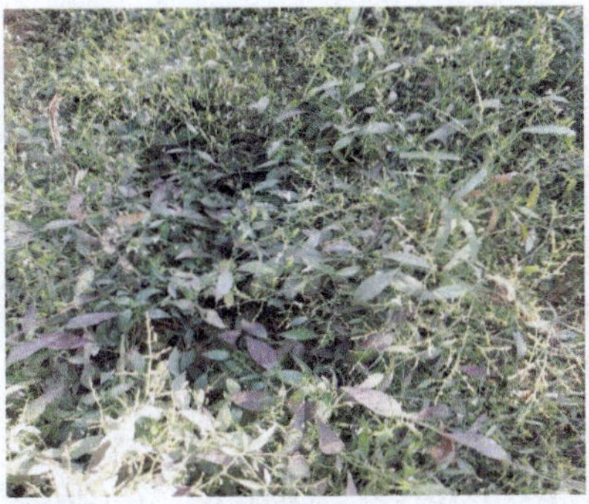

Scientific name: *Andrographis paniculata*

Common name: Creat or green chiretta

Distribution: It is used as a traditional medicine in many countries, including Hong Kong, China, Philippines, Indonesia, Malaysia and Thailand. In India, it is used by ethnic communities to treat a variety of diseases.

Part used: Leaves and stems

Bioactive principles: *Andrographis paniculata* contains a natural diterpenoid andrographolide that counts for its major anti-inflammatory activity.

Remark: Methanolic leave extract of 200 mg/kg body weight given in Wistar rats as a hepatoprotective agent.

Name of the Condition- Neurotoxicity

About the condition/Definition- Arsenic intoxication leads to damage of the nervous system, which can result in a variety of neurological and cognitive impairments.

Etiology- Oxidative stress, disruption of cellular processes, mitochondrial dysfunction.

Symptoms: Headaches, Memory loss, Dizziness, Confusion & Peripheral neuropathy.

Pathogenesis: Arsenic disrupts protein function, enzyme activity, and cellular signalling networks. Neuronal injury may result from the inhibition of vital enzymes involved in energy production, neurotransmitter metabolism, and antioxidant defense. Reactive oxygen species (ROS), which are produced by arsenic and can damage neurons lipids, proteins, and DNA, resulting in cellular malfunction and death. The cell mitochondria, can be harmed by arsenic. This hinders the synthesis of ATP, which is essential for preserving neurons' energy supply. Neuronal death and compromised synaptic function can result from a lack of energy in neurons.

General treatment: Chelating agents like DMSA (dimercaptosuccinic acid), dimercaprol (BAL) and unithiol.

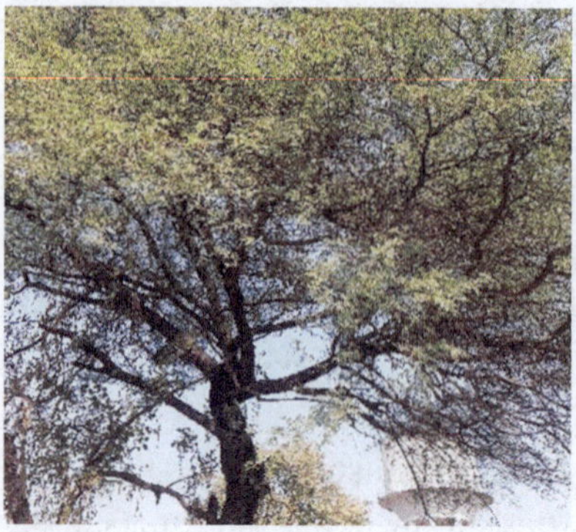

Scientific name: *Acacia nilotica*

Common name: Gum arabic tree, thorn mimosa, Egyptian acacia or thorny acacia (English) and babul (Hindi).

Distribution: It is native to Egypt, South Africa, Burma, Arabian Peninsula and to Indian subcontinent.

Part used: Pods and leaves.

Bioactive principles: *Acacia nilotica* is rich in polyphenolics like gallic acid, protocatechuic acid, pyrocatechol, catechin, epi-gallocatechin-7-gallate and also certain tannis.

Remark: Methanolic pod extract of *Acacia nilotica* at a dose of 50 mg/kg/day given in Swiss albino mice as a neuroprotective agent.

Medicinal Plants for Fluoride Toxicity

Name of the Condition- Nephrotoxicity

About the condition/Definition- Fluoride toxicity result in renal damage reflected by an increase in blood urea nitrogen, creatinine & uric acid.

Etiology- The major setback of fluoride toxicity includes Changes in urine ion excretion by the kidneys, disruption of collagen biosynthesis in the body, and immediate effects on the tubular area of the kidneys, which inhibit tubular reabsorption.

Symptoms- Proteinuria & albuminuria.

Pathogenesis- The accumulation of fluoride in renal tissues, oxidative stress, disruption of cellular functions, and inflammation all contribute to fluoride nephrotoxicity. The longevity of the body is severely jeopardized by kidney damage brought on by prolonged exposure to excessive fluoride levels. As a result, fluoride exposure should be controlled, particularly for populations that are at risk, such as individuals that live in places where drinking water has high amounts of fluoride or who are exposed to it at work.

General treatment- Fluids through a vein (by IV) and symptomatic treatments.

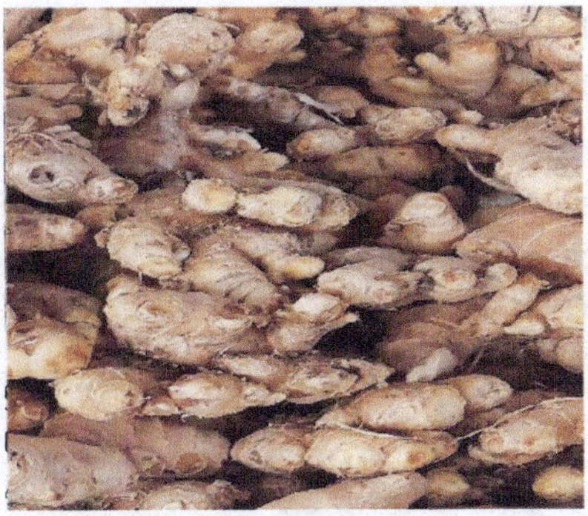

Scientific name: *Zingiber officinale*

Common name: Ginger (English), Sunthi, Srungavera, Ardraka, Vishvabheshaja, Nagara, Adrak, Sonth (Hindi).

Distribution: It is distributed throughout the tropics of Asia, America and Africa.

Part used: Rhizome

Bioactive principles: Shogaols, paradols and gingerols

Remark: Hydroalcoholic extract of *Zingiber officinale* at a dose of 300 mg/kg body weight given in Wistar rats as a nephroprotective agent.

Name of the Condition- Skeletal fluorosis

About the condition/Definition- Skeletal fluorosis is a condition that results from the accumulation of excessive fluoride in the bones over a long period.

Etiology- Fluoride has affinity for long bones and it interferes with normal collagen cross-linking, fluoride damages the collagen matrix within the bone, further eroding its integrity and structure

Symptoms- Stiffness and joint pain and limited range of motion

Pathogenesis- Fluoride impacts the activity of osteoblasts, or cells that make bones. Fluoride increases the synthesis of bone matrix by stimulating osteoblasts at low to moderate doses. Prolonged exposure to high fluoride levels, however, causes irregular bone remodelling, resulting in the production of juvenile bone (osteoid), which may not have the usual mineralization. Additionally, fluoride may increase the activity of osteoclasts, which are cells that tear down bone tissue. This results in aberrant remodelling and resorptions of bone.

General treatment - Nonsteroidal anti-inflammatory drugs (NSAIDs) like ibuprofen for pain management, applying heat or cold packs to the affected joints.

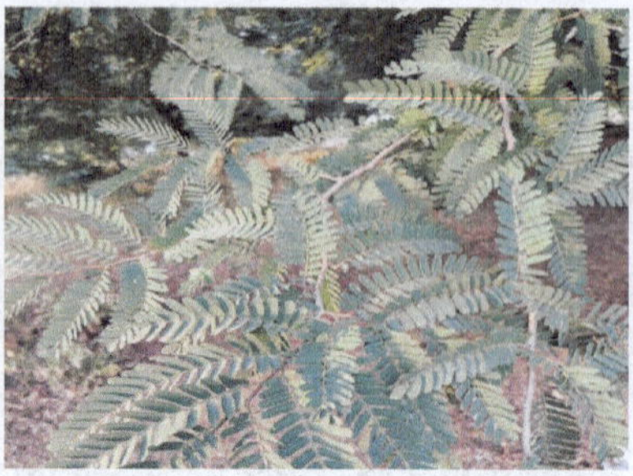

Scientific name: *Tamarindus indica*

Common name: Imli

Distribution: It is found in Asia, Australia, Brazil, Caribbean, Mexico, Pacific as well Indian Ocean, Philippine and United States.

Part used: Seed cotyledons, fruit pulp, leaves & flowers

Bioactive principles: Tartaric acid, Vitamin B and vitamin C.

Remark: 5 grams powder of seed cotyledons mixed with milk and jaggery and given orally daily for 2 months for cartilage development in humans.

Name of the Condition- Reproductive toxicity & hypothyroidism

About the condition/Definition- Fluoride toxicity leads to hypothyroidism by causing thyroid dysfunction. It also suppresses endocrine function and damages ovarian and uterine structure.

Etiology- Disruption of iodine metabolism, oxidative stress to reproductive as well endocrine organs.

Symptoms- Fatigue, sensitivity to cold, weight gain, dry skin and hair, depression & slowed heart rate motion.

Pathogenesis- Thyroid hormones (T_3 and T_4) are produced by the thyroid gland using iodine. Hypothyroidism can result from too much fluoride interfering with the thyroid's absorption of iodine, which is essential for hormone synthesis. Key enzymes involved in the manufacture of thyroid hormones, including those that convert iodide to iodine in the thyroid gland, may be inhibited by fluoride. There may be a decrease in amount of thyroid hormones levels in the bloodstream as a result of fluoride's direct effects on thyroid tissue. Increased levels of thyroid-stimulating hormone (TSH) have been linked to high fluoride exposure. In this instance, hypothyroidism may result from the elevated TSH not being sufficient to offset the decreased thyroid hormone synthesis.

General treatment- Removal of source of fluoride, symptomatic treatment and synthetic thyroid hormone.

Scientific name: *Nigella sativa*

Common name: Black caraway, black cumin & nigella (English) kalonji & charnushka (hindi)

Distribution: Commercial farming of *Nigella sativa* has extended to areas of Europe and North America, and the plant is widely distributed throughout Asia, North Africa, and the Middle East. It is grown for both culinary and medicinal purposes and is most frequently seen in areas with warm and temperate climates.

Part used: Seed (black seed oil), leaves, roots & flowers.

Bioactive principles: Thymoquinone, Nigellimine, Nigellone & Carvacrol

Remark: *Nigella sativa* seed oil at a dose of 300 mg/kg body weight given in Wistar Rats for correction of hypothyroidism and reproductive toxicity (ovarian and uterine damage).

Medicinal Plants for Strychnos Nux-Vomica Toxicity

Name of the Condition- Epilepsy

About the condition/Definition- Strychnine causes convulsions by damaging nerve cells and destructing mitochondrial function & integrity of brain's prefrontal cortex. Strychnos nux-vomica, commonly known as nux vomica, contains strychnine and brucine, which are highly toxic alkaloids. Poisoning can lead to severe symptoms, including muscle spasms, seizures, and respiratory failure. While immediate medical treatment is necessary for strychnine poisoning, some medicinal plants have been traditionally reported to offer supportive or detoxifying effects. These plants may help reduce toxicity or alleviate symptoms, but they should not replace standard medical care.

Etiology- Inhibition of glycine receptors, exaggeration of spinal reflexes & tonic clonic reflexes.

Symptoms- Anxiety, restlessness, anxiety, muscle stiffness & respiratory failure

Pathogenesis: Strychnine mainly works by inhibiting glycine receptors in the brainstem and spinal cord. By reducing excessive neuronal activity, the inhibitory neurotransmitter glycine aids in the regulation of motor function. When glycine receptors are in good working order, they can "calm down" or reduce excessive firing of neurons. Strychnine reduces inhibition in the nervous system by blocking glycine's ability to connect to its receptors. The motor neurons become hyper-excitable in the absence of this inhibitory regulation. Glycine's inhibitory effects cause the nervous system to become overstimulated, which results in convulsions and spasms. Severe muscular spasms and prolonged, widespread seizures may result from this overstimulation environment.

General treatment- Supportive care for respiratory patency, benzodiazepines, muscle relaxant & sedatives. Immediate medical attention is critical in cases of strychnine poisoning. The following plants may serve as supplementary aids in recovery, not as primary treatments.

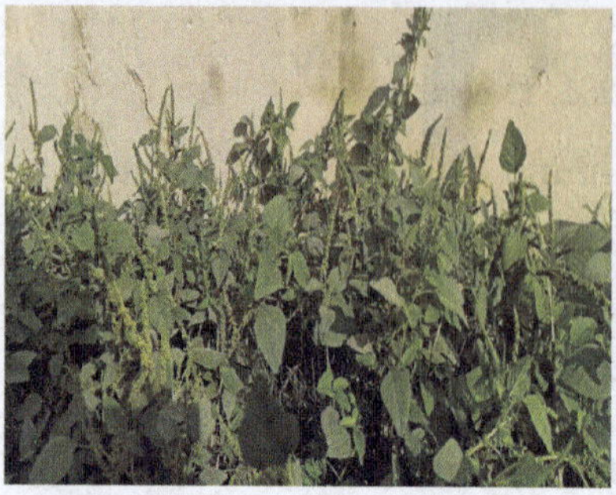

Scientific name: *Amaranthus viridis*

Common name: Slender amaranth, green amaranth (English) & Chaulai (Hindi).

Distribution: Australia and Pacific Islands, Africa, Asia & Europe.

Part used: Leaves, seeds & roots

Bioactive principles: Quercetin, kaempferol, anthocyanins & tannins

Remark: Dichloromethane extract of leaves of *Amaranthus viridis* at a dose of 400 mg/kg body weight is effective in mitigating epilepsy associated with Strychnine toxicity in Wistar rats.

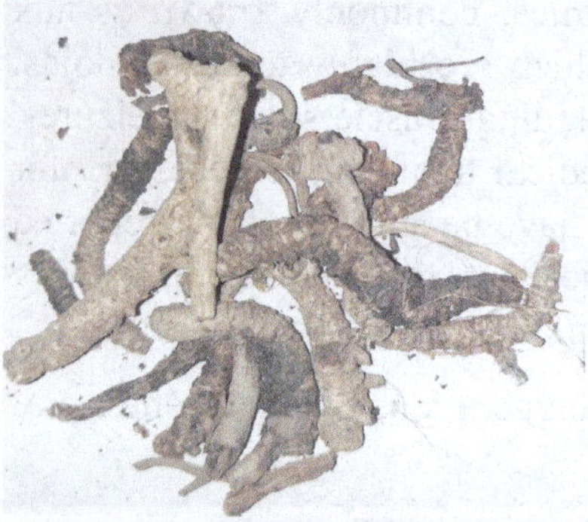

Scientific name: *Picrorhiza kurroa*

Common name: Kutki

Uses: Frequently used in Ayurvedic medicine for detoxification and liver protection. May assist in metabolizing toxic compounds.

Active Compounds: Picrosides and kutkosides, known for their hepatoprotective effects.

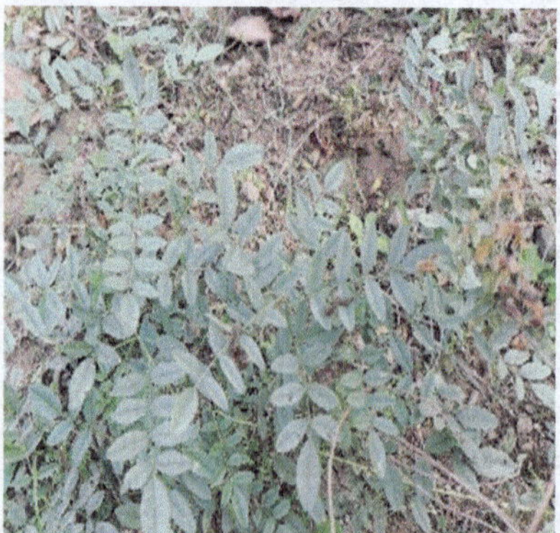

Scientific name: *Glycyrrhiza glabra*

Common name: Licorice

Uses: Soothes the gastrointestinal tract and has anti-inflammatory properties that can reduce systemic stress from toxins.

Active Compounds: Glycyrrhizin, which has antioxidant and anti-inflammatory effects.

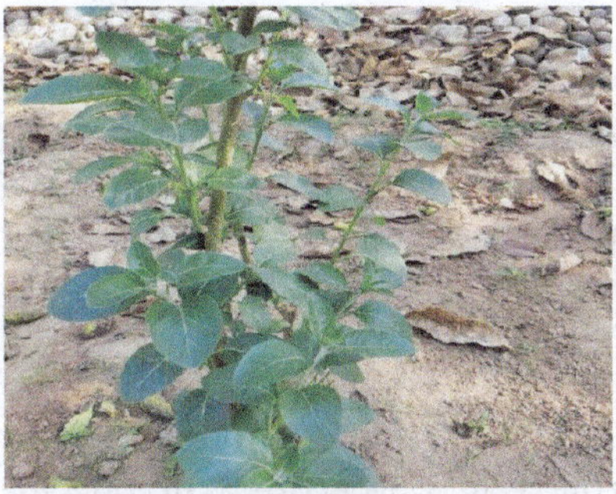

Scientific name: *Withania somnifera*

Common name: Ashwagandha

Uses: Acts as an adaptogen, potentially helping the body mitigate stress and recover from toxic stress.

Active Compounds: Withanolides, which offer neuroprotective and anti-inflammatory effects.

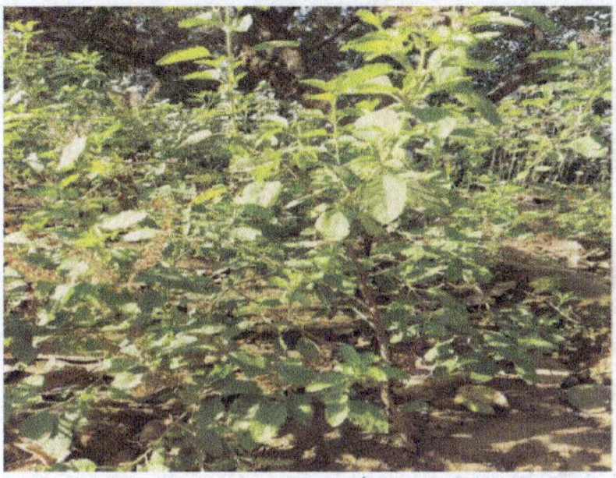

Scientific name: *Ocimum sanctum*

Common name: Holy Basil

Uses: Known for its adaptogenic, anti-inflammatory, and antioxidant properties, which may counteract oxidative stress from poisoning.

Active Compounds: Eugenol, rosmarinic acid, and flavonoids.

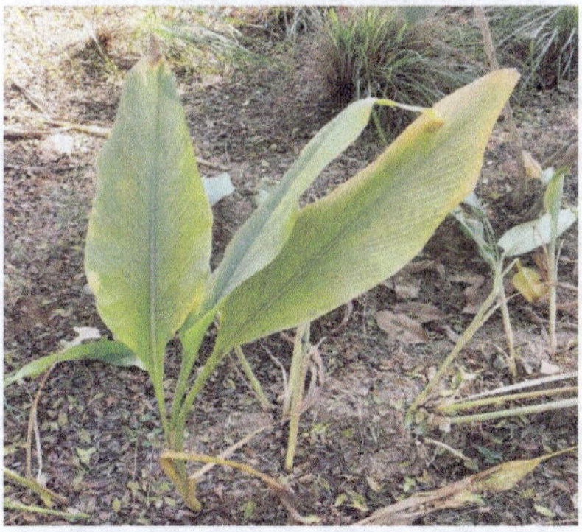

Scientific name: *Curcuma longa*

Common name: Turmeric

Uses: The anti-inflammatory and antioxidant properties of turmeric may help reduce oxidative damage caused by strychnine.

Active Compounds: Curcumin, a potent antioxidant and anti-inflammatory compound

Medicinal Plants for Organophosphorous (Ops) Toxicity

Name of the Condition- Neurotoxicity

About the condition/Definition- Organophosphate compounds cause persistent cholinergic signalling and generates excessive stimulation of the central nervous system (CNS) and peripheral nervous system (PNS).

Etiology- Inhibition of Acetylcholinesterase (AChE)

Symptoms- Muscle fasciculations, paralysis, weakness, salivation, sweating, bronchoconstriction, miosis, bradycardia, and gastrointestinal symptoms including nausea, vomiting, diarrhoea.

Pathogenesis: Organophosphates function by blocking acetylcholinesterase irreversibly. They bind to the enzyme in a covalent manner, stopping it from degrading acetylcholine. Inhibition of AChE causes acetylcholine to build up at synapses and neuromuscular junctions. This results in continuously stimulated target cell whether it is a muscle cell or another nerve cell.

General treatment- OP poisoning in animals requires immediate medical treatment, primarily involving antidotes such as atropine and oximes (2-PAM) to counteract the toxic effects. However, certain medicinal plants with detoxifying, antioxidant, and neuroprotective properties can provide supportive care or mitigate the toxic effects. Here are some medicinal plants that may have potential benefits in cases of OP poisoning:

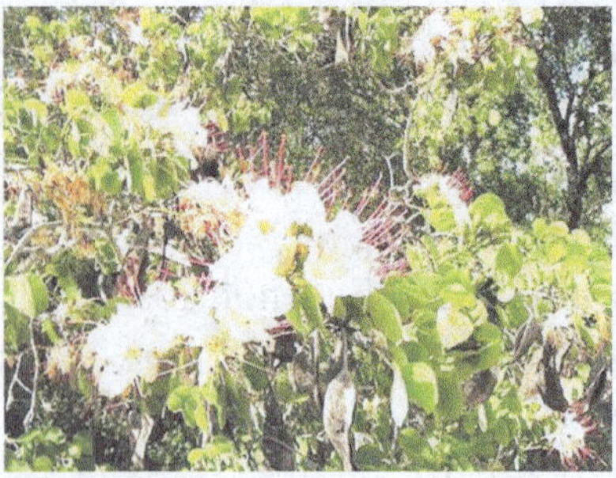

Scientific name: *Lysiphyllum strychnifolium*

Common name: Strychnine tree & toxic bark tree (English).

Distribution: Southeast Asia, Amazon, Brazil, Peru, Colombia & Ecuador.

Part used: Leaves, stems & roots

Bioactive principles: Yanangdaengin, Gallic acid, 1,2-Benzenediol, D-allose & 13-Docosenamide.

Remark: Ethanolic extract of stems of *Lysiphyllum strychnifolium* at a dose of 350 mg/kg body weight is effective in organophosphorous induced nephropathy in Wistar rats.

Name of the Condition- Hepatotoxicity

About the condition/Definition- Organophosphorous compounds can also have toxic effects on the liver which resulting in hepatotoxicity.

Etiology-Oxidative stress & cytochrome P450 enzyme induction in hepatocytes.

Symptoms- Jaundice elevated liver enzymes, hepatomegaly, fatty Liver (Steatosis) & abdominal Pain.

Pathogenesis: Oxidative stress can result from frequent production of ROS, which can overpower the liver's antioxidant defense. Lipids, proteins, DNA, and other biological components may be impacted by this damage, which will ultimately compromise liver function. OPs are mostly metabolized by cytochrome P450 enzymes (CYPs) in the liver. There are instances where this metabolic process can produce poisonous metabolites (such oxon metabolites of OPs), which are more dangerous than the parent substances and have the ability to cause direct harm to liver cells. Inflammatory reactions in the liver brought on by prolonged exposure to OP chemicals can result in hepatocyte damage, liver fibrosis, and in extreme situations, cirrhosis. Immune cells such as neutrophils and macrophages may be activated and pro-inflammatory cytokines may be released as part of the inflammatory process. In liver cells, mitochondria are essential for both energy production and detoxification. Apoptosis (programmed cell death) of hepatocyte can result from OPs' impairment of mitochondrial activity, which also causes ATP depletion and an increase in ROS generation.

General treatment- N-acetylcysteine (NAC) Atropine Sulphate & Pralidoxime (2-PAM).

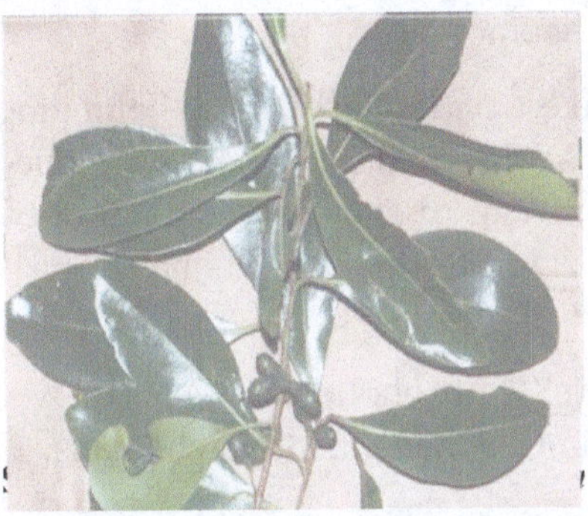

Scientific name: *Litsea martabanica*

Common name: Tetranthera martabanica Kurz (English).

Distribution: China, Indo-China, Thailand, and Myanmar.

Part used: Roots and stems

Bioactive principles: Phenols, Alkaloids and terpenes

Remark: Ethanolic extract of roots of *Litsea martabanica* at a dose of 750 mg/kg body weight is effective in organophosphorus (chlorpyrifos) induced hepatotoxicity in Wistar rats.

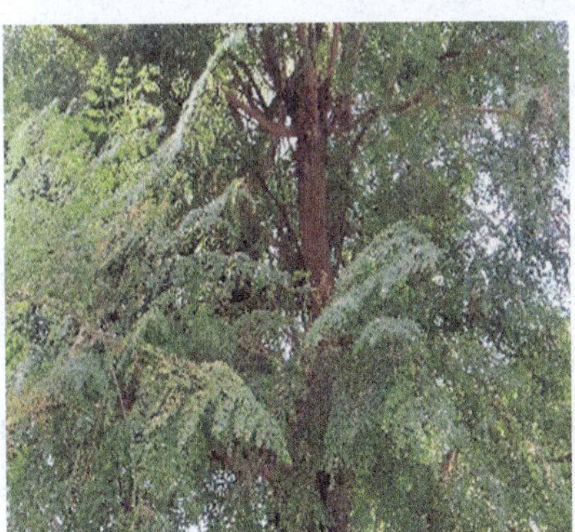

Scientific name: *Moringa oleifera*

Common name: Drumstick Tree

Uses: Antioxidant and hepatoprotective properties.

Active Compounds: Quercetin and chlorogenic acid.

Potential Benefits: Enhances liver detoxification and reduces oxidative damage from OP exposure.

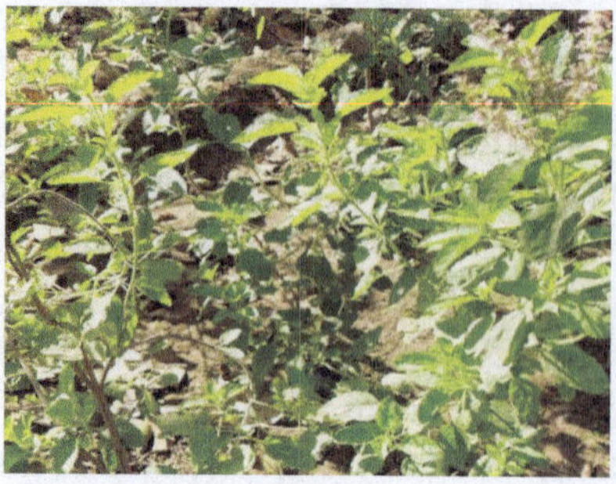

Scientific name: *Ocimum sanctum*

Common name: Holy Basil/Tulsi

Uses: An adaptogen with antioxidant and anti-inflammatory effects.

Active Compounds: Eugenol, rosmarinic acid, and flavonoids.

Potential Benefits: Protects against oxidative stress and supports the nervous system.

Medicinal Plants for Snake Bite Envenoming

Name of the Condition: Neurotoxicity and haemolysis

About the condition/Definition: Many snakes, particularly those belonging to the Elapidae family (including cobras, kraits, and sea snakes produce neurotoxins within their venom. These toxins can disrupt nerve function by affecting various elements of the nervous system. It also exhibits haemolysis effects.

Etiology: Acetylcholine receptor blockade, phospholipases A_2 (PLA_2), destruction of neurotransmitters and ligand and voltage gated ion channels.

Symptoms: Muscle weakness, respiratory distress, autonomic dysfunction, ptosis & respiratory arrest.

Pathogenesis: Certain neurotoxins inhibit the release of acetylcholine that is a crucial neurotransmitter for muscle contraction. This results in muscle paralysis, particularly affecting the diaphragm, which can lead to respiratory failure. Some toxins attach to acetylcholine receptors on muscle fibers, obstructing the usual transmission of nerve signals. Various venoms impact ion channels in nerve membranes, disrupting the transmission of nerve signals. Moreover, the phospholipid bilayer of cell membranes is hydrolysed by PLA_2 enzymes, which causes the membrane structure become unstable. As a result, the red blood cells are more susceptible to lysis or rupture.

General treatment: Supportive care, antivenom, acetylcholinesterase inhibitors and observation as well as monitoring of patients. The following plants may serve as supplementary aids in recovery, not as primary treatments.

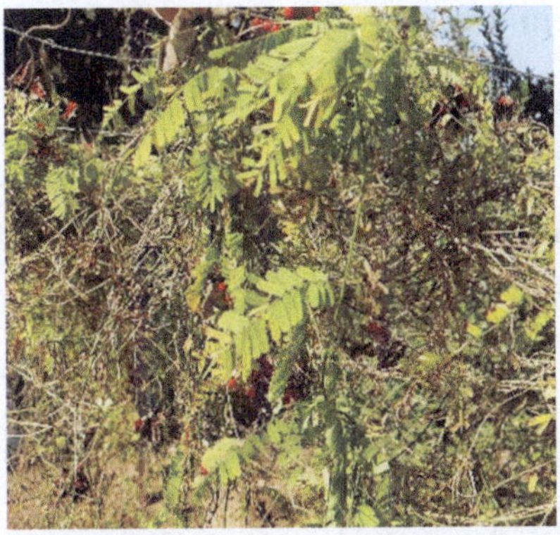

Scientific name: *Abrus precatorius*

Common name: Crab's eye, rosary pea, paternoster pea, (English) and ratti (in Hindi).

Distribution: Asia, Australia, Malesia, Africa and the Pacific Region

Part used: Seeds, leaves & roots

Bioactive principles: abrin A, B, C, I, II, III, abrol, abrasine, precasine and abruslactone

Remark: *Abrus precatorius* may be effective in treating snake bites when the powdered root is applied to the wound twice daily for duration of 5 to 7 days. Two to three grams of fresh leaves or roots with seeds are ground into a paste and eaten with cow's milk or cold water.

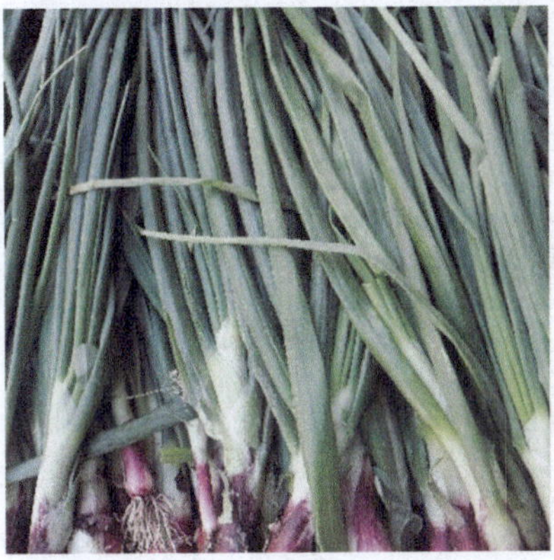

Scientific name: *Allium cepa*

Common name: Onion (English), Palandu (Sanskrit) & pyaj (in Hindi).

Distribution: India, China, United States of America, Turkey & Iran.

Part used: Bulb, stems and leaves

Bioactive principles: Onionin A, cysteine sulfoxides and quercetin

Remark: The paste is made from fresh skin bulb and applied on the bite.

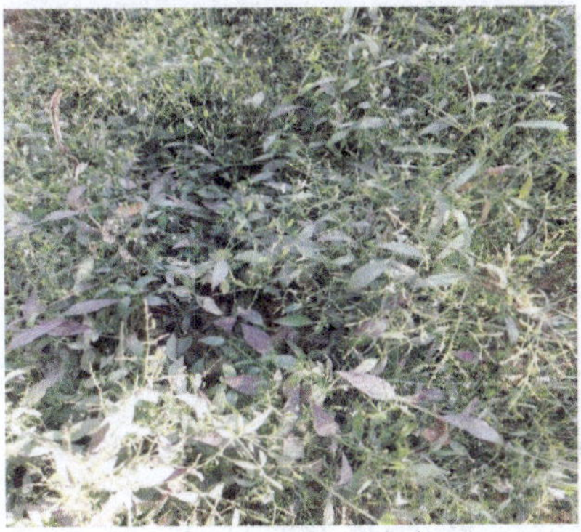

Scientific name: *Andrographis paniculata*

Common name: Bhumi neem, Neelaveppu, Nilavaembu & Periyanangai

Distribution: India, Hong Kong, China, Philippines, Indonesia, Malaysia and Thailand

Part used: Leaves and stems.

Bioactive principles: Andrographolide

Remark: The decoction of leaves is given orally and is also applied externally.

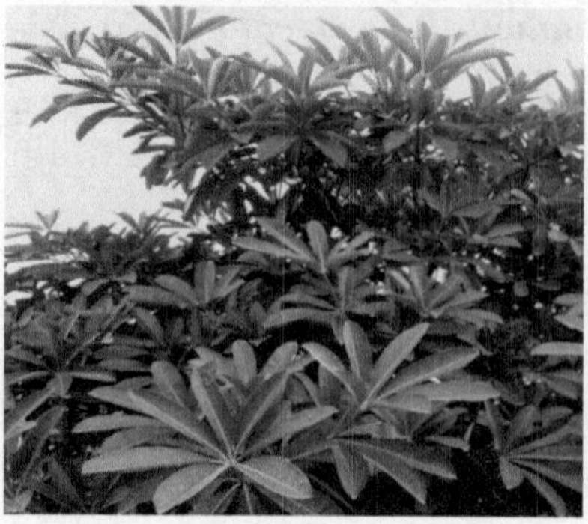

Scientific name: *Alstonia scholaris*

Common name: Devil's tree, Blackboard tree, Milkwood, Scholar's tree, White Cheesewood, Dita Bark (English) and Saptaparna (Hindi).

Distribution: Central America, Africa, Southeast Asia, Polynesia, and Australia

Part used: Bark, leaves and stems.

Bioactive principles: 19-epischolaricine, cholaricine, vallesamine, and picrinine

Remark: The decoction of bark is given orally.

References

Babu NJ, Murty PP, Rao GN. Plant Species Utilized to Treat Skeletal Fluorosis and Fluorosis Arthritis from Eastern Ghats of Andhra Pradesh, India. International Journal of Ayurvedic and Herbal Medicine. 2020;10(2):3748-57.

Bharadwaj A, Sharma A, Singh T, Pathak D, Virmani T, Kumar G, Sharma A, Alhalmi A. Attenuation of Strychnine-Induced Epilepsy Employing Amaranthus viridis L. Leaves Extract in Experimental Rats. Behavioural Neurology. 2023;2023(1):6684781.

Elghareeb MM, Elshopakey GE, Rezk S, Ateya A, El-Ashry ES, Shukry M, Ghamry HI, Alotaibi BS, Hashem NM. Nigella sativa oil restores hormonal levels, and endocrine signals among thyroid, ovarian, and uterine tissues of female Wistar rats following sodium fluoride toxicity. Biomedicine & Pharmacotherapy. 2024 Jan 1;170:116080.

Foyzun T, Mahmud AA, Ahammed MS, Manik MI, Hasan MK, Islam KM, Lopa SS, Al-Amin MY, Biswas K, Afrin MR, Alam AK. Polyphenolics with strong antioxidant activity from Acacia nilotica ameliorate some biochemical signs of arsenic-induced neurotoxicity and oxidative stress in mice. Molecules. 2022 Feb 3;27(3):1037.

Kumar V, Akhouri V, Singh SK, Kumar A. Phytoremedial effect of Tinospora cordifolia against arsenic induced toxicity in Charles Foster rats. BioMetals. 2020 Dec;33(6):379-96.

Kunnaja P, Chansakaow S, Wittayapraparat A, Yusuk P, Sireeratawong S. In vitro antioxidant activity of Litsea martabanica root extract and its hepatoprotective effect on chlorpyrifos-induced toxicity in rats. Molecules. 2021 Mar 28;26(7):1906.

Owoade AO, Alausa AO, Adetutu A, Owoade AW. Protective effects of methanolic extract of Andrographis paniculata (Burm. f.) Nees leaves against arsenic-induced damage in rats. Bulletin of the National Research Centre. 2022 May 16;46(1):141.

Sharma P, Verma PK, Sood S, Yousuf R, Kumar A, Raina R, Shabbir MA, Bhat ZF. Protective effect of quercetin and ginger (Zingiber officinale) extract against dimethoate potentiated fluoride-induced nephrotoxicity in rats. Foods. 2023 May 5;12(9):1899.

Sukprasert S, Deenonpoe R, Yimsoo T, Yingmema W, Prasopdee S, Krajang A, Kornthong N, Pattaraarchachai J, Daduang S. Antidote activity and protective effects of Lysiphyllum strychnifolium (Craib) A. Schmitz extract against organophosphate pesticide in omethoate-treated rats. Journal of Traditional and Complementary Medicine. 2021 May 1;11(3):189-96.

Upasani SV, Beldar VG, Tatiya AU, Upasani MS, Surana SJ, Patil DS. Ethnomedicinal plants used for snakebite in India: a brief overview. Integrative medicine research. 2017 Jun 1;6(2):114-30.

Scientific Index

Botanical Index